W9-CEF-996

Instructor's Resource Manual

Dental Radiography
Principles and Techniques

Third Edition

Joen M. Iannucci, DDS, MS
Professor of Clinical Dentistry
Section of Primary Care
Director, Admissions
Director, Screening Clinic
Director, Sterilization Monitoring Service
The Ohio State University
College of Dentistry
Columbus, Ohio

Laura Jansen Howerton, RDH, MS
Clinical Associate Professor
Department of Dental Ecology
The University of North Carolina at Chapel Hill
School of Dentistry
Chapel Hill, North Carolina

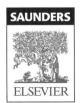

SAUNDERS

ELSEVIER

ELSEVIER
SAUNDERS

11830 Westline Industrial Drive
St. Louis, Missouri 63146

Instructor's Resource Manual,
DENTAL RADIOGRAPHY: PRINCIPLES
AND TECHNIQUES, Third Edition

ISBN 13: 978-1-4160-3100-0
ISBN 10: 1-4160-3100-6

Notice

Neither the Publisher nor the Authors assume any responsibility for any loss or injury and/or damage to persons or property arising out of or related to any use of the material contained in this book. It is the responsibility of the treating practitioner, relying on independent expertise and knowledge of the patient, to determine the best treatment and method of application for the patient.

The Publisher

Previous editions copyrighted 1996, 2000

ISBN 13 978-1-4160-1300-0
ISBN 10 1-4160-1300-6

Executive Editor: Penny Rudolph
Managing Editor: Jaime Pendill
Publishing Services Manager: Patricia Tannian
Senior Project Manager: Anne Altepeter
Cover Designer: Julia Dummitt

Printed in the United States of America
Last digit is the print number: 9 8 7 6 5 4 3 2 1

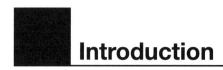

Introduction

The *Instructor's Resource Manual for Dental Radiography: Principles and Techniques,* Third Edition, is designed to save the instructor time. It is available in print format, or electronically on the Evolve website. Divided into three parts, this manual provides instructors with valuable resources that can be used in lesson planning and classroom preparation.

Chapter Features

Each chapter includes elements directly from the textbook such as the Key Terms, Learning Objectives, and chapter outlines.

Answers to Quiz Questions

This section includes answers to the quizzes presented at the end of each chapter in the textbook. Answers are only available to instructors in the *Instructor's Resource Manual*, or on the Evolve website.

Test Bank

An all-new test bank divided by chapter has been created for the third edition of *Dental Radiography: Principles and Techniques*. More than 790 questions with rationales for correct and incorrect answers are included. A printed version of the test bank with answers is included in this manual for instructor reference. The test bank is available electronically in ExamView on the Evolve website. The ExamView program allows instructors to randomize test questions.

We hope that you find this new edition of *Dental Radiography: Principles and Techniques* and its entire package of ancillary products helpful in your teaching endeavors.

Joen M. Iannucci
Laura Jansen Howerton

Contents

Chapter Features

1 Radiation History

KEY TERMS

LEARNING OBJECTIVES

1. Define the key terms listed.
2. Summarize the importance of dental radiographs.
3. List the uses of dental radiographs.
4. Summarize the discovery of x-radiation.
5. Recognize the pioneers in dental x-radiation and their contributions and discoveries.
6. List the highlights in the history of x-ray equipment and film.
7. List the highlights in the history of dental radiographic techniques.

CHAPTER OUTLINE

2 | Radiation Physics

KEY TERMS

absorption, p. 21
alpha particles, p. 13
aluminum disks, p. 16
amperage, p. 18
ampere (A), p. 18
anode, p. 17
atom, p. 13
atom, neutral, p. 13
atomic number, p. 11
atomic weight, p. 11
autotransformer, p. 18
beta particles, p. 13
binding energy, p. 11
Bremsstrahlung, p. 20
cathode, p. 13
cathode ray, p. 13
circuit, p. 17
circuit, filament, p. 18
circuit, high-voltage, p. 18
coherent scatter, p. 21
Compton electron, p. 22
Compton scatter, p. 21
control panel, p. 15
copper stem, p. 17
current, alternating (AC), p. 18
current, direct (DC), p. 18
electrical current, p. 17
electricity, p. 16
electromagnetic spectrum, p. 14
electron, p. 10
electron volt (eV), p. 12
electrostatic force, p. 11
element, p. 11
energy, p. 10
extension arm, p. 15
frequency, p. 14
insulating oil, p. 16
ion, p. 13
ion pair, p. 13
ionization, p. 10
kilo electron volt (keV), p. 12
kilovolt (kV), p. 18
kilovoltage peak, p. 18
kinetic energy, p. 13
lead collimator, p. 16
leaded-glass housing, p. 17
mass number, p. 11
matter, p. 10
metal housing, p. 16
milliamperage, p. 16

milliampere (mA), p. 18
molecule, p. 12
molybdenum cup, p. 17
nanometer, p. 14
neutron, p. 11
nucleon, p. 11
nucleus, p. 10
orbit, p. 10
periodic table of the elements, p. 11
photoelectric effect, p. 21
photon, p. 14
position-indicating device, p. 17
primary beam, p. 20
proton, p. 11
quanta, p. 14
radiation, p. 10
radiation, braking, p. 20
radiation, characteristic, p. 20
radiation, electromagnetic, p. 13
radiation, general, p. 20
radiation, ionizing, p. 10
radiation, particulate, p. 13
radiation, primary, p. 20
radiation, scatter, p. 21
radiation, secondary, p. 21
radioactivity, p. 12
recoil electron, p. 22
rectification, p. 18
scatter, p. 20
shell, p. 11
thermionic emission, p. 19
transformer, p. 16
transformer, step-down, p. 18
transformer, step-up, p. 18
tubehead, p. 15
tubehead seal, p. 16
tungsten filament, p. 17
tungsten target, p. 17
unmodified scatter, p. 22
useful beam, p. 20
velocity, p. 14
voltage, p. 16
wavelength, p. 14
x-rays, p. 10
x-ray tube, p. 10

LEARNING OBJECTIVES

1. Define the key terms listed.
2. Identify the structure of the atom.
3. Describe the process of ionization.

3

4. Discuss the difference between radiation and radioactivity.
5. List the two types of ionizing radiation and give examples of each.
6. List the characteristics of electromagnetic radiation.
7. List the properties of x-radiation.
8. Identify the component parts of the x-ray machine.
9. Label the parts of the dental x-ray tubehead and the dental x-ray tube.
10. Describe in detail how dental x-rays are produced.
11. List and describe the possible interactions of x-rays with matter.

CHAPTER OUTLINE

Fundamental Concepts
   Atomic and Molecular Structure
   Ionization, Radiation, and Radioactivity
   Ionizing Radiation
X-radiation
X-ray Machine
   Component Parts
   X-ray Tube
   X-ray Generating Apparatus
Production of X-radiation
   Production of Dental X-rays
   Types of X-rays Produced
   Forms of X-radiation
Interactions of X-radiation
   No Interaction
   Absorption of Energy and Photoelectric Effect
   Compton Scatter
   Coherent Scatter

3 | Radiation Characteristics

KEY TERMS

amperage, p. 31
ampere (A), p. 32
contrast, p. 30
density, p. 30
exposure time, p. 30
half-value layer, p. 34
impulse, p. 30
intensity (of x-ray beam), p. 29
inverse square law, p. 33
kilovolt (kV), p. 29
kilovoltage, p. 29
kilovoltage peak, p. 29
milliamperage, p. 30
milliampere (mA), p. 32
milliampere-seconds (mAs), p. 32
polychromatic x-ray beam, p. 30
quality (of x-ray beam), p. 29
quantity (of x-ray beam), p. 29
volt (V), p. 29
voltage, p. 29

LEARNING OBJECTIVES

1. Define the key terms listed.
2. Describe the effect that the kilovoltage peak has on the quality of the x-ray beam.
3. Describe how milliamperage influences the quantity of the x-ray beam.
4. Identify the range of kilovoltage and milliamperage required for dental radiography.
5. Describe how increasing and decreasing exposure factors affect the density and contrast of the film.
6. State the rules governing kilovoltage, milliamperage, distance, and exposure time that are used when changing exposure variables.
7. Describe how kilovoltage, milliamperage, exposure time, and source-to-film distance influence the intensity of the x-ray beam.
8. Calculate an example of radiation intensity using the inverse square law.
9. Explain how the half-value layer determines the penetrating quality of the x-ray beam.

CHAPTER OUTLINE

4 Radiation Biology

KEY TERMS

cell, p. 39
cell differentiation, p. 43
cell metabolism, p. 43
coulomb (C), p. 43
critical organ, p. 43
cumulative effects, p. 41
direct theory, p. 40
dose, p. 40
dose, total, p. 41
dose equivalent, p. 43
dose rate, p. 41
dose-response curve, p. 40
exposure, p. 39
free radical, p. 39
genetic cells, p. 42
genetic effects, p. 43
gray (Gy), p. 43
indirect theory, p. 40
injury, period of, p. 41
ionization, p. 39
latent period, p. 41
long-term effects, p. 42
mitotic activity, p. 41
nonstochastic effects, p. 40
quality factor (QF), p. 45
radiation, background, p. 45
radiation absorbed dose (rad), p. 43
radiation biology, p. 39
radioresistant, p. 43
radiosensitive, p. 43
recovery period, p. 41
risk, p. 39

roentgen (R), p. 43
roentgen equivalent (in) man (rem), p. 43
short-term effects, p. 42
sievert (Sv), p. 43
somatic cells, p. 43
somatic effects, p. 40
stochastic effects, p. 40

LEARNING OBJECTIVES

1. Define the key terms listed.
2. Describe the mechanisms, theories, and sequence of radiation injury.
3. Define and discuss the dose-response curve and radiation injury.
4. List the determining factors for radiation injury.
5. Discuss the short-term and long-term effects as well as the somatic and genetic effects of radiation exposure.
6. Describe the effects of radiation exposure on cells, tissues, and organs.
7. Identify the relative sensitivity of a given tissue to x-radiation.
8. Define the units of measurement used in radiation exposure.
9. List common sources of radiation exposure.
10. Discuss risk and risk estimates for radiation exposure.
11. Discuss dental radiation and exposure risks.
12. Discuss the risk versus benefit of dental radiographs.

CHAPTER OUTLINE

Radiation Injury
    Mechanisms of Injury
    Theories of Radiation Injury
    Dose-Response Curve
    Stochastic and Nonstochastic Radiation Effects
    Sequence of Radiation Injury
    Determining Factors for Radiation Injury
Radiation Effects
    Short-term and Long-term Effects
    Somatic and Genetic Effects
    Radiation Effects on Cells
    Radiation Effects on Tissues and Organs

5 | Radiation Protection

LEARNING OBJECTIVES

1. Define the key terms listed.
2. Describe in detail the basics of patient protection before x-ray exposure.
3. Discuss the different types of filtration, and state the recommended total filtration for dental x-ray machines operating above and below 70 kVp.
4. Describe the collimator used in dental x-ray machines, and state the recommended diameter of the useful beam at the patient's skin.
5. List six ways to protect the patient from excess radiation during x-ray exposure.
6. Describe the importance of film handling and processing after patient exposure to x-rays.
7. Discuss operator protection in terms of adequate distance, shielding, and avoidance of the useful beam.
8. Describe personnel and equipment monitoring devices used to detect radiation.
9. Discuss radiation exposure guidelines, including radiation safety legislation, MPD, MAD, and ALARA.
10. Discuss with the dental patient what radiation protection steps will be used before, during, and after x-ray exposure.

CHAPTER OUTLINE

Patient Protection
   Before Exposure
   During Exposure
   After Exposure
Operator Protection
   Protection Guidelines
   Radiation Monitoring
Radiation Exposure Guidelines
   Radiation Safety Legislation
   Maximum Permissible Dose
   Maximum Accumulated Dose
   ALARA Concept
Radiation Protection and Patient Education

6 Dental X-ray Equipment

KEY TERMS

beam alignment device, p. 67
collimating device, p. 69
control devices, p. 67
control panel, p. 67
exposure button, p. 67
exposure light, p. 67
extension arm, p. 67
film, extraoral, p. 67
film, intraoral, p. 67
film holder, p. 67
indicator light, p. 67
on-off switch, p. 67
tubehead, p. 67

LEARNING OBJECTIVES

1. Define the key terms listed.
2. Discuss the regulation of dental x-ray machines at the federal, state, and local levels.
3. Recognize dental x-ray machines used for intraoral and extraoral films.
4. Identify the component parts of the dental x-ray machine.
5. Describe the purpose and use of dental x-ray film holders and devices.
6. Identify commonly used dental x-ray film holders and devices.

CHAPTER OUTLINE

Dental X-ray Machines
    Performance Standards
    Types of Machines
    Component Parts
Dental X-ray Film Holders and Beam Alignment Devices
    Types of Film Holders
    Types of Beam Alignment Devices

7 Dental X-ray Film

LEARNING OBJECTIVES

1. Define the key terms listed.
2. Describe in detail film composition and latent image formation.
3. List and describe the different types of x-ray film used in dentistry.
4. Define intraoral film and describe intraoral film packaging.
5. Identify the types and sizes of intraoral film available.
6. Discuss film speed.
7. Discuss the differences between intraoral film and extraoral film.
8. Describe the difference between screen and non-screen films.
9. Describe the use of intensifying screens and cassettes.
10. Describe duplicating film.
11. Discuss proper film storage and protection.

CHAPTER OUTLINE

8 Dental X-ray Image Characteristics

KEY TERMS

contrast, p. 90
contrast, film, p. 92
contrast, high, p. 92
contrast, long-scale, p. 92
contrast, low, p. 92
contrast, scale of, p. 92
contrast, short-scale, p. 92
contrast, subject, p. 92
density, p. 90
distance, object-film, p. 96
distance, target-film, p. 96
distortion, p. 90
exposure factors, p. 91
exposure time, p. 91
focal spot, p. 94
magnification, p. 90
milliamperage (mA), p. 91
operating kilovoltage peak, p. 91
penumbra, p. 94
radiograph, diagnostic, p. 90
radiolucent, p. 90
radiopaque, p. 90
sharpness, p. 90
stepwedge, p. 92
subject thickness, p. 91

LEARNING OBJECTIVES

1. Define the key terms listed.
2. Differentiate between radiolucent and radiopaque areas on a dental radiograph.
3. Describe a diagnostic dental radiograph.
4. List the two visual characteristics of the radiographic image.
5. List the factors that influence film density and contrast.
6. Discuss the difference between high and low contrast.
7. Describe film contrast and subject contrast.
8. Describe the difference between short-scale and long-scale contrast.
9. Identify images of high contrast, low contrast, no contrast, short-scale contrast, and long-scale contrast.
10. Describe a stepwedge.
11. List the three geometric characteristics of the radiographic image.
12. List the factors that influence sharpness, magnification, and distortion.

CHAPTER OUTLINE

Overview of Image Characteristics
Visual Characteristics
   Density
   Contrast
Geometric Characteristics
   Sharpness
   Magnification
   Distortion

9 Dental X-ray Film Processing

KEY TERMS

accelerator, p. 104
acetic acid, p. 106
acidifier, p. 106
air bubbles, p. 121
ammonium thiosulfate, p. 105
compartment, developer, p. 113
compartment, fixer, p. 113
compartment, water, p. 114
darkroom, p. 102
darkroom plumbing, p. 107
darkroom storage space, p. 107
darkroom work space, p. 107
daylight loader, p. 108
developer cutoff, p. 119
developer solution, p. 103
developer spots, p. 117
developing agent, p. 104
development, p. 103
drying chamber, p. 114
elon, p. 104
film, cleaning, p. 114
film, duplicating, p. 115
film, fogged, p. 105
film, overdeveloped, p. 117
film, overlapped, p. 120
film, scratched, p. 122
film, underdeveloped, p. 116
film, yellow-brown, p. 119
film duplicator, p. 115
film feed slot, p. 113
film hangers, p. 109
film recovery slot, p. 114
fingernail artifact, p. 121
fingerprint artifact, p. 121
fixation, p. 104
fixer cutoff, p. 120
fixer solution, p. 103
fixer spots, p. 118
fixing agent, p. 105
hardening agent, p. 105
humidity level, p. 107
hydroquinone, p. 104
hypo, p. 105
latent image, p. 102
light-tight, p. 106
light leak, p. 106
oxidation, p. 108
potassium alum, p. 106
potassium bromide, p. 105
preservative, p. 104

processing, automatic, p. 108
processing, manual, p. 107
processor, automatic, p. 106
processor housing, p. 113
radiolucent, p. 103
radiopaque, p. 103
reduction, p. 102
reduction, selective, p. 102
replenisher, p. 112
replenisher pump, p. 114
replenisher solution, p. 112
restrainer, p. 104
reticulation of emulsion, p. 118
rinsing, p. 104
roller film transporter, p. 113
room lighting, p. 106
safelight filter, p. 106
safelighting, p. 106
sodium carbonate, p. 105
sodium sulfite, p. 105
sodium thiosulfate, p. 105
static electricity, p. 107
stirring paddle, p. 110
stirring rod, p. 110
sulfuric acid, p. 106
tank, insert, p. 108
tank, master, p. 108
tank, processing, p. 106
thermometer, p. 109
timer, p. 109
valve, mixing, p. 107

LEARNING OBJECTIVES

1. Define the key terms listed.
2. Describe in detail how a latent image becomes a visible image.
3. List and discuss the five steps of film processing.
4. List and describe the four basic ingredients of the developer solution.
5. List and describe the four basic ingredients of the fixer solution.
6. Discuss the location, size, lighting, and equipment requirements necessary for the darkroom.
7. Discuss safelighting.
8. Discuss the parts of the processing tank: insert tanks, master tank, and lid.
9. List and describe the equipment needed for manual film processing.

10. List and discuss the procedural steps for manual film processing.
11. Describe the care and maintenance of the processing solutions, equipment, and equipment accessories used in manual film processing.
12. Discuss the advantages of automatic film processing.
13. List and identify the component parts of the automatic film processor.
14. Describe the mechanism of automatic film processing.
15. List and discuss the procedural steps used for automatic film processing.
16. Describe the care and maintenance of the automatic film processor and automatic processing solutions.
17. Discuss the equipment requirements and procedural steps used for film duplication.
18. Describe film processing problems that result from time and temperature errors.
19. Describe film processing problems that result from chemical contamination errors.
20. Describe film processing problems that result from film handling errors.
21. Describe film processing problems that result from lighting errors.

CHAPTER OUTLINE

Film Processing
    Film Processing Fundamentals
    Film Processing Steps
    Film Processing Solutions
The Darkroom
    Room Requirements
    Equipment Requirements
Manual Film Processing
    Equipment Accessories
    Step-by-Step Procedures
    Care and Maintenance
Automatic Film Processing
    Component Parts of Automatic Processor
    Step-by-Step Procedures
    Care and Maintenance
Film Duplication
    Equipment Requirements
    Step-by-Step Procedures
Processing Problems and Solutions
    Time and Temperature
    Chemical Contamination
    Film Handling
    Lighting

13

10 Quality Assurance in the Dental Office

LEARNING OBJECTIVES

1. Define the key terms listed.
2. List quality control tests and quality administration procedures that should be included in the quality assurance plan.
3. Discuss the purpose and frequency of testing dental x-ray machines.
4. Describe the tests used to check for fresh film and adequate film-screen contact. Discuss the frequency of testing and the interpretation of test results.
5. Describe the test used to check for darkroom light leaks and proper safelighting. Discuss the frequency of testing and the interpretation of test results.
6. Describe the test used to check the automatic processor. Discuss the frequency of testing and the interpretation of test results.
7. List three tests used to check the strength of the developer solution.
8. Describe the preparation of the reference radiograph and the standard stepwedge radiograph. Discuss the use of these radiographs to compare film densities and to monitor the strength of developer solution.
9. Describe the test used to check the strength of the fixer. Discuss the frequency of testing and the interpretation of test results.
10. Discuss the basic elements of a quality administration plan.
11. Detail the importance of operator competence in dental radiographic procedures.

11 Dental Radiographs and the Dental Radiographer

LEARNING OBJECTIVES

1. Define the key terms listed.
2. Discuss the importance of dental radiographs.
3. List the uses of dental radiographs.
4. Discuss the benefits of dental radiographs.
5. List examples of common dental conditions that may be evident on a dental radiograph.
6. Discuss the knowledge and skill requirements of the dental radiographer.
7. List the responsibilities that may be assigned to the dental radiographer.
8. Discuss the professional goals of the dental radiographer.

12 Patient Relations and the Dental Radiographer

KEY TERMS

LEARNING OBJECTIVES

1. Define the key terms listed.
2. Discuss verbal, nonverbal, and listening skills, and explain how each can be used to enhance communication.
3. Discuss how facilitative skills can be used to enhance patient trust.
4. Define a relationship of trust between the dental professional and the patient.
5. Discuss the importance of first impressions, chairside manner, and attitude, and explain how each can enhance patient relations.

CHAPTER OUTLINE

16

13 Patient Education and the Dental Radiographer

LEARNING OBJECTIVES

1. Summarize the importance of educating patients about dental radiographs.
2. List three methods that can be used by the dental radiographer to educate patients about dental radiographs.
3. Answer common patient questions about the need for dental radiographs, x-ray exposure, the safety of dental x-rays, and other miscellaneous concerns.

CHAPTER OUTLINE

Importance of Patient Education
Methods of Patient Education
Common Questions and Answers
    Necessity Questions
    Exposure Questions
    Safety Questions
    Miscellaneous Questions

14 Legal Issues and the Dental Radiographer

LEARNING OBJECTIVES

1. Define the key terms listed.
2. List the federal and state regulations affecting the use of dental x-ray equipment.
3. Describe the general application of federal and state regulations as they affect the dental auxiliary.
4. Describe the licensure requirements for exposing dental radiographs.
5. Define the legal concept of informed consent.
6. Describe how to obtain informed consent from a patient.
7. Discuss the legal significance of the dental record.
8. Describe the legal implications of patient refusal to have dental radiographs exposed.
9. Discuss how confidentiality laws affect the information in the dental record.
10. Describe the patient's rights with regard to the dental record.

CHAPTER OUTLINE

15 Infection Control and the Dental Radiographer

KEY TERMS

antiseptic, p. 163
asepsis, p. 163
barrier envelope, p. 167
bloodborne pathogens, p. 163
disinfect, p. 163
disinfectant, high-level, p. 165
disinfectant, intermediate-level, p. 165
disinfectant, low-level, p. 165
disinfection, p. 164
exposure, occupational, p. 164
exposure, parenteral, p. 164
exposure incident, p. 163
infectious waste, p. 164
instrument, critical, p. 165
instrument, noncritical, p. 165
instrument, semicritical, p. 165
pathogen, p. 163
sharp, p. 164
standard precautions, p. 164
sterilization, p. 164
sterilize, p. 164
universal precautions, p. 164

LEARNING OBJECTIVES

1. Define the key terms listed.
2. Describe the rationale for infection control.
3. Describe three possible routes of disease transmission.
4. Describe the conditions that must be present for disease transmission to occur.
5. Discuss protective attire and barrier techniques, handwashing and care of hands, sterilization or disinfection of instruments, and the cleaning and disinfection of the dental unit and environmental surfaces.
6. Detail infection control procedures necessary before x-ray exposure.
7. Detail infection control procedures necessary during x-ray exposure.
8. Detail infection control procedures necessary after x-ray exposure.
9. Detail infection control procedures necessary for processing.
10. Discuss film handling in the darkroom with and without barrier envelopes.
11. Discuss film handling without barrier envelopes using the daylight loader of an automatic processor.

CHAPTER OUTLINE

Infection Control Basics
    Rationale for Infection Control
    Infection Control Terminology
Guidelines for Infection Control Practices
    Protective Attire and Barrier Techniques
    Handwashing and Care of Hands
    Sterilization or Disinfection of Instruments
    Cleaning and Disinfection of Dental Unit and Environmental Surfaces
Infection Control in Dental Radiography
    Infection Control Procedures Used Before Exposure
    Infection Control Procedures Used During Exposure
    Infection Control Procedures Used After Exposure
    Infection Control Procedures Used for Processing

16 Introduction to Radiographic Examinations

LEARNING OBJECTIVES

1. Define the key terms listed.
2. List the three types of intraoral radiographic examinations.
3. Describe the purpose and the type of film and technique used for each of the three types of intraoral radiographic examinations.
4. List the films that constitute a complete mouth radiographic series (CMRS).
5. List the general diagnostic criteria for intraoral radiographs.
6. List examples of extraoral radiographic examinations.
7. Discuss the prescribing of dental radiographs.
8. Describe when prescribing a CMRS for a new patient is warranted.

CHAPTER OUTLINE

Intraoral Radiographic Examination
    Types of Intraoral Radiographic Examinations
    Complete Mouth Radiographic Series
    Diagnostic Criteria for Intraoral Radiographs
Extraoral Radiographic Examination
Prescribing of Dental Radiographs

20

17 Paralleling Technique

LEARNING OBJECTIVES

1. Define the key terms listed.
2. State the basic principle of the paralleling technique and illustrate the placement of the film, film holder, position-indicating device (PID), and central ray.
3. Discuss how object-film distance affects the radiographic image and how target-film distance is used to compensate for such changes.
4. List the film holders that can be used with the paralleling technique.
5. Describe why a film holder is necessary with the paralleling technique.
6. Identify and label the parts of the Rinn XCP instruments.
7. Describe the different sizes of film used with the paralleling technique and how each film is placed in the bite-block.
8. State the five basic rules of the paralleling technique.
9. Describe the patient and equipment preparations that are necessary before using the paralleling technique.
10. Discuss the exposure sequence for 15 periapical film placements using the paralleling technique.
11. Describe each of the 15 periapical film placements recommended for use with the XCP instruments.
12. Summarize the guidelines for periapical film positioning.
13. Explain the modifications in the paralleling technique that are used for a patient with a shallow palate, bony growths, or a sensitive premolar region.
14. List the advantages and disadvantages of the paralleling technique.

CHAPTER OUTLINE

18 Bisecting Technique

KEY TERMS

angle, p. 217
angulation, p. 219
angulation, horizontal, p. 220
angulation, vertical, p. 219
bisect, p. 218
bisecting technique, p. 217
bisector, imaginary, p. 218
central ray, p. 217
elongation, p. 222
exposure sequence, p. 217
film holder, p. 219
film placement, p. 217
finger-holding method, p. 219
foreshortening, p. 222
hypotenuse, p. 217
isometry, p. 217
isometry, rule of, p. 217
long axis (tooth), p. 217
teeth, anterior, p. 224
teeth, posterior, p. 225
triangle, p. 217
triangle, equilateral, p. 217
triangle, right, p. 217
triangles, congruent, p. 217

LEARNING OBJECTIVES

1. Define the key terms listed.
2. State the rule of isometry.
3. State the basic principles of the bisecting technique, and illustrate the location of the film, tooth, imaginary bisector, central ray, and position-indicating device (PID).
4. List the film holders that can be used with the bisecting technique.
5. Describe the finger-holding method of film stabilization.
6. List the disadvantages of the finger-holding method.
7. Describe the film size used with the bisecting technique.
8. Describe correct and incorrect horizontal angulation.
9. Describe correct and incorrect vertical angulation.
10. State each of the recommended vertical angulation ranges used for periapical exposures in the bisecting technique.
11. State the basic rules of the bisecting technique.
12. Describe the patient and equipment preparations necessary before using the bisecting technique.
13. Discuss the exposure sequence used for the 14 periapical film placements used in the bisecting technique.
14. Describe each of the 14 periapical film placements recommended for use with the bisecting technique.
15. List the advantages and disadvantages of the bisecting technique.

CHAPTER OUTLINE

Basic Concepts
   Terminology
   Principles of Bisecting Technique
   Film Stabilization
   Film for Bisecting Technique
   Angulation of Position-Indicating Device
   Rules for Bisecting Technique
Step-by-Step Procedures
   Patient Preparation
   Equipment Preparation
   Exposure Sequence for Film Placements
   Film Placement for Bisecting Technique
Advantages and Disadvantages
   Advantages of Bisecting Technique
   Disadvantages of Bisecting Technique

19 Bite-Wing Technique

LEARNING OBJECTIVES

1. Define the key terms listed.
2. Describe the purpose and use of the bite-wing film.
3. Describe the appearance of opened and overlapped contact areas on a dental radiograph.
4. State the basic principles of the bite-wing technique.
5. List the two ways a film can be stabilized in the bite-wing technique, and identify which one is recommended for bite-wing exposures.
6. List the four film sizes that can be used in the bite-wing technique, and identify which film size is recommended for exposures in the adult patient.
7. Describe correct and incorrect horizontal angulation.
8. Describe the difference between positive and negative vertical angulation.
9. State the recommended vertical angulation for all bite-wing exposures.
10. State the basic rules for the bite-wing technique.
11. Describe the patient and equipment preparations that are necessary before using the bite-wing technique.
12. Discuss the exposure sequence for a complete mouth radiographic series (CMRS) that includes both periapical and bite-wing exposures.
13. Describe the premolar and molar bite-wing film placements.
14. Describe the purpose and use of vertical bite-wings. List the number of exposures and the size of film used in the vertical bite-wing technique.

CHAPTER OUTLINE

Basic Concepts
  Terminology
  Principles of Bite-Wing Technique
  Film Holder and Bite-Wing Tab
  Film for Bite-Wing Technique
  Angulation of Position-Indicating Device
  Rules for Bite-Wing Technique
Step-by-Step Procedures
  Patient Preparation
  Equipment Preparation
  Exposure Sequence for Film Placements
  Film Placement for Bite-Wing Technique
Vertical Bite-Wings
Modifications in Bite-Wing Technique
  Edentulous Spaces
  Bony Growths

20 Exposure and Technique Errors

KEY TERMS

angulation, p. 273
angulation, horizontal, p. 274
angulation, vertical, p. 274
cone-cut, p. 275
contacts, overlapped, p. 274
elongated images, p. 275
film, overexposed, p. 272
foreshortened images, p. 275
herringbone pattern, p. 280
phalangioma, p. 279

LEARNING OBJECTIVES

1. Define the key terms listed.
2. Identify and describe the appearance of the following film exposure errors: unexposed film, film exposed to light, underexposed film, and overexposed film.
3. Describe horizontal and vertical angulation.
4. Identify and describe the appearance of the following periapical technique errors: incorrect horizontal angulation, incorrect vertical angulation (foreshortened images and elongated images), and incorrect beam alignment (cone-cut images).
5. Describe and identify proper film placement for bite-wing radiographs.
6. Identify and describe the appearance of the following bite-wing technique errors: incorrect horizontal angulation, incorrect vertical angulation, and incorrect position-indicating device (PID) alignment (cone-cut images).
7. Identify and describe the appearance of the following miscellaneous technique errors: film bending, film creasing, phalangioma, double exposure, movement, and reversed film.

CHAPTER OUTLINE

Film Exposure Errors
  Exposure Problems
  Time and Exposure Factor Problems
Technique Errors (Periapical Films)
  Film Placement Problems
  Angulation Problems
  PID Alignment Problems
Technique Errors (Bite-Wing Films)
  Film Placement Problems
  Angulation Problems
  PID Alignment
Miscellaneous Technique Errors
  Film Bending
  Film Creasing
  Phalangioma
  Double Exposure
  Movement
  Reversed Film

21 Occlusal and Localization Techniques

LEARNING OBJECTIVES

1. Define the key terms listed.
2. Describe the purpose of the occlusal examination.
3. List the uses of the occlusal examination.
4. Describe the patient and equipment preparations necessary before using the occlusal technique.
5. State the recommended vertical angulations for the following maxillary occlusal projections: topographic, lateral (right or left), and pediatric.
6. State the recommended vertical angulations for the following mandibular occlusal projections: topographic, cross-sectional, and pediatric.
7. State the purpose of localization techniques.
8. Describe the buccal object rule.
9. Describe the right-angle technique.
10. List the patient and equipment preparations that are necessary before using the buccal object rule or the right-angle technique.
11. Describe the film placements for the buccal object rule and compare the resulting radiographs.
12. Describe the film placements for the right-angle technique and compare the resulting radiographs.

CHAPTER OUTLINE

Occlusal Technique
    Basic Concepts
    Step-by-Step Procedures
Localization Techniques
    Basic Concepts
    Step-by-Step Procedures

22 Panoramic Radiography

LEARNING OBJECTIVES

1. Define the key terms listed.
2. Describe the purpose and uses of panoramic radiography.
3. Describe the fundamentals of panoramic radiography.
4. Describe the equipment used in panoramic radiography.
5. Describe the patient preparations, equipment preparations, and patient positioning procedures needed before exposing a panoramic film.
6. Identify the patient preparation and positioning errors seen on panoramic radiographs.
7. Discuss the causes of patient preparation and positioning errors and the necessary measures needed to correct such errors.
8. Discuss the advantages and disadvantages of panoramic radiography.

23 Extraoral Radiography

KEY TERMS

LEARNING OBJECTIVES

1. Define the key terms listed.
2. Describe the purpose and uses of extraoral radiography.
3. Describe the equipment used in extraoral radiography.
4. Detail the equipment and patient preparations necessary before exposing an extraoral film.
5. Identify the specific purpose of each of the extraoral film projections.
6. Describe the head position, film placement, and beam alignment for each of the following extraoral films: lateral jaw projection—body of the mandible, lateral jaw projection—ramus of the mandible, lateral cephalometric projection, posteroanterior projection, Waters projection, submentovertex projection, reverse Towne projection, and transcranial projection.

CHAPTER OUTLINE

24 Digital Radiography

KEY TERMS

analog image, p. 342
bit-depth image, p. 342
charge-coupled device, p. 342
charge injection device, p. 345
complementary metal oxide semiconductor/active pixel sensor, p. 345
digital image, p. 342
digital radiography, p. 342
digital subtraction, p. 342
digitize, p. 342
direct digital imaging, p. 342
indirect digital imaging, p. 342
line pairs/millimeter (lp/ml), p. 342
pixel, p. 342
sensor, p. 342
storage phosphor imaging, p. 342

LEARNING OBJECTIVES

1. Define the key terms listed.
2. Describe the purpose and use of digital radiography.
3. Discuss the fundamentals of digital radiography.
4. List and describe the equipment used in digital radiography.
5. List and describe the two types of digital imaging.
6. Describe the patient and equipment preparations required for digital radiography.
7. List and discuss the advantages and disadvantages of digital radiography.

CHAPTER OUTLINE

Basic Concepts
 Terminology
 Purpose and Use
 Fundamentals
 Radiation Exposure
 Equipment
Types of Digital Imaging
 Direct Digital Imaging
 Indirect Digital Imaging
Step-by-Step Procedures
 Sensor Preparation
 Sensor Placement
Advantages and Disadvantages
 Advantages of Digital Radiography
 Disadvantages of Digital Radiography

25 Radiography of Patients with Special Needs

LEARNING OBJECTIVES

1. Define the key terms listed.
2. List the areas of the oral cavity that are most likely to elicit the gag reflex when stimulated.
3. List two precipitating factors responsible for initiating the gag reflex.
4. Describe how to control the gag reflex using operator attitude, patient and equipment preparations, exposure sequencing, film placement and technique, and helpful hints.
5. Describe common physical disabilities and what modifications in technique may be necessary during the radiographic examination.
6. Describe common developmental disabilities and what modifications in technique may be necessary during the radiographic examination.
7. List helpful hints that can be used when treating a person with a disability.
8. Describe the prescribing of dental radiographs, patient and equipment preparations, recommended techniques, and patient management as they pertain to the pediatric dental patient.
9. Describe the use of the dental radiograph, film placement modifications, and recommended periapical technique during root canal procedures.
10. Describe the purposes of the radiographic examination in the edentulous patient.
11. List and describe the three types of radiographic examination that may be used for the edentulous patient.

Chapter **25** **Radiography of Patients with Special Needs**

26 Normal Anatomy: Intraoral Films

KEY TERMS

alveolar bone, p. 373
alveolar crest, p. 387
alveolar process, p. 381
anterior nasal spine, p. 369
body of mandible, p. 381
canal, p. 369
cancellous, p. 367
coronoid process, p. 368
cortical, p. 367
dentin, p. 386
dentinoenamel junction, p. 386
enamel, p. 386
external oblique ridge, p. 385
floor of nasal cavity, p. 375
foramen, p. 369
fossa, p. 369
genial tubercles, p. 369
hamulus, p. 369
incisive foramen, p. 371
inferior nasal conchae, p. 375
internal oblique ridge, p. 369
inverted Y, p. 378
lamina dura, p. 388
lateral fossa, p. 373
lingual foramen, p. 381
mandibular canal, p. 369
maxillary sinus, p. 369
maxillary tuberosity, p. 369
median palatal suture, p. 371
mental foramen, p. 369
mental fossa, p. 382
mental ridge, p. 382
mylohyoid ridge, p. 383
nasal cavity, p. 372
nasal septum, p. 370
nutrient canal(s), p. 378
periodontal ligament space, p. 387
process, p. 368

pulp cavity, p. 386
ramus, p. 381
ridge, p. 368
septum, septa, p. 378
sinus, p. 369
spine, p. 369
submandibular fossa, p. 369
superior foramina of incisive canal, p. 372
suture, p. 370
tubercle, p. 369
tuberosity, p. 369
zygoma, p. 379
zygomatic process of maxilla, p. 379

LEARNING OBJECTIVES

1. Define the key terms listed.
2. State the difference between cortical and cancellous bone.
3. Define the general terms that describe prominences, spaces, and depressions in bone.
4. Identify and describe the normal anatomic landmarks of the maxilla on a human skull.
5. Identify and describe the normal anatomic landmarks of the maxilla on dental radiographs.
6. Identify and describe the normal anatomic landmarks of the mandible on a human skull.
7. Identify and describe the normal anatomic landmarks of the mandible on dental radiographs.
8. Identify and describe the radiographic appearance of tooth anatomy.
9. Identify each normal radiographic landmark of the maxilla and mandible as either radiolucent or radiopaque.
10. Identify each normal anatomic landmark of a tooth as radiolucent or radiopaque.

27 Film Mounting and Viewing

LEARNING OBJECTIVES

1. Define the key terms listed.
2. List the individuals who are qualified to mount and view dental radiographs.
3. Describe when and where films are mounted.
4. List five reasons to use a film mount.
5. Describe what information is placed on a film mount.
6. Discuss the importance of normal anatomy in film mounting.
7. Describe how the identification dot is used to determine film orientation.
8. List and describe two methods of film mounting and identify the preferred method.
9. List and describe the step-by-step procedures for film mounting.
10. List and describe the necessary equipment for film viewing.
11. Discuss the importance of masking extraneous viewbox light seen around a film mount.
12. Describe optimal viewing conditions, as well as when and where films should be viewed.
13. Explain the importance of examining films in an established viewing sequence.
14. List and describe the step-by-step procedures for film viewing.
15. Explain why multiple viewings of dental radiographs are necessary, and list the areas, diseases, and abnormalities that must be included in the examinations.

CHAPTER OUTLINE

Film Mounting
    Basic Concepts
    Normal Anatomy and Film Mounting
    Film Mounting Methods
    Step-by-Step Procedure
Film Viewing
    Basic Concepts
    Step-by-Step Procedure

KEY TERMS

LEARNING OBJECTIVES

1. Define the key terms listed.
2. Identify and describe the bony landmarks of the maxilla and surrounding structures as viewed on the panoramic radiograph.
3. Identify and describe the bony landmarks of the mandible and surrounding structures as viewed on the panoramic radiograph.
4. Identify air space images as viewed on the panoramic radiograph.
5. Identify soft tissue images as viewed on the panoramic radiograph.

CHAPTER OUTLINE

Normal Anatomic Landmarks
    Bony Landmarks of Maxilla and Surrounding Structures
    Bony Landmarks of Mandible and Surrounding Structures
Air Space Images Seen on Panoramic Radiographs
Soft Tissue Images Seen on Panoramic Radiographs

29 Introduction to Radiographic Interpretation

LEARNING OBJECTIVES

1. Define the key terms listed.
2. Summarize the importance of radiographic interpretation.
3. Define the roles of the dentist and dental auxiliary in the interpretation of dental radiographs.
4. Discuss the difference between interpretation and diagnosis.
5. Describe who is able to interpret dental radiographs.
6. Describe when and where dental radiographs are interpreted.
7. Describe how radiographic interpretation can be used to educate the dental patient about the importance and use of dental radiographs.

CHAPTER OUTLINE

30 Descriptive Terminology

KEY TERMS

LEARNING OBJECTIVES

1. Identify the categories of information that should be documented for all lesions viewed radiographically.
2. Define descriptive terminology and describe why the dental professional should use descriptive terms.
3. Define the terms *radiograph, x-ray, radiolucent,* and *radiopaque*.
4. Differentiate between radiograph and x-ray.
5. Differentiate between radiolucent and radiopaque.
6. Define the terms *unilocular* and *multilocular*.
7. Define periapical, inter-radicular, edentulous zone, pericoronal, and alveolar bone loss.
8. Identify radiolucent lesions on a radiograph in terms of appearance, location, and size.
9. Define focal opacity, target lesion, multifocal confluent, irregular/ill-defined, ground glass, mixed lucent-opaque, and soft tissue opacity.
10. Identify radiopaque lesions on a radiograph in terms of appearance, location, and size.

CHAPTER OUTLINE

Definitions and Uses
    What Is Descriptive Terminology?
    Why Use Descriptive Terminology?
    Descriptive Terminology versus Diagnosis
Review of Basic Terms
    Radiograph versus X-Ray
    Radiolucent versus Radiopaque
    Terms Used to Describe Radiolucent Lesions
    Terms Used to Describe Radiopaque Lesions

31 Identification of Restorations, Dental Materials, and Foreign Objects

LEARNING OBJECTIVES

1. Define the key terms listed.
2. Discuss the importance of interpreting radiographs while the patient is present.
3. Identify and describe the radiographic appearance of the following restorations: amalgam, gold, stainless steel and chrome, post and core, porcelain, porcelain-fused-to-metal, composite, and acrylic.
4. Identify and describe the radiographic appearance of the following dental materials and devices: base materials, metallic pins, gutta percha, silver points, removable partial dentures, complete dentures, orthodontic bands, brackets and wires, fixed retainers, implants, suture wires, splints, and stabilizing arches and wires.
5. Identify and describe the radiographic appearance of the following miscellaneous objects: jewelry, eyeglasses, and patient napkin chains.

CHAPTER OUTLINE

32 Interpretation of Dental Caries

KEY TERMS

LEARNING OBJECTIVES

1. Define the key terms listed.
2. Describe dental caries.
3. Explain why caries appears radiolucent on a dental radiograph.
4. Discuss interpretation tips for evaluating caries on a dental radiograph.
5. Discuss the factors that may influence the radiographic interpretation of dental caries.
6. Detail the radiographic classification of caries.
7. Identify and describe the radiographic appearance of the following: incipient, moderate, advanced, and severe interproximal caries.
8. Identify and describe the radiographic appearance of the following: incipient, moderate, and severe occlusal caries.
9. Identify and describe the radiographic appearance of the following: buccal, lingual, root surface, recurrent, and rampant caries.

CHAPTER OUTLINE

33 Interpretation of Periodontal Disease

LEARNING OBJECTIVES

1. Define the key terms listed.
2. Describe the healthy periodontium.
3. Briefly describe periodontal disease.
4. Discuss the importance of the clinical and radiographic examinations in the diagnosis of periodontal disease.
5. Describe the limitations of radiographs in the detection of periodontal disease.
6. Describe the type of radiographs that should be used to document periodontal disease and the preferred exposure technique.
7. State the difference between horizontal and vertical bone loss.
8. State the difference between localized and generalized bone loss.
9. State the differences among mild, moderate, and severe bone loss.
10. List each of the four American Dental Association (ADA) case types and describe the corresponding radiographic appearance.
11. Recognize each of the four ADA case types on dental radiographs.
12. List two predisposing factors for periodontal disease.
13. Recognize and describe the radiographic appearance of calculus.

34 Interpretation of Trauma and Pulpal and Periapical Lesions

KEY TERMS

avulsion, p. 482
condensing osteitis, p. 489
extrusion, p. 482
fracture, p. 482
hypercementosis, p. 489
intrusion, p. 482
luxation, p. 483
periapical abscess, p. 487
periapical cyst, p. 487
periapical granuloma, p. 487
periapical lesion, p. 482
periodontal abscess, p. 488
pulp stones, p. 485
pulpal obliteration, p. 485
pulpal sclerosis, p. 485
resorption, external, p. 484
resorption, internal, p. 485
resorption, pathologic, p. 484
resorption, physiologic, p. 484

sclerotic bone, p. 489
trauma, p. 482

LEARNING OBJECTIVES

1. Define the key tems listed.
2. Describe and identify the radiographic appearance of crown, root, and jaw fractures.
3. Describe and identify the radiographic appearance of an avulsion.
4. Describe and identify the radiographic appearance of internal and external resorption.
5. Describe and identify the radiographic appearance of pulpal sclerosis, pulpal obliteration, and pulp stones.
6. Describe and identify the radiographic appearance of a periapical granuloma, cyst, and abscess.
7. Describe and identify the radiographic appearance of condensing osteitis, sclerotic bone, and hypercementosis.

CHAPTER OUTLINE

Radiographic Changes Caused by Trauma
    Fractures
    Injuries
Radiographic Changes Caused by Resorption
    External Resorption
    Internal Resorption
Radiographic Features of Pulpal Lesions
    Pulpal Sclerosis
    Pulpal Obliteration
    Pulp Stones
Radiographic Features of Periapical Lesions
    Periapical Radiolucencies
    Periapical Radiopacities

Answers to Quiz Questions

CHAPTER 1

Answers to Matching

1. c
2. i
3. a
4. d
5. e
6. h
7. g
8. f
9. b
10. c
11. h
12. j
13. a
14. g
15. d
16. i
17. b
18. f
19. e

Answers to Essay

Because of the nature of questions 20 and 21, correct answers are subject to the discretion of individual instructors.

CHAPTER 2

Answers to Multiple Choice

1. d
2. b
3. c
4. b
5. b
6. d
7. a
8. b
9. a
10. b

Answers to Identification

11. filament
12. molybdenum cup
13. electron stream
14. tungsten target
15. copper sleeve
16. vacuum
17. x-ray beam
18. leaded glass
19. aluminum filter
20. lead collimator
21. position-indicating device
22. tubehead seal
23. x-ray tube
24. oil
25. unleaded window
26. metal housing

Answers to Multiple Choice

27. b
28. a
29. c
30. b
31. c
32. a
33. b
34. a
35. c
36. a

Answers to Identification

37. absorption
38. Compton scatter
39. coherent scatter
40. no interaction

Answers to Multiple Choice

41. b
42. d
43. c
44. a

CHAPTER 3

Answers to Multiple Choice

1. a
2. c
3. d
4. b
5. a
6. d
7. d
8. c
9. b
10. a
11. a
12. c
13. a
14. c
15. a
16. b
17. c
18. c
19. a
20. d

CHAPTER 4

Answers to Multiple Choice

1. d
2. e
3. a
4. c
5. c
6. e
7. d
8. b

9. b
10. d
11. c
12. a
13. e
14. c
15. b
16. a
17. a
18. e
19. e
20. c
21. b
22. e
23. b
24. d
25. a

CHAPTER 5

Answers to True/False

1. True
2. False
3. True
4. False
5. False

Answers to Multiple Choice

6. b
7. c
8. b
9. b
10. b
11. a
12. d
13. a
14. b
15. c

Answers to Fill in the Blank

16. a. 1.5; b. 2.5
17. 90-135
18. $(N - 18) \times 5$ rem/year (0.05 Sv/year)
19. 5.0 rem/year (0.05 Sv/year)
20. 0.1 rem/year (0.001 Sv/year)

CHAPTER 6

Answers to Multiple Choice

1. c
2. a
3. b
4. b
5. a
6. b
7. c
8. a

CHAPTER 7

Answers to Fill in the Blank

1. protective layer
2. film base
3. halides
4. latent image

Answers to Identification

5. dot on label side of film packet
6. outer package wrapping on label side of film packet
7. lead foil sheet
8. black paper film wrapper
9. identification dot on tube side of film packet
10. intraoral film
11. outer package wrapping on tube side of film packet

Answers to Multiple Choice

12. c
13. d
14. a
15. c
16. b
17. c
18. a
19. b
20. a
21. a
22. a
23. b
24. d
25. b
26. c
27. a
28. c
29. c
30. a

CHAPTER 8

Answers to Multiple Choice

1. b
2. b
3. d
4. d
5. a
6. a
7. a
8. a
9. d
10. b
11. b
12. a
13. b
14. a
15. a
16. b
17. c

18. a
19. d
20. c
21. a
22. c
23. d
24. b

Answers to Fill in the Blank
25. increase
26. decrease
27. increase
28. increase
29. decrease
30. decrease
31. increase
32. decrease
33. decrease
34. decrease
35. increase

CHAPTER 9

Answers to Multiple Choice
1. a
2. c
3. c
4. e
5. b
6. c
7. a
8. d
9. d
10. a
11. a
12. d
13. c
14. e
15. d
16. d
17. c
18. d

Answers to Matching
19. h
20. a
21. g
22. b
23. d
24. j
25. c
26. e
27. f
28. i

Answers to Fill in the Black
29. film duplicator and duplicating film
30. The longer duplicating film is exposed to light, the *lighter* it appears.

Answers to Matching
31. e
32. d
33. a
34. c
35. b
36. c

Answers to Identification
37. contamination with the developer
38. contamination with the fixer; air bubbles
39. exhausted developer or fixer; insufficient fix time; insufficient rinse time
40. reticulation of emulsion
41. developer cutoff
42. fixer cutoff
43. fingernail artifact
44. static electricity
45. scratch marks on film

Answers to True/False
46. True
47. False
48. False
49. True
50. True

CHAPTER 10

Answers to Multiple Choice
1. b
2. a
3. a
4. b
5. a
6. b
7. d
8. a
9. e
10. c
11. a
12. a
13. d
14. d
15. b
16. a

CHAPTER 11

Answers to True/False
1. False
2. False
3. True
4. False
5. True
6. True
7. False
8. True
9. True
10. False

CHAPTER 12

Answers to True/False
1. False
2. False
3. True
4. True
5. False
6. False
7. False
8. True
9. False
10. True

CHAPTER 13

Answers to Essay
Because of the nature of questions 1 and 2, correct answers are subject to the discretion of individual instructors.

Answers to Short Answer
Because of the nature of questions 3 to 17, correct answers are subject to the discretion of individual instructors.

CHAPTER 14

Answers to Multiple Choice
1. c
2. c
3. a
4. a
5. c
6. b
7. b
8. d
9. c
10. a

CHAPTER 15

Answers to Matching
1. b
2. e
3. j
4. i
5. a
6. g
7. h
8. f
9. d
10. c

Answers to Fill in the Blank
11. to prevent disease transmission
12. direct contact with pathogens, indirect contact with pathogens, and direct contact with airborne contaminants
13. susceptible host, pathogen with sufficient infectivity and numbers to cause infection, and portal of entry through which the pathogen may enter the host

Answers to Multiple Choice
14. c
15. b
16. d
17. a
18. d
19. d
20. c

Answers to Essay
Because of the nature of questions 21 to 25, correct answers are subject to the discretion of individual instructors.

CHAPTER 16

Answers to Matching
1. f
2. l
3. b
4. j
5. e
6. d
7. g
8. a
9. h
10. c

Answers to Short Answer
Because of the nature of questions 11 to 15, correct answers are subject to the discretion of individual instructors.

CHAPTER 17

Answers to Matching
1. h
2. g
3. f
4. e
5. a
6. b
7. c
8. d

Answers to Fill in the Blank
9. image magnification, loss of definition
10. film holder
11. X= extension; C= cone (PID); P= paralleling
12. size 1
13. size 2
14. Precision film holders; Rinn XCP instruments with snap-on collimators
15. upper arch parallel to the floor; midsagittal plane perpendicular to the floor

Answers to Multiple Choice
16. a
17. b
18. c

19. a
20. b
21. c
22. b
23. b
24. b
25. a

Answers to Essay
Because of the nature of questions 26 to 33, correct answers are subject to the discretion of individual instructors.

CHAPTER 18

Answers to Matching
1. d
2. b
3. c
4. a

Answers to Identification
5. c
6. b
7. b
8. none
9. c
10. b

Answers to Fill in the Blank
11. magnification results
12. size 2
13. Rinn BAI instruments
14. maxillary arch parallel to the floor; midsagittal plane perpendicular to the floor
15. mandibular arch parallel to the floor; midsagittal plane perpendicular to the floor

Answers to Multiple Choice
16. d
17. a
18. d
19. a

Answer to Essay
Because of the nature of questions 20 to 30, correct answers are subject to the discretion of individual instructors.

CHAPTER 19

Answers to Fill in the Blank
1. patient "bites" on a "wing" (tab) to stabilize film
2. size 2
3. size 0
4. upper arch parallel to the floor; midsagittal plane perpendicular to the floor
5. caries
6. size 3
7. vertical angulation

8. horizontal angulation
9. overlapped contacts
10. if the beam is not centered over the film

Answers to Multiple Choice
11. c
12. c
13. a
14. b
15. d

Answers to Essay
Because of the nature of questions 16 to 23, correct answers are subject to the discretion of individual instructors.

CHAPTER 20

Answers to Identification
1. underexposed film (Figure 20-27)
2. patient movement (Figure 20-28)
3. elongated images (Figure 20-29)
4. reversed film (Figure 20-30)
5. cone-cut (Figure 20-31)
6. overlapped contacts (Figure 20-32)
7. overexposed film (Figure 20-33)
8. incorrect premolar film placement (Figure 20-34)
9. foreshortened images (Figure 20-35)
10. incorrect film placement: no apices (Figure 20-36)

Answers to Matching
11. d
12. c
13. b
14. a
15. c

Answers to Multiple Choice
16. b
17. a
18. c
19. d
20. a

CHAPTER 21

Answers to Fill in the Blank
1. chewing surfaces of the posterior teeth
2. size 4
3. size 2
4. upper arch parallel to the floor
5. See text for uses.
6. +65 degrees
7. +60 degrees
8. −55 degrees
9. 90 degrees
10. maxillary = +60 degrees; mandibular = −55 degrees

Answers to Short Answer
11. BUCCAL. In the second film *(B)*, PID was shifted down, and amalgam moved up (opposite = buccal).

12. BUCCAL. In the second film *(B)*, PID was shifted distally, and fragment moved mesially (opposite = buccal).
13. BUCCAL. In the second film *(B)*, PID was shifted down, and canine moved up (opposite = buccal).
14. LINGUAL. In the second film *(B)*, PID was shifted distally, and gutta percha moved distally (same = lingual).
15. LINGUAL. In the second film *(B)*, PID was shifted mesially, and impacted canine moved mesially (same = lingual).

CHAPTER 22

Answers to Multiple Choice
1. c
2. a
3. c
4. a
5. b

Answers to Matching
6. a
7. a
8. a
9. c
10. a
11. b
12. b
13. a
14. a
15. a
16. a
17. b
18. a
19. c
20. a

Answers to Essay
Because of the nature of questions 21 to 25, correct answers are subject to the discretion of individual instructors.

Answer to Identification
26. This is a pediatric patient exhibiting mixed dentition.

CHAPTER 23

Answers to Essay
Because of the nature of questions 1 to 8, correct answers are subject to the discretion of individual instructors.

Answers to Multiple Choice
9. c
10. a
11. d
12. b
13. a
14. c
15. d

CHAPTER 24

Answers to Matching
1. h
2. a
3. i
4. d
5. e
6. g
7. f
8. c
9. b

Answers to True/False
10. False
11. False
12. True
13. True
14. False
15. True
16. True
17. True
18. True

Answers to Multiple Choice
19. c
20. d
21. b
22. b
23. a
24. a
25. c

CHAPTER 25

Answers to True/False
1. False
2. False
3. True
4. True
5. True
6. False
7. False
8. False
9. True
10. False
11. True
12. True
13. True
14. False
15. False
16. False
17. False
18. True
19. False
20. False
21. False
22. False
23. True
24. False
25. True

CHAPTER 26

Answers to Matching
1. b
2. d
3. a
4. c
5. f
6. g
7. h
8. e

Answers to Identification
9. zygomatic process of the maxilla
10. floor of the maxillary sinus
11. incisive foramen
12. coronoid process
13. lingual foramen
14. internal oblique ridge
15. mandibular canal
16. mental foramen

CHAPTER 27

Answers to True/False
1. True
2. False
3. False
4. False
5. True
6. True
7. True
8. True
9. False
10. False
11. False
12. True
13. False
14. True
15. True
16. False
17. True
18. True
19. True
20. False

Answers to Short Answer
Because of the nature of questions 21 to 25, correct answers are subject to the discretion of individual instructors.

CHAPTER 28

Answers to Identification
Question 1
1. glenoid fossa
2. mandibular condyle
3. coronoid process
4. maxillary tuberosity
5. infraorbital foramen
6. mental foramen
7. lingual foramen
8. genial tubercles
9. incisive foramen
10. nasal cavity
11. hard palate
12. zygomatic process of the maxilla
13. mylohyoid ridge
14. internal oblique ridge
15. external oblique ridge

Question 2
1. palatoglossal air space
2. hard palate
3. infraorbital foramen
4. floor of the orbit
5. zygomatic process of the maxilla
6. posterior wall of the maxillary sinus
7. zygomaticotemporal suture
8. external auditory meatus
9. lateral pterygoid plate
10. maxillary tuberosity
11. styloid process
12. ear
13. mandibular canal
14. cervical spine
15. hyoid bone
16. mental foramen

CHAPTER 29

Answers to Short Answer
Because of the nature of questions 1 to 6, correct answers are subject to the discretion of individual instructors.

Answers to True/False
7. True
8. True
9. True
10. False
11. False
12. False
13. False
14. True
15. True

CHAPTER 30

Answers to Short Answer
Because of the nature of questions 1 to 3, correct answers are subject to the discretion of individual instructors.

Answers to Matching
4. d
5. b
6. e

7. a
8. f
9. g
10. c

CHAPTER 31

Answers to Identification
1. gutta percha (Figure 31-45)
2. amalgam (Figure 31-46)
3. gold (Figure 31-47)
4. all-porcelain crowns (Figure 31-48)
5. implant with a porcelain-fused-to-metal crown (Figure 31-49)
6. removable partial denture with a metallic framework (Figure 31-50)
7. necklace of the patient (Figure 31-51)
8. a maxillary denture is in place (Figure 31-52)

Answers to Multiple Choice
9. Radiopaque ranking:
   (3) gutta percha
   (4) acrylic restorations
   (1) amalgam
   (2) stainless steel
10. a
11. a
12. d
13. c

Answers to Short Answer
Because of the nature of questions 14 to 16, correct answers are subject to the discretion of individual instructors.

CHAPTER 32

Answers to Identification
1. rampant severe caries (Figure 32-25)
2. incipient interproximal caries (Figure 32-26)
3. root surface caries (Figure 32-27)
4. moderate interproximal caries (Figure 32-28)
5. severe interproximal caries (Figure 32-29)

Answers to Matching
6. e
7. a
8. b
9. d
10. c
11. g
12. f

Answers to Short Answer
Because of the nature of questions 13 to 20, correct answers are subject to the discretion of individual instructors.

CHAPTER 33

Answers to Identification
1. horizontal, moderate, ADA Case Type III (Figure 33-30)
2. horizontal, mild, ADA Case Type II (Figure 33-31)
3. horizontal, severe, ADA Case Type IV (Figure 33-32)
4. none, none (Figure 33-33}
5. none, none (Figure 33-34)

Answers to Matching
6. c
7. a
8. d
9. b

Answers to Fill in the Blank
10. periodontium
11. periodontal
12. furcation
13. periapical
14. paralleling technique
15. horizontal
16. vertical
17. periodontal disease
18. localized
19. generalized
20. calculus

CHAPTER 34

Answers to Matching
1. b
2. e
3. a
4. f
5. d
6. c

Answers to Identification
7. pulp stone (Figure 34-23)
8. hypercementosis (Figure 34-24)
9. pulpal obliteration (Figure 34-25)
10. condensing osteitis (Figure 34-26)
11. external resorption (Figure 34-27)
12. pulpal sclerosis (Figure 34-28)

Test Bank

MULTIPLE CHOICE

1. Radiation is defined as:
    a. A form of energy carried by waves or streams of particles.
    b. A beam of energy that has the power to penetrate substances and record image shadows on photographic film.
    c. A high-energy radiation produced by the collision of a beam of electrons with a metal target in an x-ray tube.
    d. A branch of medicine that deals with the use of x-rays.

Answer: a
Correct: Radiation is a form of energy carried by waves or streams of particles.
Incorrect:
    (b) An *x-ray* is a beam of energy that has the power to penetrate substances and record image shadows on photographic film.
    (c) *X-radiation* is a high-energy radiation produced by the collision of a beam of electrons with a metal target in an x-ray tube.
    (d) *Radiology* is a branch of medicine that deals with the use of x-rays.
REF: p. 3

2. A radiograph is defined as:
    a. A beam of energy that has the power to penetrate substances and record image shadows on photographic film.
    b. A picture on film produced by the passage of x-rays through an object or body.
    c. The art and science of making radiographs by the exposure of film to x-rays.
    d. A form of energy carried by waves or a stream of particles.

Answer: b
Correct: A radiograph is a picture on film produced by the passage of x-rays through an object or body.
Incorrect:
    (a) An *x-ray* is a beam of energy that has the power to penetrate substances and record image shadows on photographic film.
    (c) *Radiography* is the art and science of making radiographs by the exposure of film to x-rays.
    (d) *Radiation* is a form of energy carried by waves or streams of particles.
REF: p. 3

3. Which of the following statements is *true* regarding the importance of dental radiographs?
    a. An oral examination with dental radiographs limits the practitioner to what is seen clinically.
    b. All dental diseases and conditions produce clinical signs and symptoms.
    c. Dental radiographs are not a necessary component of comprehensive patient care.
    d. Many dental diseases are typically discovered only through the use of dental radiographs.

Answer: d
Correct: Many dental diseases are typically discovered only through the use of dental radiographs.
Incorrect:
    (a) An oral examination *without* dental radiographs limits the practitioner to what is seen clinically.
    (b) Many dental diseases and conditions produce *no* clinical signs and symptoms.
    (c) Dental radiographs *are* a necessary component of comprehensive patient care.
REF: p. 3

4. The x-ray was discovered by:
    a. Heinrich Geissler
    b. Wilhelm Roentgen
    c. Johann Hittorf
    d. William Crookes

Answer: b
Correct: Wilhelm Roentgen discovered the x-ray on November 8, 1895.
Incorrect:
    (a) Heinrich Geissler built the first vacuum tube in 1838.
    (c) Johann Hittorf observed in 1870 that discharges emitted from the negative electrode of a vacuum tube travelled in straight lines, produced heat, and resulted in a greenish fluorescence.
    (d) William Crookes discovered that cathode rays were streams of charged particles in the late 1870s.
REF: p. 3

5. _____ exposed the first dental radiograph in the United States using a live person.
    a. Otto Walkoff
    b. Wilhelm Roentgen
    c. C. Edmund Kells
    d. Weston Price

Answer: c
Correct: C. Edmund Kells exposed the first dental radiograph in the United States using a live person.
Incorrect:
    (a) Otto Walkoff was a German dentist who made the first dental radiograph.
    (b) Wilhelm Roentgen was a Bavarian physicist who discovered the x-ray.
    (d) Weston Price introduced the bisecting technique in 1904.
REF: p. 5

6. William Rollins:
   a. Established the first college course in radiography for dental students.
   b. Was the first to use film in intraoral radiography.
   c. Developed the first dental x-ray unit.
   d. Developed the first hot cathode x-ray tube.

Answer: c
Correct: William Rollins developed the first dental x-ray unit.
Incorrect:
   (a) Howard Riley Raper developed the first college course in radiography for dental students.
   (b) Frank Van Woert was the first dentist to use film in intraoral radiography.
   (d) William D. Coolidge developed the first hot cathode x-ray tube.
REF: p. 5

7. The variable kilovoltage x-ray machine was introduced in:
   a. 1895
   b. 1913
   c. 1923
   d. 1957

Answer: d
Correct: The variable kilovoltage x-ray machine was introduced in 1957.
Incorrect:
   (a) Wilhelm Roentgen discovered the x-ray in 1895.
   (b) William Coolidge developed the first hot cathode x-ray tube in 1913.
   (c) A miniature version of the x-ray tube was placed inside the head of an x-ray machine and immersed in oil by the Victor X-Ray Corporation in 1923.
REF: p. 6

8. Current fast radiographic film requires less than _____ % the initial exposure times used in 1920.
   a. 25
   b. 10
   c. 5
   d. 2

Answer: d
Correct: Current fast radiographic film requires less than 2% the initial exposure times used in 1920.
Incorrect:
   (a) The exposure time has been reduced to less than 2% of what it was in 1920.
   (b) The exposure time has been reduced to less than 2% of what it was in 1920.
   (c) The exposure time has been reduced to less than 2% of what it was in 1920.
REF: p. 6

CHAPTER 2   RADIATION PHYSICS

MULTIPLE CHOICE

1. The fundamental unit of matter is the:
   a. Proton
   b. Neutron
   c. Electron
   d. Atom

Answer: d
Correct: The fundamental unit of matter is the atom.
Incorrect:
   (a) A proton is a subatomic particle; the fundamental unit of matter is the atom.
   (b) A neutron is a subatomic particle; the fundamental unit of matter is the atom.
   (c) An electron is a subatomic particle; the fundamental unit of matter is the atom.
REF: p. 10

2. The nucleus of an atom contains:
   a. Protons
   b. Neutrons
   c. Protons and neutrons
   d. Electrons

Answer: c
Correct: The nucleus of an atom contains protons and neutrons.
Incorrect:
   (a) The nucleus of an atom contains neutrons as well as protons.
   (b) The nucleus of an atom contains protons as well as neutrons.
   (d) The nucleus of an atom does not contain electrons; it contains protons and neutrons.
REF: pp. 10-11

3. Which subatomic particle carries a negative electrical charge?
   a. Neutron
   b. Proton
   c. Electron
   d. Nucleon

Answer: c
Correct: An electron carries a negative electrical charge.
Incorrect:
   (a) A neutron does not carry an electrical charge.
   (b) A proton carries a positive electrical charge.
   (d) A nucleon carries a positive (proton) or no (neutron) electrical charge.
REF: p. 11

4. Which of the following elements is the simplest atom, with an atomic number of 1?
   a. Hydrogen
   b. Helium
   c. Nitrogen
   d. Oxygen

Answer: a
Correct: Hydrogen is the simplest atom; with a single proton, it has an atomic number of 1.
Incorrect:
  (b) Helium has an atomic number of 2.
  (c) Nitrogen has an atomic number of 7.
  (d) Oxygen has an atomic number of 8.
REF: p. 11

5. Which of the following statements is *true* of orbits or shells in the atom?
  a. Protons travel around the nucleus in well-defined shells.
  b. An atom contains innumerable shells.
  c. The energy level within each shell is the same.
  d. The K shell is closest to the nucleus and has the highest energy level.

Answer: c
Correct: The energy level within each shell is the same.
Incorrect:
  (a) Electrons travel around the nucleus in well-defined shells.
  (b) An atom contains a maximum of seven shells.
  (d) The K shell is located closest to the nucleus and has the lowest energy level.
REF: p. 11

6. The binding energy or binding force of an electron is:
  a. Determined by the distance between the neutrons and protons within the nucleus.
  b. Weaker for electrons located in outer shells than for inner shells.
  c. Weaker for electrons located in inner shells than for outer shells.
  d. Both a and c.

Answer: b
Correct: The binding energy or binding force of an electron is weaker for electrons located in outer shells than for inner shells.
Incorrect:
  (a) The binding energy or binding force of an electron is determined by the distance between the nucleus and the orbiting electron.
  (c) The binding energy or binding force of an electron is stronger for electrons located in inner shells than for outer shells.
  (d) Neither a nor c is correct.
REF: pp. 11–12

7. Which of the following statements is/are *true* of ionization?
  a. An atom that gains an electron will have a negative charge.
  b. An atom that loses an electron will have a negative charge.
  c. An atom that loses an electron will have a positive charge.
  d. Both a and c.

Answer: d
Correct: An atom that gains an electron will have a negative charge, and an atom that loses an electron will have a positive charge.
Incorrect:
  (a) This statement is true; however, choice c is also correct.
  (b) An atom that loses an electron will have a positive charge.
  (c) This statement is true; however, choice a is also correct.
REF: p. 12

8. An ion pair results when:
  a. A proton is removed from an atom.
  b. An electron is removed from an atom.
  c. A neutron is removed from an atom.
  d. Two atoms share a pair of electrons.

Answer: b
Correct: An ion pair results when an electron is removed from an atom.
Incorrect:
  (a) An ion pair results when an *electron* is removed from an atom rather than a proton.
  (c) An ion pair results when an *electron* is removed from an atom rather than a neutron.
  (d) An ion pair results when an *electron* is removed from an atom.
REF: p. 13

9. *Radiation* is the emission and propagation of energy through space or a substance in the form of waves or particles. *Radioactivity* can be defined as the process by which certain unstable atoms or elements undergo spontaneous disintegration, or decay, in an effort to attain a more balanced nuclear state.
  a. Both statements are true.
  b. Both statements are false.
  c. The first statement is true; the second is false.
  d. The first statement is false; the second is true.

Answer: a
Correct: Both the statements about radiation and radioactivity are true.
Incorrect:
  (b) Both statements are true.
  (c) Both statements are true.
  (d) Both statements are true.
REF: p. 13

10. Radioactivity is:
  a. The emission and propagation of energy through space or a substance in the form of waves.
  b. The emission and propagation of energy through space or a substance in the form of particles.
  c. The process by which certain unstable atoms or elements undergo spontaneous disintegration, or decay, in an effort to attain a more balanced nuclear state.

53

d. The process by which certain unstable atoms or elements undergo spontaneous disintegration, or decay, in an effort to attain a less balanced nuclear state.

Answer: c

Correct: Radioactivity is the process by which certain unstable atoms or elements undergo spontaneous disintegration, or decay, in an effort to attain a more balanced nuclear state.

Incorrect:
(a) *Radiation* is the emission and propagation of energy through space or a substance in the form of waves or particles.
(b) *Radiation* is the emission and propagation of energy through space or a substance in the form of waves or particles.
(d) Radioactivity is the process by which certain unstable atoms or elements undergo spontaneous disintegration, or decay, in an effort to attain a *more* balanced nuclear state.

REF: p. 13

11. Which of the following statements is/are *true* of ionizing radiation?
    a. It is radiation that is capable of producing ions by removing or adding an electron to an atom.
    b. It is strictly an electromagnetic radiation and does not involve particles that have mass.
    c. It may be classified as to whether it is particulate or electromagnetic radiation.
    d. Both a and c.

Answer: d

Correct: Ionizing radiation is radiation that is capable of producing ions by removing or adding an electron to an atom, and it may be classified as to whether it is particulate or electromagnetic radiation.

Incorrect:
(a) This answer is true, but answer c is also true, making answer d the correct answer.
(b) Ionizing radiation involves both particulate and electromagnetic radiation.
(c) This answer is true, but answer a is also true, making answer d the correct answer.

REF: p. 13

12. Particulate radiations:
    a. Are tiny particles of matter.
    b. Do not possess mass.
    c. Travel in curved lines at low speeds.
    d. Do not transmit kinetic energy.

Answer: a

Correct: Particulate radiations are tiny particles of matter.

Incorrect:
(b) Particulate radiations *do* possess mass.
(c) Particulate radiations travel in *straight* lines at *high* speeds.
(d) Particulate radiations *do* transmit kinetic energy.

REF: p. 13

13. Cathode rays are derived from which of the following types of particulate radiation?
    a. Electrons
    b. Alpha particles
    c. Protons
    d. Neutrons

Answer: a

Correct: Cathode rays are derived from electrons.

Incorrect:
(b) Alpha particles are emitted from the nuclei of heavy metals.
(c) Protons are accelerated particles with a mass of 1 and a charge of +1.
(d) Neutrons are accelerated particles with a mass of 1 and no electrical charge.

REF: p. 13

14. Which of the following types of particulate radiation are emitted from the nucleus of radioactive atoms?
    a. Alpha particles
    b. Beta particles
    c. Protons
    d. Neutrons

Answer: b

Correct: Beta particles are emitted from the nucleus of radioactive atoms.

Incorrect:
(a) Alpha particles are emitted from the nuclei of heavy metals.
(c) Protons are accelerated particles, specifically hydrogen nuclei, with a mass of 1 and a charge of +1.
(d) Neutrons are accelerated particles with a mass of 1 and no electrical charge.

REF: p. 13

15. Electromagnetic radiations:
    a. Are entirely man-made.
    b. Include x-rays and visible light.
    c. Are a form of particulate radiation.
    d. Have mass.

Answer: b

Correct: Electromagnetic radiations include x-rays and visible light.

Incorrect:
(a) Electromagnetic radiations are man-made *or* occur naturally.
(c) Electromagnetic radiations are *not* a form of particulate radiation.
(d) Electromagnetic radiations do *not* have mass.

REF: p. 14

16. Which of the following forms of electromagnetic radiation are capable of ionization?
    a. Radio waves
    b. Visible light
    c. Ultraviolet light
    d. X-rays

Answer: d
Correct: Of the forms of electromagnetic radiation listed, only x-rays are capable of ionization.
Incorrect:
  (a) Radio waves are not capable of ionization.
  (b) Visible light is not capable of ionization.
  (c) Ultraviolet light is not capable of ionization.
REF: p. 14

17. Photons are:
    a. Bundles of energy with mass and weight.
    b. Bundles of energy that travel at the speed of sound.
    c. A component of the particle concept of electromagnetic radiation.
    d. A component of the wave concept of electromagnetic radiation.

Answer: c
Correct: Photons are a component of the particle concept of electromagnetic radiation.
Incorrect:
  (a) Photons are bundles of energy *without* mass or weight.
  (b) Photons are bundles of energy that travel at the speed of *light*.
  (d) Photons are a component of the *particle* concept of electromagnetic radiation.
REF: p. 14

18. Which of the following statements is *true* of the wave concept of electromagnetic radiation?
    a. *Wavelength* refers to the speed of the wave.
    b. The *velocity* refers to the number of wavelengths that pass a given point in a certain amount of time.
    c. The *frequency* is defined as the distance between the crest of one wave and the crest of the next.
    d. Frequency and wavelength are inversely related.

Answer: d
Correct: Frequency and wavelength are inversely related; if the frequency of the wave is high, the wavelength will be short, and if the frequency is low, the wavelength will be long.
Incorrect:
  (a) *Velocity* refers to the speed of the wave.
  (b) The *frequency* refers to the number of wavelengths that pass a given point in a certain amount of time.
  (c) The *wavelength* is defined as the distance between the crest of one wave and the crest of the next.
REF: pp. 14-15

19. Which of the following forms of electromagnetic radiation has the shortest wavelength?
    a. Radio wave
    b. Television wave

    c. Radar wave
    d. Dental x-ray wave

Answer: d
Correct: The dental x-ray wave has a wavelength of 0.1 nanometer, or 0.00000000001 meter.
Incorrect:
  (a) A radio wave has a wavelength as long as 100 meters.
  (b) A television wave has a wavelength of approximately 1 meter.
  (c) A radar wave has a wavelength of 1/100 of a meter.
REF: p. 15

20. Which of the following components of the x-ray machine would have an indicator light for the on-off switch and an indicator light for the exposure button?
    a. X-ray tube
    b. X-ray tubehead
    c. The control panel
    d. The extension arm

Answer: c
Correct: The control panel has an indicator light for the on-off switch and an indicator light for the exposure button.
Incorrect:
  (a) The control panel has the indicator lights, rather than the x-ray tube.
  (b) The control panel has the indicator lights, rather than the x-ray tubehead.
  (d) The control panel has the indicator lights, rather than the extension arm.
REF: p. 16

21. Which component of the x-ray tubehead absorbs heat created by the production of x-rays?
    a. Metal housing
    b. Insulating oil
    c. Aluminum disks
    d. Lead collimator

Answer: b
Correct: Insulating oil absorbs heat created by the production of x-rays.
Incorrect:
  (a) The metal housing protects the x-ray tube and grounds the high-voltage components.
  (c) Aluminum disks filter out nonpenetrating, longer wavelength x-rays.
  (d) The lead collimator restricts the size of the x-ray beam.
REF: p. 16

22. Which component of the tubehead aims and shapes the x-ray beam?
    a. Metal housing
    b. Tubehead seal
    c. Aluminum disks
    d. Position-indicating device

Answer: d
Correct: The position-indicating device aims and shapes the x-ray beam.
Incorrect:
  (a) The metal housing protects the x-ray tube and grounds the high-voltage components.
  (b) The tubehead seal seals the oil in the tubehead and acts as a filter to the x-ray beam.
  (c) Aluminum disks filter out the nonpenetrating, longer wavelength x-rays.
REF: p. 17

23. Within the x-ray tube, electrons are generated by the:
  a. Tungsten filament in the cathode
  b. Tungsten filament in the anode
  c. Molybdenum cup
  d. Copper stem

Answer: a
Correct: Within the x-ray tube, electrons are generated by the tungsten filament in the cathode.
Incorrect:
  (b) Within the x-ray tube, electrons are generated by the tungsten filament in the *cathode*.
  (c) The molybdenum cup focuses the electrons into a narrow beam and directs the beam across the tube toward the tungsten target of the anode.
  (d) The copper stem functions to dissipate heat away from the tungsten target.
REF: p. 17

24. The purpose of the anode is to:
  a. Produce electrons when heated.
  b. Convert electrons into x-ray photons.
  c. Absorb heat created by the production of x-rays.
  d. Filter out nonpenetrating, longer wavelength x-rays.

Answer: b
Correct: The purpose of the anode is to convert electrons into x-ray photons.
Incorrect:
  (a) The purpose of the *cathode* is to produce electrons when heated.
  (c) The purpose of *insulating oil* is to absorb heat created by the production of x-rays.
  (d) The purpose of *aluminum disks* is to filter out nonpenetrating, longer wavelength x-rays.
REF: p. 17

25. _____ is the measurement of the number of electrons moving through a conductor.
  a. Alternating current
  b. Direct current
  c. Amperage
  d. Voltage

Answer: c
Correct: Amperage is the measurement of the number of electrons moving through a conductor.

Incorrect:
  (a) Alternating current describes a current in which the electrons flow in two opposite directions.
  (b) Direct current describes a current in which the electrons flow in one direction through a conductor.
  (d) Voltage is the measurement of electrical force that causes electrons to move from a negative pole to a positive one.
REF: p. 18

26. Which transformer in the x-ray machine is used to increase the voltage from the incoming 110- or 220-line voltage to the 65,000 to 100,000 volts required?
  a. Step-down transformer
  b. Step-up transformer
  c. Autotransformer
  d. Both a and c

Answer: b
Correct: The step-up transformer is used to increase the voltage to the 65,000 to 100,000 required.
Incorrect:
  (a) A step-down transformer is used to decrease the voltage from the incoming 110- or 220-line voltage to the 3 to 5 volts required.
  (c) An autotransformer serves as a voltage compensator that corrects for minor fluctuations in the current.
  (d) Neither a nor c is correct.
REF: p. 18

27. Thermionic emission of electrons occurs at the:
  a. Tungsten filament in the anode
  b. Tungsten filament in the cathode
  c. Copper stem
  d. Molybdenum cup

Answer: b
Correct: Thermionic emission of electrons occurs at the tungsten filament in the cathode.
Incorrect:
  (a) Thermionic emission of electrons occurs at the tungsten filament in the *cathode*.
  (c) Thermionic emission of electrons occurs at the tungsten filament in the *cathode;* the copper stem functions as a heat sink for the tungsten target.
  (d) Thermionic emission of electrons occurs at the tungsten filament in the *cathode;* the molybdenum cup focuses the electrons into a narrow beam.
REF: p. 19

28. Approximately what percentage of the kinetic energy of the electrons is converted to x-rays at the anode?
  a. Less than 1%
  b. 25%
  c. 50%
  d. 100%

Answer: a

Correct: Less than 1% of the kinetic energy of the electrons is converted to x-rays at the anode.

Incorrect:
  (b) 25% is incorrect; less than 1% of the kinetic energy of the electrons is converted to x-rays at the anode.
  (c) 50% is incorrect; less than 1% of the kinetic energy of the electrons is converted to x-rays at the anode.
  (d) 100% is incorrect; less than 1% of the kinetic energy of the electrons is converted to x-rays at the anode.

REF: p. 19

29. The lead collimator:
   a. Carries away the heat produced during the production of x-rays.
   b. Permits a small number of x-rays to exit from the x-ray tube.
   c. Filters the longer wavelength x-rays from the beam.
   d. Restricts the size of the x-ray beam.

Answer: d

Correct: The lead collimator restricts the size of the x-ray beam.

Incorrect:
  (a) The copper stem carries away the heat produced during the production of x-rays.
  (b) The unleaded glass window portion of the tube permits a small number of x-rays to exit from the x-ray tube.
  (c) The aluminum disk filters the longer wavelength x-rays from the beam.

REF: p. 19

30. Which of the following statements is *true* of general radiation?
   a. It is also known as braking (bremsstrahlung) radiation.
   b. It is also known as characteristic radiation.
   c. It is the source of the majority of x-rays that are produced.
   d. Both a and c.

Answer: d

Correct: General radiation is also known as braking (bremsstrahlung) radiation, and it is the source of the majority of x-rays produced.

Incorrect:
  (a) This is true, but choice c is also correct.
  (b) This is not true; general radiation is *not* the same as characteristic radiation.
  (c) This is true, but choice a is also correct.

REF: p. 20

31. Which form of the x-ray beam is most detrimental to the patient and operator?
   a. Primary radiation
   b. Secondary radiation

   c. Scatter radiation
   d. Useful beam

Answer: c

Correct: Scatter radiation is the most detrimental to the patient and operator.

Incorrect:
  (a) Primary radiation is the penetrating x-ray beam produced at the target of the anode.
  (b) Secondary radiation is created when the primary beam interacts with matter.
  (d) The *useful beam* is another term for primary radiation.

REF: p. 21

32. Which is the most common possibility when an x-ray photon interacts with matter?
   a. No interaction
   b. Absorption or photoelectric effect
   c. Compton scatter
   d. Coherent scatter

Answer: c

Correct: Compton scatter accounts for 62% of interactions with matter that occur in diagnostic radiography.

Incorrect:
  (a) No interaction means the photon passed through matter without any interaction.
  (b) Absorption (photoelectric effect) accounts for 30% of the interactions with matter of the dental x-ray beam.
  (d) Coherent scatter accounts for only 8% of the interactions with matter of the dental x-ray beam.

REF: p. 22

33. Which of the following four possibilities that can occur when an x-ray photon interacts with matter is responsible for producing densities on film that make dental radiography possible?
   a. No interaction
   b. Absorption or photoelectric effect
   c. Compton scatter
   d. Coherent scatter

Answer: a

Correct: X-ray photons that pass through a patient without interaction are responsible for producing the densities on film that make dental radiography possible.

Incorrect:
  (b) Absorption or photoelectric effect is incorrect; x-ray photons that pass through a patient without interaction are responsible for producing densities on film that make dental radiography possible.
  (c) Compton scatter is incorrect; x-ray photons that pass through a patient without interaction are responsible for producing densities on film that make dental radiography possible.

(d) Coherent scatter is incorrect; x-ray photons that pass through a patient without interaction are responsible for producing densities on film that make dental radiography possible.

REF: p. 21

CHAPTER 3   RADIATION CHARACTERISTICS

MULTIPLE CHOICE

1. In dental radiography, the term _____ is used to describe the mean energy or penetrating ability of the x-ray beam.
   a. *quality*
   b. *quantity*
   c. *intensity*
   d. *wavelength*

Answer: a
Correct: The term *quality* is used to describe the mean energy or penetrating ability of the x-ray beam.
Incorrect:
   (b) *Quantity* refers to the number of x-rays produced.
   (c) *Intensity* is defined as the product of the quantity and quality per unit of area per time of exposure.
   (d) *Wavelength* determines the energy and penetrating power of radiation.
REF: p. 29

2. Which of the following statements is/are *true* of wavelength in reference to radiation?
   a. X-rays with longer wavelength have less penetrating power.
   b. X-rays with longer wavelength have more penetrating power.
   c. X-rays with longer wavelengths are more likely to be absorbed by matter.
   d. Both a and c.

Answer: d
Correct: X-rays with longer wavelength have less penetrating power and are more likely to be absorbed by matter.
Incorrect:
   (a) Choice a is true, however, choice c is also correct.
   (b) X-rays with longer wavelengths have *less* penetrating power.
   (c) Choice c is true, however, choice a is also correct.
REF: p. 29

3. _____ is a measurement of force that refers to the potential difference between two electrical charges.
   a. Exposure time
   b. Wavelength
   c. Voltage
   d. Ampere

Answer: c
Correct: Voltage is a measurement of force that refers to the potential difference between two electrical charges

Incorrect:
   (a) Exposure time refers to the interval of time during which x-rays are produced.
   (b) Wavelength can be defined as the distance between the crest of one wave and the crest of the next wave.
   (d) Ampere is the unit of measure used to describe the number of electrons, or current flowing through the cathode filament.
REF: p. 29

4. When the voltage is increased:
   a. Electrons move from the anode to the cathode with more speed.
   b. Photons move from the anode to the cathode with more speed.
   c. Electrons move from the cathode to the anode with more speed.
   d. Photons move from the cathode to the anode with more speed.

Answer: c
Correct: When the voltage is increased, electrons move from the cathode to the anode with more speed.
Incorrect:
   (a) Electrons move from the *cathode* to the *anode*.
   (b) *Electrons* move from the cathode to the anode.
   (d) *Electrons* move from the cathode to the anode.
REF: p. 29

5. Which of the following statements is *true* of the use of voltage in dental x-ray equipment?
   a. Dental x-ray equipment requires the use of 3 to 5 volts.
   b. Dental x-ray equipment requires the use of less than 65 kilovolts.
   c. Dental x-ray equipment requires the use of more than 100 kilovolts.
   d. Dental x-ray equipment requires the use of 65 to 100 kilovolts.

Answer: d
Correct: Dental x-ray equipment requires use of 65 to 100 kilovolts (kV).
Incorrect:
   (a) The filament circuit requires 3 to 5 volts, however, an exposure requires the use of 65 to 100 kV.
   (b) The use of less than 65 kV does not allow adequate penetration.
   (c) The use of more than 100 kV results in overpenetration.
REF: p. 29

6. When contrasted with the use of 65 to 75 kV for dental x-rays, the use of 85 to 100 kV produces:
   a. More penetrating dental x-rays with longer wavelength.
   b. Less penetrating dental x-rays with longer wavelength.
   c. More penetrating dental x-rays with shorter wavelength.

d. Less penetrating dental x-rays with shorter wave-length.

Answer: c

Correct: The use of 85 to 100 kV for dental x-rays produces more penetrating dental x-rays with shorter wavelength.

Incorrect:

(a) The use of 85 to 100 kV for dental x-rays produces more penetrating dental x-rays with *shorter* wavelength.

(b) The use of 85 to 100 kV for dental x-rays produces *more* penetrating dental x-rays with *shorter* wavelength.

(d) The use of 85 to 100 kV for dental x-rays produces *more* penetrating dental x-rays with shorter wavelength.

REF: p. 29

7. The kVp represents _____ of an alternating current.
   a. The mean x-ray tube voltage
   b. The mean filament voltage
   c. The maximum or peak voltage
   d. The milliamperage

Answer: c

Correct: The kVp represents the maximum or peak x-ray tube voltage of an alternating current.

Incorrect:

(a) The kVp represents the *maximum* or *peak* x-ray tube voltage, not the mean.

(b) The filament voltage is low voltage circuit used to illuminate the indicator light and exposure button.

(d) Milliamperage represents quantity, whereas kVp represents the quality or voltage peak.

REF: p. 29

8. When kilovolt peak is increased, a:
   a. Lower energy x-ray beam with increased penetrating ability results.
   b. Lower energy x-ray beam with decreased penetrating ability results.
   c. Higher energy x-ray beam with increased penetrating ability results.
   d. Higher energy x-ray beam with decreased penetrating ability results.

Answer: c

Correct: When kilovolt peak is increased, a higher energy x-ray beam with increased penetrating ability results.

Incorrect:

(a) *Higher* energy x-ray beam with increased penetrating ability results.

(b) *Higher* energy x-ray beam with *increased* penetrating ability results.

(d) Higher energy x-ray beam with *increased* penetrating ability results.

REF: p. 30

9. *Density* is the overall darkness or blackness of a film. *When* the kilovolt peak is increased while other exposure factors remain constant, the resultant film exhibits a decreased density and appears lighter.
   a. Both statements are true.
   b. Both statements are false.
   c. The first statement is true; the second statement is false.
   d. The first statement is false; the second statement is true.

Answer: c

Correct: Density is the overall darkness or blackness of a film. When the kilovolt peak is increased while other exposure factors remain constant, the resultant film exhibits an *increased* density and appears *darker*.

Incorrect:

(a) The first statement is true. However, when the kilovolt peak is increased while other exposure factors remain constant, the resultant film exhibits an *increased* density and appears *darker*.

(b) The second statement is false. However, the first statement is true.

(d) The first statement is true; the second statement is false.

REF: p. 30

10. When low kilovoltage peak settings are used (65 to 70 kVp), a film with _____ will result.
    a. high contrast
    b. low contrast
    c. many shades of gray
    d. Both a and c

Answer: a

Correct: When low kilovoltage peak settings are used (65 to 70 kVp), a film with high contrast will result.

Incorrect:

(b) When low kilovoltage peak settings are used (65 to 70 kVp), a film with *high* contrast will result.

(c) When low kilovoltage peak settings are used (65 to 70 kVp), a film with *few* shades of gray will result.

(d) Choice a is true, but choice c is not correct.

REF: p. 30

11. A film with "low" contrast (greater or equal to 90kVp):
    a. Is useful for the detection of periodontal or periapical disease.
    b. Is useful for the detection and progression of dental caries.
    c. Has many shades of gray.
    d. Both a and c.

Answer: d

Correct: A film with "low" contrast is useful for the detection of periodontal or periapical disease and has many shades of gray.

Incorrect:

(a) Choice a is true, but choice c is also correct.

(b) A film with "high" contrast is useful for the detection and progression of dental caries.

(c) Choice c is true, but choice a is also correct.

REF: p. 30

12. Exposure time is measured in:
    a. kVp
    b. Milliamperage
    c. Density
    d. Impulses

Answer: d

Correct: Exposure time is measured in impulses; one impulse occurs every 1/60 of a second because of the use of alternating current.

Incorrect:

(a) kVp is a measure of the maximum or peak voltage.

(b) Milliamperage is a measure of the number of electrons flowing through the cathode filament.

(c) Density is a measure of the darkness of the film.

REF: p. 30

13. The quantity of the x-rays produced is controlled by:
    a. Voltage
    b. Kilovoltage
    c. Kilovoltage peak
    d. Milliamperage

Answer: d

Correct: The quantity of the x-rays produced is controlled by milliamperage.

Incorrect:

(a) Voltage controls the maximum penetrating power of the electrons.

(b) Kilovoltage is the term for 1000 volts as dental exposures requires large amounts of voltage.

(c) Kilovoltage peak represents the maximum voltage available.

REF: p. 32

14. Milliamperage regulates the _____ of electrons produced at the cathode filament.
    a. quality
    b. quantity
    c. speed
    d. power

Answer: b

Correct: Milliamperage regulates the quantity of electrons produced at the cathode filament.

Incorrect:

(a) Voltage regulates the quality (speed or power) of electrons produced at the cathode filament.

(c) Voltage regulates the quality (speed or power) of electrons produced at the cathode filament.

(d) Voltage regulates the quality (speed or power) of electrons produced at the cathode filament.

REF: p. 32

15. Milliampere-seconds is a combination of milliamperes and:
    a. Density
    b. Contrast
    c. Voltage
    d. Exposure time

Answer: d

Correct: Milliampere-seconds is a combination of milliamperes and exposure time.

Incorrect:

(a) Density is the overall darkness or blackness of a film.

(b) Contrast is how sharply dark and light areas are differentiated.

(c) Voltage is a measure of force.

REF: p. 32

16. Using 10 mA with an exposure time of 3 seconds would result in 30 mAs. If the milliamperage is increased to 15, the time must be decreased to _____ seconds to maintain the same density of the exposed radiograph.
    a. 0.5
    b. 1
    c. 1.5
    d. 2

Answer: d

Correct: If the milliamperage is increased to 15, the time must be decreased to 2 seconds to maintain the same density of the exposed radiograph (15 mA $\times$ 2.0 seconds = 30 mAs).

Incorrect:

(a) If the milliamperage is increased to 15, the time must be decreased to 2 seconds to maintain the same density of the exposed radiograph.

(b) If the milliamperage is increased to 15, the time must be decreased to 2 seconds to maintain the same density of the exposed radiograph.

(c) If the milliamperage is increased to 15, the time must be decreased to 2 seconds to maintain the same density of the exposed radiograph.

REF: p. 32

17. In regard to increasing density:
  a. An increase in either kVp or mA will increase density.
  b. An increase in kVp will increase density, but an increase in mA will not increase density.
  c. An increase in mA will increase density, but an increase in kVp will not increase density.
  d. Neither an increase in kVp nor an increase in mA will increase density.

Answer: a
Correct: In regard to increasing density, an increase in either kVp or mA will increase density.
Incorrect:
  (b) An increase in either kVp or mA will increase density.
  (c) An increase in either kVp or mA will increase density.
  (d) An increase in either kVp or mA will increase density.
REF: p. 32

18. Which of the following changes will increase x-ray beam intensity?
  a. Decreasing the kilovoltage peak
  b. Decreasing the milliamperage
  c. Decreasing the exposure time
  d. Decreasing the source-to-film distance

Answer: d
Correct: Decreasing the source-to-film distance will increase x-ray beam intensity.
Incorrect:
  (a) Decreasing the kilovoltage peak will *decrease* x-ray beam intensity.
  (b) Decreasing the milliamperage will *decrease* x-ray beam intensity.
  (c) Decreasing the exposure time will *decrease* x-ray beam intensity.
REF: p. 33

19. According to the inverse square law, the intensity of radiation is _____ proportional to the _____ from the source of radiation.
  a. directly; distance
  b. directly; square of the distance
  c. inversely; distance
  d. inversely; square of the distance

Answer: d
Correct: The intensity of radiation is *inversely* proportional to the *square of the distance* from the source of radiation.
Incorrect:
  (a) The intensity of radiation is *inversely* proportional to the *square of the distance* from the source of radiation.
  (b) The intensity of radiation is *inversely* proportional to the *square of the distance* from the source of radiation.

(c) The intensity of radiation is *inversely* proportional to the *square of the distance* from the source of radiation.
REF: p. 33

20. According to the inverse square law, if the length of the PID is doubled, the resultant beam is _____ as intense.
  a. four times
  b. twice
  c. half
  d. one quarter

Answer: d
Correct: According to the inverse square law, if the length of the PID is doubled, the resultant beam is one quarter as intense.
Incorrect:
  (a) According to the inverse square law, if the length of the PID is doubled, the resultant beam is *one quarter* as intense.
  (b) According to the inverse square law, if the length of the PID is doubled, the resultant beam is *one quarter* as intense.
  (c) According to the inverse square law, if the length of the PID is doubled, the resultant beam is *one quarter* as intense.
REF: p. 34

21. Aluminum filters are used to remove _____-energy, _____ wavelength x-rays.
  a. low; longer
  b. high; longer
  c. low; shorter
  d. high; shorter

Answer: a
Correct: Aluminum filters are used to remove *low*-energy, *longer* wavelength x-rays.
Incorrect:
  (b) Aluminum filters are used to remove *low*-energy, *longer* wavelength x-rays.
  (c) Aluminum filters are used to remove *low*-energy, *longer* wavelength x-rays.
  (d) Aluminum filters are used to remove *low*-energy, *longer* wavelength x-rays.
REF: p. 34

22. Aluminum filters:
  a. Remove more penetrating x-rays from the beam.
  b. Decrease the mean penetrating ability of the x-ray beam.
  c. Remove high-energy x-rays from the beam.
  d. Reduce the intensity of the x-ray beam.

Answer: d
Correct: Aluminum filters reduce the intensity of the x-ray beam.

Incorrect:

   (a) Aluminum filters remove *less* penetrating x-rays from the beam.

   (b) Aluminum filters *increase* the mean penetrating ability of the x-ray beam.

   (c) Aluminum filters remove *low-energy* x-rays from the beam.

REF: p. 34

CHAPTER 4   RADIATION BIOLOGY

MULTIPLE CHOICE

1. (1) All ionizing radiations are harmful and produce biologic changes in living tissue. (2) The amount of radiation used in dental radiography is small, but biologic damage does occur.

   a. Both statements are true.

   b. Both statements are false.

   c. The first statement is true; the second statement is false.

   d. The first statement is false; the second statement is true.

Answer: a

Correct: All ionizing radiations are harmful and produce biologic changes in living tissue. The amount of radiation used in dental radiography is small, but biologic damage does occur.

Incorrect:

   (b) All ionizing radiations *are* harmful and produce biologic changes in living tissue. The amount of radiation used in dental radiography is small, but biologic damage *does* occur.

   (c) The amount of radiation used in dental radiography is small, but biologic damage *does* occur.

   (d) All ionizing radiations *are* harmful and produce biologic changes in living tissue.

REF: p. 39

2. What specific mechanism of radiation injury may result in the formation of hydrogen peroxide when x-ray energy is absorbed by patient tissues?

   a. An ejected high-speed electron may interact with other atoms within absorbing tissues.

   b. Free radical formation created by the ionization of water.

   c. Unequal charge distribution may result in negative electrical potential.

   d. Creation of a magnetic field may cause polarization.

Answer: b

Correct: Hydrogen peroxide may be formed as a result of free radical formation created by the ionization of water.

Incorrect:

   (a) This is an example of ionization; hydrogen peroxide may be formed as a result of free radical formation.

   (c) Hydrogen peroxide may be formed as a result of free radical formation created by the ionization of water.

   (d) Hydrogen peroxide may be formed as a result of free radical formation created by the ionization of water.

REF: p. 39

3. Which of the following mechanisms of radiation injury may occur when x-ray energy is absorbed by patient tissues?

   a. Ionization

   b. Free radical formation

   c. Negative electrical potential

   d. Both a and b

Answer: d

Correct: Ionization and free radical formation may occur when x-ray energy is absorbed by patient tissues.

Incorrect:

   (a) Choice a is correct, but choice b is also true.

   (b) Choice b is correct, but choice a is also true.

   (c) Ionization and free radical formation may occur when x-ray energy is absorbed by patient tissues.

REF: p. 39

4. Which of the following statements is *true* regarding the direct theory of radiation injury?

   a. It involves absorption of an x-ray photon by water within a cell.

   b. It involves the combination of free radicals to form toxins.

   c. It involves a direct hit and absorption of an x-ray photon within a cell.

   d. Both a and b.

Answer: c

Correct: The direct theory of radiation injury involves a direct hit and absorption of an x-ray photon within a cell.

Incorrect:

   (a) The *indirect* theory of radiation injury involves absorption of an x-ray photon by water within a cell.

   (b) The *indirect* theory of radiation injury involves the combination of free radicals to form toxins.

   (d) Neither a nor b is correct.

REF: p. 40

5. The indirect theory proposes that:

   a. Free radicals combine to form toxins.

   b. Ionizing radiation directly hits critical areas within cells.

   c. Direct injuries occur more frequently than indirect injuries.

   d. Both a and c.

Answer: a

Correct: The indirect theory proposes that free radicals combine to form toxins.

Incorrect:

    (b) The *direct* theory proposes that ionizing radiation directly hits critical areas within cells.

    (c) Indirect injuries occur more frequently than direct injuries.

    (d) Choice a is correct, but choice c is not true.

REF: p. 40

6. According to the dose-response curve, when dose and damage are plotted on a graph, a _____ relationship is seen.
    a. nonlinear, nonthreshold
    b. linear, nonthreshold
    c. nonlinear, threshold
    d. linear, threshold

Answer: b

Correct: When dose and damage are plotted on a graph, a linear, nonthreshold relationship is seen.

Incorrect:

    (a) When dose and damage are plotted on a graph a *linear*, nonthreshold relationship is seen.

    (c) When dose and damage are plotted on a graph a *linear, nonthreshold* relationship is seen.

    (d) When dose and damage are plotted on a graph a linear, *nonthreshold* relationship is seen.

REF: p. 40

7. A nonthreshold dose-response curve suggests that:
    a. Below a threshold amount of radiation, no biologic damage occurs.
    b. Below a threshold amount of radiation, a safe amount of biologic damage occurs.
    c. Above a threshold amount of radiation, some biologic damage occurs.
    d. No matter how small the amount of radiation received, some biologic damage occurs.

Answer: d

Correct: A nonthreshold dose-response curve suggests that no matter how small the amount of radiation received, some biologic damage occurs.

Incorrect:

    (a) A nonthreshold dose-response curve suggests that no matter how small the amount of radiation received, some biologic damage occurs.

    (b) A nonthreshold dose-response curve suggests that no matter how small the amount of radiation received, some biologic damage occurs.

    (c) A nonthreshold dose-response curve suggests that no matter how small the amount of radiation received, some biologic damage occurs.

REF: p. 40

8. Stochastic biologic effects from radiation:
    a. Do not occur as a direct function of dose.
    b. Occur as a direct function of dose.
    c. Have a dose threshold.
    d. Both a and c.

Answer: b

Correct: Stochastic biologic effects from radiation occur as a direct function of dose.

Incorrect:

    (a) Stochastic biologic effects from radiation *occur* as a direct function of dose.

    (c) Stochastic biologic effects from radiation *do not* have a dose threshold.

    (d) Neither a nor c is correct.

REF: p. 40

9. Examples of nonstochastic effects include:
    a. Erythema
    b. Cancer
    c. Loss of hair
    d. Both a and c

Answer: d

Correct: Examples of nonstochastic effects include erythema and loss of hair.

Incorrect:

    (a) Choice a is true, but choice c is also correct.

    (b) Cancer is an example of a stochastic effect.

    (c) Choice c is true, but choice a is also correct.

REF: p. 40

10. The _____ radiation received and the _____ the dose rate, the shorter the latent period.
    a. less; slower
    b. less; faster
    c. more; slower
    d. more; faster

Answer: d

Correct: The more radiation received and the faster the dose rate, the shorter the latent period.

Incorrect:

    (a) The *less* radiation received and the *slower* the dose rate, the longer the latent period.

    (b) *Less* radiation received at a faster dose rate would result in a latent period longer than more radiation at a faster dose rate.

    (c) More radiation received at a *slower* dose rate would result in a longer latent period than more radiation at a faster dose rate.

REF: p. 41

11. Cellular injuries following the latent period may include (1) cell death, (2) cessation of mitotic activity, and/or (3) abnormal mitotic activity.
    a. 1, 2, 3
    b. 1, 2
    c. 1, 3
    d. 1 only

Answer: a

Correct: Cellular injuries following the latent period may include cell death, cessation of mitotic activity, or abnormal mitotic activity.

Incorrect:
  (b) Cellular injuries following the latent period may include cell death, cessation of mitotic activity, or *abnormal mitotic activity.*
  (c) Cellular injuries following the latent period may include cell death, *cessation of mitotic activity,* or abnormal mitotic activity.
  (d) Cellular injuries following the latent period may include cell death, *cessation of mitotic activity,* or *abnormal mitotic activity.*
REF: p. 41

12. _____ refers to the quantity of radiation received or the total amount of radiation energy absorbed.
  a. Total dose
  b. Dose rate
  c. Amount of tissue irradiated
  d. Cell sensitivity

Answer: a
Correct: *Total dose* refers to the quantity of radiation received or the total amount of radiation energy absorbed.
Incorrect:
  (b) Dose rate is the rate at which exposure to radiation occurs and absorption takes place.
  (c) Amount of tissue irradiated refers to the areas of the body exposed.
  (d) Cell sensitivity refers to the susceptibility of the particular type of cell to radiation.
REF: p. 41

13. (1) More radiation damage takes place with high dose rates, (2) because a rapid delivery of radiation does not allow time for cellular damage to be repaired.
  a. Both statements are true.
  b. Both statements are false.
  c. The first statement is true; the second statement is false.
  d. The first statement is false; the second statement is true.

Answer: a
Correct: More radiation damage takes place with high dose rates, because a rapid delivery of radiation does not allow time for cellular damage to be repaired.
Incorrect:
  (b) *More* radiation damage takes place with high dose rates, because a rapid delivery of radiation *does not* allow time for cellular damage to be repaired.
  (c) More radiation damage takes place with high dose rates, because a rapid delivery of radiation *does not* allow time for cellular damage to be repaired.
  (d) *More* radiation damage takes place with high dose rates, because a rapid delivery of radiation does not allow time for cellular damage to be repaired.
REF: pp. 41-42

14. Which types of cells are more sensitive to radiation: (1) rapidly dividing, (2) slowly dividing, (3) young, and/or (4) old?
  a. 1 and 3
  b. 1 and 4
  c. 2 and 3
  d. 2 and 4

Answer: a
Correct: Rapidly dividing, young cells are most sensitive to radiation.
Incorrect:
  (b) Rapidly dividing, *young* cells are most sensitive to radiation.
  (c) *Rapidly* dividing, young cells are most sensitive to radiation.
  (d) *Rapidly* dividing, *young* cells are most sensitive to radiation.
REF: p. 42

15. Short-term radiation effects are associated with:
  a. Large amounts of radiation absorbed in a short time.
  b. Small amounts of radiation absorbed over a long time.
  c. Acute radiation syndrome.
  d. Both a and c.

Answer: d
Correct: Short-term radiation effects are associated with large amounts of radiation absorbed in a short time and with acute radiation syndrome.
Incorrect:
  (a) Choice a is correct, but choice c is also true.
  (b) Long-term radiation effects are associated with small amounts of radiation absorbed over a long period.
  (c) Choice c is correct, but choice a is also true.
REF: p. 42

16. Which of the following is considered a short-term effect of radiation exposure?
  a. Genetic defects
  b. Birth abnormalities
  c. Hair loss
  d. Cancer

Answer: c
Correct: Hair loss is considered a short-term effect of radiation exposure.
Incorrect:
  (a) Genetic defects are considered a long-term effect of radiation exposure.
  (b) Birth abnormalities are considered a long-term effect of radiation exposure.
  (d) Cancer is considered a long-term effect of radiation exposure.
REF: p. 42

17. Which of the following statements is *true* of somatic effects of irradiation?
    a. Changes are not transmitted to future generations.
    b. Changes are in the genetic cells of the individual.
    c. Mutations occur that affect the health of offspring.
    d. Damage cannot be repaired.

Answer: a
Correct: Somatic effects are not transmitted to future generations.
Incorrect:
    (b) Changes in genetic cells of the individual are a genetic effect.
    (c) Mutations that affect the health of offspring are a genetic effect.
    (d) Genetic damage cannot be repaired.
REF: p. 42

18. Which of the following types of cells is most radiosensitive?
    a. Nerve
    b. Bone
    c. Muscle
    d. Blood

Answer: d
Correct: Blood cells are more radiosensitive than bone, muscle, or nerve cells.
Incorrect:
    (a) A nerve cell is more *radioresistant* than a blood cell.
    (b) A bone cell is more *radioresistant* than a blood cell.
    (c) A muscle cell is more *radioresistant* than a blood cell.
REF: p. 43

19. Which of the following are considered to be radioresistant tissues?
    a. Bone marrow
    b. Salivary glands
    c. Lymphoid tissue
    d. Intestines

Answer: b
Correct: Salivary glands are considered to be radioresistant tissues.
Incorrect:
    (a) Bone marrow is considered to be *radiosensitive.*
    (c) Lymphoid tissue is considered to be *radiosensitive.*
    (d) Intestines are considered to be *radiosensitive.*
REF: p. 43

20. Critical organs exposed during dental radiographic procedures in the head and neck region include (1) skin, (2) thyroid gland, (3) lens of the eye, and/or (4) bone marrow.
    a. 1, 2, 3, 4
    b. 1, 2, 3
    c. 1, 2, 4
    d. 2, 4

Answer: a
Correct: Critical organs exposed during dental radiographic procedures in the head and neck region include: skin, thyroid gland, lens of the eye, and bone marrow.
Incorrect:
    (b) Skin, thyroid gland, and lens of the eye are true; however, bone marrow is also correct.
    (c) Skin, thyroid gland, and bone marrow are true; however, lens of the eye is also correct.
    (d) Thyroid gland and bone marrow are true; however, skin and lens of the eye are also correct.
REF: p. 43

21. The traditional unit of dose is called:
    a. The roentgen (R)
    b. The radiation absorbed dose (rad)
    c. The roentgen equivalent in man (rem)
    d. The gray (Gy)

Answer: b
Correct: The traditional unit of dose is called the rad.
Incorrect:
    (a) The roentgen is the traditional unit of exposure for x-rays; the traditional unit of dose is the rad.
    (c) The rem is the traditional unit of the dose equivalent; the traditional unit of dose is the rad.
    (d) The gray is the SI unit equivalent to the rad; the traditional unit of dose is the rad.
REF: p. 43

22. One gray is equivalent to _____ rad(s).
    a. 1
    b. 10
    c. 100
    d. 1000

Answer: c
Correct: One gray is equivalent to 100 rads.
Incorrect:
    (a) One gray is equivalent to *100* rads.
    (b) One gray is equivalent to *100* rads.
    (d) One gray is equivalent to *100* rads.
REF: p. 44

23. The SI equivalent of the rem is:
    a. The rad
    b. The gray
    c. The sievert
    d. The roentgen

Answer: c
Correct: The SI equivalent of the rem is the sievert.
Incorrect:
    (a) The SI equivalent of the rem is the *sievert;* the rad is a traditional unit of radiation measurement.
    (b) The SI equivalent of the rem is the *sievert;* the gray is the SI equivalent of the rad.
    (d) The SI equivalent of the rem is the *sievert;* the roentgen is a traditional unit of radiation measurement.
REF: p. 45

65

24. Naturally occurring background radiation includes:
    a. Cosmic radiation
    b. Consumer products
    c. Terrestrial radiation
    d. Both a and c

Answer: d
Correct: Naturally occurring background radiation includes cosmic radiation and terrestrial radiation.
Incorrect:
    (a) Choice a is correct, but choice c is also true.
    (b) Naturally occurring background radiation includes cosmic radiation and terrestrial radiation; consumer products are a form of artificial radiation.
    (c) Choice c is correct, but choice a is also true.
REF: p. 45

25. Uranium is an example of _____ radiation.
    a. terrestrial
    b. cosmic
    c. artificial
    d. Both a and c

Answer: a
Correct: Uranium is an example of terrestrial radiation.
Incorrect:
    (b) Uranium is an example of *terrestrial* radiation; cosmic radiation originates from the stars and sun.
    (c) Uranium is a form of naturally occurring *terrestrial* background radiation.
    (d) Choice a is correct, but choice c is not true.
REF: p. 45

26. _____ is/are the single largest contributor to artificial radiation exposure (0.00053 Sv/year).
    a. Consumer products
    b. Medical radiation
    c. Fallout from atomic weapons
    d. The nuclear fuel cycle

Answer: b
Correct: Medical radiation is the single largest contributor to artificial radiation exposure.
Incorrect:
    (a) Consumer products contribute 0.00009 Sv/year less than medical radiation.
    (c) Fallout from atomic weapons contributes <0.00001 Sv/year less than medical radiation.
    (d) The nuclear fuel cycle contributes <0.00001 Sv/year less than medical radiation.
REF: p. 45

27. Which of the following statements is/are true of the average dose of background radiation received by an individual in the United States?
    a. The average dose ranges from 150 to 300 millirads.
    b. Geographic areas at higher elevations are associated with increased amounts of cosmic radiation.

c. Geographic areas that contain more radioactive materials are associated with increased amounts of cosmic radiation.
    d. Both a and b.

Answer: d
Correct: The average dose received by an individual in the United States ranges from 150 to 300 millirads, and geographic areas at higher elevations are associated with increased amounts of cosmic radiation.
Incorrect:
    (a) Choice a is correct, but choice b is also true.
    (b) Choice b is correct, but choice a is also true.
    (c) Geographic areas that contain more radioactive materials are associated with increased amounts of *terrestrial* radiation.
REF: p. 45

28. The potential risk of dental radiography inducing a fatal cancer in an individual is about _____ the risk of a person developing cancer spontaneously.
    a. 1/10
    b. 1/100
    c. 1/1000
    d. 1/1,000,000

Answer: c
Correct: The potential risk of dental radiography inducing a fatal cancer in an individual is about 1/1000 the risk of a person developing cancer spontaneously.
Incorrect:
    (a) The potential risk of dental radiography inducing a fatal cancer in an individual is about 1/1000 the risk of a person developing cancer spontaneously.
    (b) The potential risk of dental radiography inducing a fatal cancer in an individual is about 1/1000 the risk of a person developing cancer spontaneously.
    (d) The potential risk of dental radiography inducing a fatal cancer in an individual is about 1/1000 the risk of a person developing cancer spontaneously.
REF: p. 45

29. A 1 in 1 million risk of a fatal outcome is associated with which of the following activities?
    a. Riding 10 miles on a bike
    b. Riding 300 miles in an auto
    c. Riding 1000 miles in an airplane.
    d. Choices a, b, and c

Answer: d
Correct: A 1 in 1 million risk of a fatal outcome is associated with riding 10 miles on a bike, 300 miles in an auto, or 1000 miles in an airplane.
Incorrect:
    (a) Choice a is correct, but choices b and c are also true.
    (b) Choice b is correct, but choices a and c are also true.
    (c) Choice c is correct, but choices a and b are also true.
REF: pp. 45-46

30. Risk estimates suggest (1) that death is more likely to occur from common activities than from dental radiographic procedures, and (2) that cancer is much more likely to be unrelated to radiation exposure.
   a. Both statements are true.
   b. Both statements are false.
   c. The first statement is true; the second statement is false.
   d. The first statement is false; the second statement is true.

Answer: a
Correct: Risk estimates suggest that death is more likely to occur from common activities than from dental radiographic procedures, and that cancer is much more likely to be unrelated to radiation exposure.
Incorrect:
   (b) Risk estimates suggest that death is more likely to occur from common activities than from dental radiographic procedures, and that cancer is much more likely to be unrelated to radiation exposure.
   (c) Risk estimates suggest that death is more likely to occur from common activities than from dental radiographic procedures, and that cancer is much more likely to be unrelated to radiation exposure.
   (d) Risk estimates suggest that death is more likely to occur from common activities than from dental radiographic procedures, and that cancer is much more likely to be unrelated to radiation exposure.
REF: p. 46

31. The use of F-speed film instead of D-speed film reduces the absorbed dose by _____%.
   a. 10
   b. 25
   c. 50
   d. 60

Answer: d
Correct: The use of F-speed film instead of D-speed film reduces the absorbed dose by 60%.
Incorrect:
   (a) The use of F-speed film instead of D-speed film reduces the absorbed dose by *60%*.
   (b) The use of F-speed film instead of D-speed film reduces the absorbed dose by *60%*.
   (c) The use of F-speed film instead of D-speed film reduces the absorbed dose by *60%*.
REF: p. 46

32. Which of the following modifications in technique will reduce patient exposure to radiation during dental radiographic procedures?
   a. Use of D-speed rather than F-speed film
   b. Round rather than rectangular collimation
   c. A longer source-to-film distance
   d. A lower kilovoltage peak

Answer: c
Correct: A longer source-to-film distance will reduce patient exposure to radiation during dental radiographic procedures.
Incorrect:
   (a) Use of D-speed rather than F-speed film will *increase* patient exposure to radiation during dental radiographic procedures.
   (b) Round rather than rectangular collimation will *increase* patient exposure to radiation during dental radiographic procedures.
   (d) A lower kilovoltage peak will *increase* patient exposure to radiation during dental radiographic procedures.
REF: p. 46

33. Which of the following combinations will result in the lowest absorbed dose for the patient from a 20-film series of dental radiographs?
   a. Round collimation with F-speed film
   b. Rectangular collimation with F-speed film
   c. Round collimation with D-speed film
   d. Rectangular collimation with D-speed film

Answer: b
Correct: The lowest absorbed dose for the patient from a 20-film series of dental radiographs will result from the use of rectangular collimation with F-speed film.
Incorrect:
   (a) The lowest absorbed dose for the patient from a 20-film series of dental radiographs will result from the use of *rectangular* collimation with F-speed film.
   (c) The lowest absorbed dose for the patient from a 20-film series of dental radiographs will result from the use of *rectangular* collimation with *F-speed* film.
   (d) The lowest absorbed dose for the patient from a 20-film series of dental radiographs will result from the use of rectangular collimation with *F-speed* film.
REF: p. 46

CHAPTER 5   RADIATION PROTECTION

MULTIPLE CHOICE

1. _____ is an example of a patient protection technique used before x-ray exposure.
   a. Proper film processing
   b. Proper prescribing of radiographs
   c. A lead apron
   d. A thyroid collar

Answer: b
Correct: Proper prescribing of radiographs is an example of a patient protection technique used before x-ray exposure.

Incorrect:
- (a) Proper film processing is an example of a patient protection technique used *after* x-ray exposure.
- (c) A lead apron is an example of a patient protection technique used *during* x-ray exposure.
- (d) A thyroid collar is an example of a patient protection technique used *during* x-ray exposure.

REF: p. 52

2. The "Guidelines for Prescribing Dental Radiographs" state that:
   - a. Dentulous adults should have posterior bite-wing examinations at 12- to 36-month intervals.
   - b. The recommendations do not need to be altered because of pregnancy.
   - c. Edentulous adults should have posterior bite-wing examinations at 12- to 36-month intervals.
   - d. Both a and b.

Answer: d

Correct: The "Guidelines for Prescribing Dental Radiographs" state that dentulous adults should have posterior bite-wing examinations at 12- to 36-month intervals, and that the recommendations do not need to be altered because of pregnancy.

Incorrect:
- (a) Choice a is true, but choice b is also correct.
- (b) Choice b is true, but choice a is also correct.
- (c) Posterior bite-wing examinations are not applicable for edentulous adults.

REF: p. 54

3. Inherent filtration in the dental x-ray tubehead:
   - a. Includes filtration that takes place when the primary beam passes through the glass window of the x-ray tube, the insulating oil, and the tubehead seal.
   - b. Includes the placement of aluminum disks in the path of the x-ray beam between the collimator and the tubehead seal.
   - c. Alone meets the standards regulated by state and federal law.
   - d. Is equivalent to approximately 5.0 mm of aluminum.

Answer: a

Correct: Inherent filtration in the dental x-ray tubehead includes filtration that takes place when the primary beam passes through the glass window of the x-ray tube, the insulating oil, and the tubehead seal.

Incorrect:
- (b) *Added filtration* includes the placement of aluminum disks in the path of the x-ray beam between the collimator and the tubehead seal.
- (c) Inherent filtration alone *does not meet* the standards regulated by state and federal law.

- (d) Inherent filtration is equivalent to approximately *0.5 to 1.0 mm* of aluminum.

REF: p. 52

4. Added filtration in the dental x-ray tubehead:
   - a. Refers to the placement of tungsten disks in the path of the x-ray beam between the collimator and the tubehead seal.
   - b. Filters out shorter wavelength x-rays from the x-ray beam.
   - c. Results in a lower energy beam.
   - d. Results in a more penetrating useful beam.

Answer: d

Correct: Added filtration in the dental x-ray tubehead results in a more penetrating useful beam.

Incorrect:
- (a) Refers to the placement of *aluminum* disks in the path of the x-ray beam between the collimator and the tubehead seal.
- (b) Filters out *longer* wavelength x-rays from the x-ray beam.
- (c) Results in a *higher* energy beam.

REF: p. 52

5. State and federal laws require that dental x-ray machines operating above 70 kVp have a minimum total (inherent plus added filtration) of _____ mm of aluminum filtration.
   - a. 1.5
   - b. 2.0
   - c. 2.5
   - d. 5.0

Answer: c

Correct: State and federal laws require that dental x-ray machines operating above 70 kVp have a minimum total (inherent plus added filtration) of 2.5 mm of aluminum filtration.

Incorrect:
- (a) State and federal laws require that dental x-ray machines operating above 70 kVp have a minimum total (inherent plus added filtration) of *2.5* mm of aluminum filtration.
- (b) State and federal laws require that dental x-ray machines operating above 70 kVp have a minimum total (inherent plus added filtration) of *2.5* mm of aluminum filtration.
- (d) State and federal laws require that dental x-ray machines operating above 70 kVp have a minimum total (inherent plus added filtration) of *2.5* mm of aluminum filtration.

REF: pp. 52-53

6. The collimator:
   - a. Is always round
   - b. Restricts the size and shape of the x-ray beam
   - c. Is a solid piece of aluminum
   - d. Is fitted within the copper stem beneath the molybdenum cup

Answer: b
Correct: The collimator restricts the size and shape of the x-ray beam.
Incorrect:
    (a) The collimator may have either a round or a rectangular opening.
    (c) The collimator is a lead plate; the filter is aluminum.
    (d) The collimator is fitted directly over the opening of the machine housing where the x-ray beam exits the tubehead.
REF: p. 53

7. A circular collimator produces a cone-shaped beam that is _____ inch(es) in diameter.
    a. less than 1
    b. 1.25
    c. 2.75
    d. 5.0

Answer: c
Correct: A circular collimator produces a cone-shaped beam that is 2.75 inches in diameter.
Incorrect:
    (a) A circular collimator produces a cone-shaped beam that is *2.75* inches in diameter.
    (b) A circular collimator produces a cone-shaped beam that is *2.75* inches in diameter.
    (d) A circular collimator produces a cone-shaped beam that is *2.75* inches in diameter.
REF: p. 53

8. A rectangular collimator:
    a. Restricts the beam more than a circular collimator.
    b. Restricts the beam less than a circular collimator.
    c. Significantly reduces patient exposure.
    d. Both a and c

Answer: d
Correct: A rectangular collimator restricts the beam more than a circular collimator and significantly reduces patient exposure.
Incorrect:
    (a) Choice a is true, but choice c is also correct.
    (b) A rectangular collimator restricts the beam *more* than a circular collimator.
    (c) Choice c is true, but choice a is also correct.
REF: p. 53

9. Which of the following types of position-indicating devices (PIDs) do *not* produce scatter radiation?
    a. Rectangular
    b. Conical
    c. Round
    d. Both a and c

Answer: d
Correct: Rectangular and round PIDs do not produce scatter radiation.
Incorrect:
    (a) Choice a is true, but choice c is also correct.

    (b) Conical PIDs *do* produce scatter radiation.
    (c) Choice c is true, but choice a is also correct.
REF: p. 53

10. Which type of PID would be most effective in reducing patient exposure?
    a. Conical
    b. 16-inch round PID
    c. 8-inch rectangular PID
    d. 16-inch rectangular PID

Answer: d
Correct: A 16-inch rectangular PID would be most effective in reducing patient exposure.
Incorrect:
    (a) A conical PID would be *least* effective in reducing patient exposure.
    (b) A 16-inch round PID would not be as effective in reducing patient exposure as a 16-inch rectangular PID.
    (c) An 8-inch rectangular PID would not be as effective as a 16-inch rectangular PID in reducing patient exposure.
REF: p. 53

11. The thyroid collar:
    a. Is recommended for all intraoral films
    b. Is recommended for all extraoral films
    c. May exist as a separate shield or as part of the lead apron
    d. Both a and c

Answer: d
Correct: The thyroid collar is recommended for all intraoral films and may exist as a separate shield or as part of the lead apron.
Incorrect:
    (a) Choice a is true, but choice c is also correct.
    (b) The thyroid collar is *not* recommended for extraoral films.
    (c) Choice c is true, but choice a is also correct.
REF: p. 53

12. The lead apron:
    a. Is recommended for intraoral films
    b. Is not recommended for extraoral films
    c. Is an option; use is not mandated by any state or federal law
    d. Is used to protect the thyroid gland

Answer: a
Correct: The lead apron is recommended for intraoral films (and extraoral films as well).
Incorrect:
    (b) The lead apron *is* recommended for extraoral films.
    (c) The lead apron is *not* an option; many state laws mandate the use of a lead apron on all patients.
    (d) The thyroid collar is used to protect the thyroid gland.
REF: p. 56

13. _____ -speed film is currently the fastest intraoral film available.
   a. D
   b. E
   c. F
   d. G

Answer: c

Correct: F-speed film is currently the fastest intraoral film available.

Incorrect:
   (a) D-speed film (ultra-speed) is the oldest and slowest intraoral film available.
   (b) E-speed film (ektaspeed) is faster than D-speed film but slower than F-speed film.
   (d) G-speed film does not exist at this time.

REF: p. 58

14. On some dental x-ray machines, only the _____ can be altered; the other parameters are preset by the manufacturer.
   a. kilovoltage peak
   b. exposure time
   c. PID length
   d. milliamperage

Answer: b

Correct: On some dental x-ray machines, only the exposure time can be altered; the other parameters are preset by the manufacturer.

Incorrect:
   (a) On some dental x-ray machines, only the _exposure time_ can be altered; the kilovoltage peak is preset by the manufacturer.
   (c) On some dental x-ray machines, only the _exposure time_ can be altered; the PID length is preset by the manufacturer.
   (d) On some dental x-ray machines, only the _exposure time_ can be altered; the milliamperage is preset by the manufacturer.

REF: p. 58

15. Which of the following occurrences during and after x-ray film exposure reduce(s) the amount of x-radiation a patient receives?
   a. Artifacts caused by improper film handling
   b. Retakes
   c. Proper film processing
   d. Nondiagnostic films

Answer: c

Correct: Proper film processing reduces the amount of x-radiation a patient receives.

Incorrect:
   (a) Artifacts caused by improper film handling _increase_ the amount of x-radiation a patient receives.

   (b) Retakes _increase_ the amount of x-radiation a patient receives.
   (d) Nondiagnostic films _increase_ the amount of x-radiation a patient receives.

REF: p. 58

16. The primary dictum of operator protection guidelines is that the operator must:
   a. Remain in the room with the patient while the film is being exposed.
   b. Avoid the primary beam.
   c. Hold the film in the patient's mouth with their own finger.
   d. Hold the tubehead during x-ray exposure.

Answer: b

Correct: The primary dictum of operator protection guidelines is that the operator must avoid the primary beam.

Incorrect:
   (a) The operator must stand at least 6 feet away from the x-ray tubehead during x-ray exposure.
   (c) The operator _must never_ hold a film in place for a patient during x-ray exposure.
   (d) The dental radiographer _must never_ hold the tubehead during x-ray exposure.

REF: p. 59

17. To avoid the primary beam, the dental radiographer must be positioned at a _____ -degree to _____ -degree angle to the beam.
   a. 0; 45
   b. 45; 90
   c. 90; 135
   d. 135; 180

Answer: c

Correct: To avoid the primary beam, the dental radiographer must be positioned at a 90-degree to 135-degree angle to the beam.

Incorrect:
   (a) To avoid the primary beam, the dental radiographer must be positioned at a _90_-degree to _135_-degree angle to the beam.
   (b) To avoid the primary beam, the dental radiographer must be positioned at a _90_-degree to _135_-degree angle to the beam.
   (d) To avoid the primary beam, the dental radiographer must be positioned at a _90_-degree to _135_-degree angle to the beam.

REF: p. 59

18. Radiation monitoring can be used to protect the dental radiographer and includes monitoring of:
   a. Equipment
   b. Personnel
   c. Both equipment and personnel
   d. Drywall for residual radiation

Answer: c

Correct: Radiation monitoring can be used to protect the dental radiographer and includes monitoring of both equipment and personnel.

Incorrect:
- (a) Choice a is true, but choice b is also correct.
- (b) Choice b is true, but choice c is also correct.
- (d) Radiation monitoring can be used to protect the dental radiographer and includes monitoring of both equipment and personnel; however, drywall is not monitored for residual radiation because it does not exist.

REF: p. 60

19. A film badge:
    a. Is worn at waist level by the patient
    b. Is worn at waist level by the operator
    c. Is clipped to the shirt pocket of the operator
    d. Is clipped to the shirt pocket of the patient

Answer: b

Correct: A film badge is worn at waist level by the operator, close to the critical reproductive organs.

Incorrect:
- (a) A film badge is worn at waist level by the *operator,* not by the patient.
- (c) A film badge is worn at *waist level* by the operator, not on a shirt pocket.
- (d) A film badge is worn at *waist level* by the *operator,* not by the patient on a shirt pocket.

REF: p. 60

20. Radiation legislation varies greatly from state to state. For example, in some states a dental radiographer must successfully complete a radiation safety examination before he or she may expose dental x-rays.
    a. Both statements are true.
    b. Both statements are false.
    c. The first statement is true; the second statement is false.
    d. The first statement is false; the second statement is true.

Answer: a

Correct: Radiation legislation varies greatly from state to state. For example, in some states a dental radiographer must successfully complete a radiation safety examination before he or she may expose dental x-rays.

Incorrect:
- (b) Radiation legislation varies greatly from state to state. For example, in some states a dental radiographer must successfully complete a radiation safety examination before he or she may expose dental x-rays.
- (c) Radiation legislation varies greatly from state to state. For example, in some states a dental radiographer must successfully complete a radiation

safety examination before he or she may expose dental x-rays.
- (d) Radiation legislation varies greatly from state to state. For example, in some states a dental radiographer must successfully complete a radiation safety examination before he or she may expose dental x-rays.

REF: p. 61

21. According to the current recommendations (2003) of the National Council on Radiation Protection and Measurements, the current MPD for occupationally exposed persons is _____/year.
    a. 500 millirem
    b. 5.0 rem
    c. 50 rem
    d. 5000 rem

Answer: b

Correct: According to the current recommendations (2003) of the National Council on Radiation Protection and Measurements, the current MPD for occupationally exposed persons is 5.0 rem/year.

Incorrect:
- (a) The current MPD for occupationally exposed persons is *5.0 rem*/year.
- (c) The current MPD for occupationally exposed persons is *5.0 rem*/year.
- (d) The current MPD for occupationally exposed persons is *5.0 rem*/year.

REF: p. 61

22. According to the current recommendations (2003) of the National Council on Radiation Protection and Measurements, the current MPD for an occupationally exposed pregnant women is the same as that for:
    a. An occupationally exposed nonpregnant women
    b. An occupationally exposed male
    c. An occupationally exposed child under 18
    d. A nonoccupationally exposed person

Answer: d

Correct: The current MPD for an occupationally exposed pregnant women is the same as that for a nonoccupationally exposed person.

Incorrect:
- (a) The current MPD for an occupationally exposed pregnant women is the same as that for *a nonoccupationally exposed person.*
- (b) The current MPD for an occupationally exposed pregnant women is the same as that for *a nonoccupationally exposed person.*
- (c) The current MPD for an occupationally exposed pregnant women is the same as that for *a nonoccupationally exposed person.*

REF: p. 61

71

23. The acronym for the permitted lifetime accumulated dose is:
  a. MPD—maximum permissible dose
  b. MPD—maximum possible dose
  c. MAD—maximum accumulated dose
  d. MAD— maximum allowed dose

Answer: c
Correct: The acronym for the permitted lifetime accumulated dose is MAD—maximum accumulated dose.
Incorrect:
  (a) The acronym for the permitted lifetime accumulated dose is MAD—maximum accumulated dose.
  (b) The acronym for the permitted lifetime accumulated dose is MAD—maximum accumulated dose.
  (d) The acronym for the permitted lifetime accumulated dose is MAD—maximum accumulated dose.
REF: p. 61

24. The ALARA concept states that all radiation must be kept:
  a. As long as readily achievable
  b. As low as reasonably allowable
  c. As low as reasonably achievable
  d. As long as reliably achievable

Answer: c
Correct: The ALARA concept states that all radiation must be kept as low as reasonably achievable.
Incorrect:
  (a) The ALARA concept states that all radiation must be kept *as low as reasonably achievable*.
  (b) The ALARA concept states that all radiation must be kept *as low as reasonably achievable*.
  (d) The ALARA concept states that all radiation must be kept *as low as reasonably achievable*.
REF: p. 61

CHAPTER 6   DENTAL X-RAY EQUIPMENT

MULTIPLE CHOICE
  1. _____ regulate(s) the manufacture and installation of dental x-ray equipment.
  a. The federal government
  b. State governments
  c. Local governments
  d. Municipal governments

Answer: a
Correct: The federal government regulates the manufacture and installation of dental x-ray equipment.
Incorrect:
  (b) State governments may regulate how dental x-ray equipment is used, but it is the *federal* government that regulates the manufacture and installation of dental x-ray equipment.
  (c) Only the *federal* government regulates the manufacture and installation of dental x-ray equipment.
  (d) Only the *federal* government regulates the manufacture and installation of dental x-ray equipment.
REF: p. 67

2. The position-indicating device (PID) is an extension of the:
  a. Tubehead
  b. Extension arm
  c. Control panel
  d. Exposure button

Answer: a
Correct: The PID is an extension of the tubehead.
Incorrect:
  (b) The *extension arm* supports the x-ray tubehead.
  (c) The *control panel* allows the dental radiographer to regulate the x-ray beam.
  (d) The *exposure button* activates the machine to produce x-rays.
REF: p. 67

3. The _____ allow(s) for positioning of the tubehead.
  a. control devices
  b. extension arm
  c. control panel
  d. exposure button

Answer: b
Correct: The extension arm allows for positioning of the tubehead.
Incorrect:
  (a) The *control devices* regulate the x-ray beam.
  (c) The *control panel* allows the dental radiographer to regulate the x-ray beam.
  (d) The *exposure button* activates the machine to produce x-rays.
REF: p. 67

4. The _____ activate(s) the machine to produce x-rays.
  a. on-off switch
  b. exposure button
  c. exposure light
  d. control devices

Answer: b
Correct: The exposure button activates the machine to produce x-rays.
Incorrect:
  (a) The *on-off switch* turns the machine off and on.
  (c) The *exposure light* is illuminated during x-ray exposure.
  (d) The *control devices* include the timer and kVp and milliamperage selectors.
REF: p. 67

5. During an exposure:
  a. The exposure button is briefly depressed and then released to initiate the exposure.
  b. The exposure button is firmly depressed until the preset exposure time is completed.
  c. The exposure light on control panel is illuminated to signal the completion of the exposure.

d. A beep sounds to signal the initiation of the exposure.

Answer: b

Correct: The exposure button is firmly depressed until the preset exposure time is completed.

Incorrect:

(a) The exposure button is firmly depressed until the preset exposure time is completed.

(c) The exposure light on the control panel is lit for the duration of the exposure.

(d) The beep sounds to signal completion of the exposure.

REF: p. 67

6. Which of the following statements is *true* of the film holder?

a. It is used to align an extraoral dental x-ray film.

b. It requires the patient to stabilize the film in the mouth.

c. It is required when using the intraoral paralleling technique.

d. It is required when using the intraoral bisecting technique.

Answer: c

Correct: The film holder is required when using the intraoral paralleling technique.

Incorrect:

(a) It is used to align an *intraoral* dental x-ray film.

(b) It *does not* require the patient to stabilize the film in the mouth.

(d) It is required when using the intraoral *paralleling* technique.

REF: p. 69

7. A _____ eliminates the need for the patient to stabilize the film.

a. PID (position-indicating device)

b. film holder

c. control panel

d. beam alignment device

Answer: b

Correct: A film holder eliminates the need for the patient to stabilize the film.

Incorrect:

(a) A *film holder* eliminates the need for the patient to stabilize the film.

(c) A *film holder* eliminates the need for the patient to stabilize the film.

(d) A *film holder* eliminates the need for the patient to stabilize the film.

REF: p. 69

8. Which of the following intraoral film holders is a disposable Styrofoam bite-block?

a. EEZEE-Grip

b. Stabe bite-block

c. EndoRay

d. Uni-bite

Answer: b

Correct: The Stabe bite-block is a disposable Styrofoam bite-block.

Incorrect:

(a) The *EEZEE-Grip* is a double-ended instrument that holds the film between two serrated plastic grips.

(c) The *EndoRay* is used during root canal procedures.

(d) The *uni-bite* is a plastic holder.

REF: p. 69

9. Features of the Stabe bite-block include:

a. Disposable

b. Slot for film retention

c. Molded plastic that can be sterilized

d. Both a and b

Answer: d

Correct: Features of the Stabe bite-block include that it is disposable and it has a slot for film retention.

Incorrect:

(a) Choice a is true, but choice b is also correct.

(b) Choice b is true, but choice a is also correct.

(c) The Stabe bite-block is a disposable Styrofoam bite-block.

REF: p. 69

10. Which of the following are beam alignment devices?

a. Stabe bite-block

b. XCP bite-block

c. EEZEE-Grip

d. Precision film holders

Answer: d

Correct: Precision film holders are beam alignment devices.

Incorrect:

(a) A *Stabe bite-block* is a Styrofoam film holder.

(b) An *XCP bite-block* is a Styrofoam film holder.

(c) An *EEZEE-Grip* is a plastic film holder.

REF: pp. 69-71

11. A beam alignment device can be used to help the dental radiographer position the PID in relation to the _____ and film.

a. control panel

b. extension arm

c. collimator

d. tooth

Answer: d

Correct: A beam alignment device can be used to help the dental radiographer position the PID in relation to the tooth and film.

Incorrect:
(a) A beam alignment device can be used to help the dental radiographer position the PID in relation to the *tooth* and film.
(b) A beam alignment device can be used to help the dental radiographer position the PID in relation to the *tooth* and film.
(c) A beam alignment device can be used to help the dental radiographer position the PID in relation to the *tooth* and film.

REF: p. 69

12. The Rinn XCP system includes a:
    a. Beam alignment device
    b. Styrofoam bite-block
    c. Snap-on metal collimating device
    d. Both a and c

Answer: d

Correct: The Rinn XCP system includes a beam alignment device and a snap-on metal collimating device.

Incorrect:
(a) Choice a is true, but choice c is also correct.
(b) The Rinn XCP system does not include a Styrofoam bite-block.
(c) Choice c is true, but a is also correct.

REF: p. 71

CHAPTER 7   DENTAL X-RAY FILM

MULTIPLE CHOICE

1. Which of the following statements is *true* regarding dental x-ray film and formation of the latent image?
    a. The film is placed to the buccal of the teeth.
    b. The film is placed to the lingual of the teeth on the inside of the mouth.
    c. A periapical film is an extraoral film.
    d. A bite-wing film is an extraoral film.

Answer: b

Correct: The film is placed to the lingual of the teeth on the inside of the mouth.

Incorrect:
(a) The film is placed to the *lingual* of the teeth.
(c) A periapical film is an *intraoral* film.
(d) A bite-wing film is an *intraoral* film.

REF: p. 75

2. Which component of x-ray film provides a stable support for the emulsion?
    a. Film base
    b. Adhesive layer
    c. Gelatin
    d. Halide crystals

Answer: a

Correct: The film base provides a stable support for the emulsion.

Incorrect:
(b) The adhesive layer serves to attach the emulsion to the base.
(c) The gelatin is used to suspend and evenly disperse millions of microscopic silver halide crystals.
(d) The halide crystals absorb radiation during x-ray exposure.

REF: p. 75

3. The film base is a flexible piece of:
    a. Shellac
    b. Cardboard
    c. Acetate
    d. Polyester plastic

Answer: d

Correct: The film base is a flexible piece of polyester plastic.

Incorrect:
(a) The film base is a flexible piece of *polyester plastic*.
(b) The film base is a flexible piece of *polyester plastic*.
(c) The film base is a flexible piece of *polyester plastic*.

REF: p. 75

4. The film base is transparent with a slight _____ tint used to emphasize contrast and enhance image quality.
    a. amber
    b. red
    c. blue
    d. green

Answer: c

Correct: The film base is transparent with a slight blue tint used to emphasize contrast and enhance image quality.

Incorrect:
(a) The film base is transparent with a slight *blue* tint used to emphasize contrast and enhance image quality.
(b) The film base is transparent with a slight *blue* tint used to emphasize contrast and enhance image quality.
(d) The film base is transparent with a slight *blue* tint used to emphasize contrast and enhance image quality.

REF: p. 75

5. The film base is _____ mm thick.
    a. 0.02
    b. 0.2
    c. 2.0
    d. 20

Answer: b

Correct: The film base is 0.2 mm thick.

Incorrect:
  (a) The film base is *0.2* mm thick.
  (c) The film base is *0.2* mm thick.
  (d) The film base is *0.2* mm thick.
REF: p. 75

6. The adhesive layer is added to the _____ before the _____ is applied.
  a. gelatin; halide crystals
  b. halide crystals; gelatin
  c. film base; emulsion
  d. emulsion; film base

Answer: c
Correct: The adhesive layer is added to the film base before the emulsion is applied.
Incorrect:
  (a) The adhesive layer is added to the *film base* before the *emulsion* is applied.
  (b) The adhesive layer is added to the *film base* before the *emulsion* is applied.
  (d) The adhesive layer is added to the *film base* before the *emulsion* is applied.
REF: p. 75

7. The film emulsion is:
  a. Attached to both sides of the film
  b. Attached to one side of the film
  c. Made of polyester plastic
  d. Opaque to block out the passage of light

Answer: a
Correct: The film emulsion is attached to both sides of the film.
Incorrect:
  (b) The film emulsion is *attached to both sides of the film.*
  (c) The film emulsion is *attached to both sides of the film.*
  (d) The film emulsion is *attached to both sides of the film.*
REF: p. 75

8. The film emulsion is composed of a homogenous mixture of:
  a. Calcium tungstate and lead salt crystal
  b. Gelatin and barium salt crystals
  c. Gelatin and silver halide crystals
  d. Primer and silver halide crystals

Answer: c
Correct: The film emulsion is composed of a homogenous mixture of gelatin and silver halide crystals.
Incorrect:
  (a) The film emulsion is composed of a homogenous mixture of *gelatin and silver halide crystals.*
  (b) The film emulsion is composed of a homogenous mixture of gelatin and *silver halide crystals.*

  (d) The film emulsion is composed of a homogenous mixture of *gelatin* and silver halide crystals.
REF: p. 75

9. The halide in dental x-ray film is primarily silver:
  a. Iodide
  b. Bromide
  c. Chloride
  d. Fluoride

Answer: b
Correct: The halide in dental x-ray film is primarily silver bromide.
Incorrect:
  (a) The halide in dental x-ray film is primarily silver *bromide*.
  (c) The halide in dental x-ray film is primarily silver *bromide*.
  (d) The halide in dental x-ray film is primarily silver *bromide*.
REF: p. 76

10. The latent image is stored by the _____ in dental x-ray film.
  a. gelatin
  b. film base
  c. adhesive layer
  d. silver halide crystals

Answer: d
Correct: The latent image is stored by the silver halide crystals in dental x-ray film.
Incorrect:
  (a) The latent image is stored by the *silver halide crystals* in dental x-ray film.
  (b) The latent image is stored by the *silver halide crystals* in dental x-ray film.
  (c) The latent image is stored by the *silver halide crystals* in dental x-ray film.
REF: p. 76

11. The areas of the film that are _____ energized will be _____ when the film is processed.
(1) more; darker
(2) more; lighter
(3) less; darker
(4) less; lighter
  a. 1 and 3
  b. 1 and 4
  c. 2 and 3
  d. 2 and 4

Answer: b
Correct: The areas of the film that are more energized will be darker when the film is processed. The areas of the film that are less energized will be lighter when the film is processed.

(a) The areas of the film that are *more* energized will be *darker* when the film is processed. The areas of the film that are *less* energized will be *lighter* when the film is processed.

(c) The areas of the film that are *more* energized will be *darker* when the film is processed. The areas of the film that are *less* energized will be *lighter* when the film is processed.

(d) The areas of the film that are *more* energized will be *darker* when the film is processed. The areas of the film that are *less* energized will be *lighter* when the film is processed.

REF: p. 76

12. The invisible pattern of stored energy on the exposed film is called the:
    a. Variable density pattern
    b. Latent image
    c. X-ray photon
    d. Emulsion

Answer: b
Correct: The invisible pattern of stored energy on the exposed film is called the latent image.
Incorrect:

(a) The invisible pattern of stored energy on the exposed film is called the *latent image*.

(c) The invisible pattern of stored energy on the exposed film is called the *latent image*.

(d) The invisible pattern of stored energy on the exposed film is called the *latent image*.

REF: p. 76

13. Latent image centers are aggregates of:
    a. Silver bromide crystals
    b. Bromine atoms
    c. Neutral silver atoms
    d. Gelatin

Answer: c
Correct: Latent image centers are aggregates of neutral silver atoms.
Incorrect:

(a) Latent image centers are aggregates of *neutral silver atoms*.

(b) Latent image centers are aggregates of *neutral silver atoms*.

(d) Latent image centers are aggregates of *neutral silver atoms*.

REF: p. 76

14. During formation of the latent image, irregularities in the lattice structure of the exposed crystal, known as _____, attract silver atoms.
    a. the protective layer
    b. the emulsion
    c. sensitivity specks
    d. the adhesive layer

Answer: c
Correct: During formation of the latent image, irregularities in the lattice structure of the exposed crystal, known as *sensitivity specks*, attract silver atoms.
Incorrect:

(a) During formation of the latent image, irregularities in the lattice structure of the exposed crystal, known as *sensitivity specks*, attract silver atoms.

(b) During formation of the latent image, irregularities in the lattice structure of the exposed crystal, known as *sensitivity specks*, attract silver atoms.

(d) During formation of the latent image, irregularities in the lattice structure of the exposed crystal, known as *sensitivity specks*, attract silver atoms.

REF: p. 76

15. Which of the following types of dental x-ray film is placed inside the mouth?
    a. Intraoral film
    b. Extraoral film
    c. Duplicating film
    d. Screen film

Answer: a
Correct: Intraoral film is placed inside the mouth.
Incorrect:

(b) Extraoral film is placed outside the mouth.

(c) Duplicating film is used to copy radiographs, it is not used inside the mouth.

(d) Screen film is used for panoramic films, which are extraoral.

REF: p. 77

16. Which of the following statements is *true* of a two-film packet?
    a. It requires twice the amount of exposure to produce a single radiograph.
    b. Two-film packet film has a single emulsion, whereas one-film packet film has a double emulsion.
    c. Two-film packet film has a double emulsion, whereas a one-film packet film has a single emulsion.
    d. Intraoral x-ray film is a double-emulsion type of film regardless of whether the film packet contains one or two films.

Answer: d
Correct: Intraoral x-ray film is a double-emulsion type of film regardless of whether the film packet contains one or two films.
Incorrect:

(a) A two-film packet requires the same amount of exposure to produce the films as a one-film packet.

(b) Intraoral x-ray film is a double-emulsion type of film regardless of whether the film packet contains one or two films.

(c) Intraoral x-ray film is a double-emulsion type of film regardless of whether the film packet contains one or two films.

REF: p. 78

17. A two-film packet requires _____ exposure time as a one-film packet.
   a. half the
   b. the same
   c. twice the
   d. four times the

Answer: b
Correct: A two-film packet requires the same exposure time as a one-film packet.
Incorrect:
   (a) A two-film packet requires *the same* exposure time as a one-film packet.
   (c) A two-film packet requires *the same* exposure time as a one-film packet.
   (d) A two-film packet requires *the same* exposure time as a one-film packet.
REF: p. 78

18. The two-film packet may be used:
   a. For maxillary radiographs where the bone is denser than in the mandible.
   b. To prevent more photons from passing through the film into patient tissue.
   c. When a duplicate record of a radiographic examination is needed.
   d. Routinely for adults; however, a one-film packet should be used for children and adolescents.

Answer: c
Correct: The two-film packet may be used when a duplicate record of a radiographic examination is needed.
Incorrect:
   (a) The two-film packet may be used *when a duplicate record of a radiographic examination is needed.*
   (b) The two-film packet may be used *when a duplicate record of a radiographic examination is needed.*
   (d) The two-film packet may be used *when a duplicate record of a radiographic examination is needed.*
REF: p. 78

19. The identification dot is used to:
   a. Determine film orientation.
   b. Identify whether or not a film has been exposed.
   c. Indicate the side of the film with an emulsion.
   d. Identify whether the film is D-speed film or F-speed film.

Answer: a
Correct: The identification dot is used to determine film orientation.
Incorrect:
   (b) The identification dot is used to *determine film orientation;* it is not used to determine whether or not a film has been exposed.

   (c) The identification dot is used to *determine film orientation;* it is not used to determine which side of the film has an emulsion as both sides have an emulsion.
   (d) The identification dot is used to *determine film orientation;* it is not used to determine the speed of the film.
REF: p. 78

20. What is the purpose of the lead foil sheet found within the film packet?
   a. To cover the film and shield the film from light.
   b. To protect the film from moisture.
   c. To shield the film from primary radiation emitted by the x-ray tubehead.
   d. To shield the film from secondary backscattered radiation.

Answer: d
Correct: The purpose of the lead foil sheet found within the film packet is to shield the film from secondary backscattered radiation.
Incorrect:
   (a) The purpose of the paper film wrapper is to cover the film and shield the film from light.
   (b) The purpose of the outer package wrapping is to protect the film from exposure to light and saliva.
   (c) The purpose of the lead foil sheet within the film packet is to shield the film from secondary backscattered radiation.
REF: p. 78

21. The thin lead foil sheet is positioned:
   a. Behind the film
   b. In front of the film
   c. Behind the paper film wrapper
   d. In front of the paper film wrapper

Answer: a
Correct: The thin lead foil sheet is positioned behind the film.
Incorrect:
   (b) The thin lead foil sheet is positioned *behind the film.*
   (c) The thin lead foil sheet is positioned *behind the film.*
   (d) The thin lead foil sheet is positioned *behind the film.*
REF: p. 78

22. The embossed pattern placed on the lead foil sheet by the manufacturer will reveal:
   a. Whether or not the film has been exposed
   b. If the film has been exposed to moisture
   c. If the film packet is inadvertently positioned in the mouth backward and then exposed
   d. If the film packet is inadvertently opened before the film is processed

77

Test Bank

Answer: c

Correct: The embossed pattern placed on the lead foil sheet by the manufacturer will reveal if the film packet is inadvertently positioned in the mouth backward and then exposed.

Incorrect:
- (a) The embossed pattern placed on the lead foil sheet by the manufacturer will not reveal whether the film has been exposed.
- (b) The embossed pattern placed on the lead foil sheet by the manufacturer will not reveal whether the film has been exposed to moisture.
- (d) The embossed pattern placed on the lead foil sheet by the manufacturer will not reveal whether the film packet was inadvertently opened before the film was processed.

REF: p. 78

23. The tube side of the dental film packet:
   - a. Has the flap used to open the dental film
   - b. Is solid white
   - c. Should face the patient's tongue
   - d. Is color-coded

Answer: b

Correct: The tube side of the dental film packet is solid white.

Incorrect:
- (a) The *label side* of the dental film packet has a flap used to open the dental film; the tube side of the dental film packet is solid white.
- (c) The *label side* of the dental film packet should face the patient's tongue; the tube side of the dental film packet is solid white.
- (d) The *label side* of the dental film packet is color-coded; the tube side of the dental film packet is solid white.

REF: p. 78

24. The label side of the dental film packet:
   - a. Is solid white
   - b. Has a raised bump in one corner that corresponds to the identification dot
   - c. The label side of the dental film packet *should face the tubehead when placed in the mouth.*
   - d. Is color-coded to distinguish between one-film and two-film packets and between film speeds

Answer: d

Correct: The label side of the dental film packet is color-coded to distinguish between one-film and two-film packets and between film speeds.

Incorrect:
- (a) The label side of the dental film packet *is color-coded to distinguish between one-film and two-film packets and between film speeds.*
- (b) The label side of the dental film packet *is color-coded to distinguish between one-film and two-film packets and between film speeds.*

- (c) The label side of the dental film packet *should not face the tubehead when placed in the mouth.*

REF: p. 79

25. Which type of intraoral film is used to examine the crowns of both the maxillary and the mandibular teeth on one film?
   - a. Maxillary periapical film
   - b. Mandibular periapical film
   - c. Bite-wing film
   - d. Occlusal film

Answer: c

Correct: The bite-wing film is used to examine the crowns of both the maxillary and the mandibular teeth on one film.

Incorrect:
- (a) The maxillary periapical film would show the crown and roots of maxillary teeth without showing mandibular teeth.
- (b) The mandibular periapical film would show the crown and roots of mandibular teeth without showing maxillary teeth.
- (d) The occlusal film would show maxillary or mandibular teeth on one film.

REF: p. 79

26. The apex (tip) of the tooth roots may be seen on which type(s) of intraoral film?
   - a. Periapical
   - b. Bite-wing
   - c. Occlusal
   - d. Periapical and occlusal

Answer: d

Correct: The apex (tip) of the tooth roots may be seen on periapical and occlusal films.

Incorrect:
- (a) The apex (tip) of the tooth roots may be seen on *periapical and occlusal* films.
- (b) The bite-wing film is used to examine the crowns of both the maxillary and the mandibular teeth on one film. It shows crowns and not the tip of the tooth root.
- (c) The apex (tip) of the tooth roots may be seen on *periapical and occlusal* films.

REF: pp. 79-80

27. Which type of intraoral film is best for visualizing interproximal surfaces?
   - a. Periapical
   - b. Bite-wing
   - c. Occlusal
   - d. Periapical and occlusal

Answer: b

Correct: The bite-wing film is best for visualizing interproximal surfaces.

Incorrect:
- (a) The *bite-wing film* is best for visualizing interproximal surfaces.
- (c) The *bite-wing film* is best for visualizing interproximal surfaces.
- (d) The *bite-wing film* is best for visualizing interproximal surfaces.

REF: p. 79

28. Which type of intraoral film is best for examination of large areas of the maxilla or mandible?
- a. Periapical
- b. Bite-wing
- c. Occlusal
- d. Periapical and occlusal

Answer: c

Correct: The occlusal film is best for examination of large areas of the maxilla or mandible.

Incorrect:
- (a) The *occlusal* film is best for examination of large areas of the maxilla or mandible.
- (b) The *occlusal* film is best for examination of large areas of the maxilla or mandible.
- (d) The *occlusal* film is best for examination of large areas of the maxilla or mandible.

REF: p. 79

29. A # _____ size film is a standard adult periapical film.
- a. 0
- b. 1
- c. 2
- d. 4

Answer: c

Correct: A #2 size film is a standard adult periapical film.

Incorrect:
- (a) A *#0* size film is used for very small children.
- (b) A *#1* size film is used primarily to examine the anterior teeth in adults.
- (d) A *#4* size film is used to show large regions of the upper or lower jaw.

REF: p. 80

30. Which size of bite-wing film is used to examine posterior teeth in very small children?
- a. 0
- b. 1
- c. 2
- d. 3

Answer: a

Correct: A #0 bite-wing film is used to examine posterior teeth in very small children.

Incorrect:
- (b) A *#0* bite-wing film is used to examine posterior teeth in very small children.
- (c) A *#0* bite-wing film is used to examine posterior teeth in very small children.

- (d) A *#0* bite-wing film is used to examine posterior teeth in very small children.

REF: p. 80

31. A size # _____ film is the most frequently used bite-wing film.
- a. 0
- b. 1
- c. 2
- d. 3

Answer: c

Correct: Size #2 film is the most frequently used bite-wing film.

Incorrect:
- (a) Size *#2* film is the most frequently used bite-wing film.
- (b) Size *#2* film is the most frequently used bite-wing film.
- (d) Size *#2* film is the most frequently used bite-wing film.

REF: p. 81

32. A fast film responds more quickly than a slow film, because:
- a. The tubehead shutter opens wider.
- b. The exposure times are longer for fast films.
- c. The silver halide crystals in the emulsion are larger.
- d. Different processing chemistry is used.

Answer: c

Correct: A fast film responds more quickly than a slow film, because the silver halide crystals in the emulsion are larger.

Incorrect:
- (a) This is not the correct choice because the tubehead does not have a shutter.
- (b) This is not the correct choice because the exposure times are shorter for fast films.
- (d) This is not the correct choice because the same processing chemistry is used for fast or slow film.

REF: p. 81

33. Which of the following film speed is the fastest film currently available?
- a. C
- b. D
- c. E
- d. F

Answer: d

Correct: F-speed film is the fastest film currently available.

Incorrect:
- (a) *C-speed* film is no longer available.
- (b) *D-speed* film is slower than F-speed film.
- (c) *E-speed* film is slower than F-speed film.

REF: p. 81

34. Which of the following types of film exhibits the bony and soft tissue areas of the facial profile?
a. Periapical
b. Bite-wing
c. Panoramic
d. Cephalometric

Answer: d
Correct: The cephalometric type of film exhibits the bony and soft tissue areas of the facial profile.
Incorrect:
  (a) The *periapical* type of film exhibits the crown and root of the tooth.
  (b) The *bite-wing* type of film exhibits the crowns of maxillary and mandibular teeth.
  (c) The *panoramic* type of film exhibits the entire skull and jaw in frontal and side views.
REF: p. 82

35. Which of the following types of film shows a wide view of the upper and lower jaws on a single radiograph?
a. Periapical
b. Bite-wing
c. Panoramic
d. Cephalometric

Answer: c
Correct: The panoramic film shows a wide view of the upper and lower jaws on a single radiograph.
Incorrect:
  (a) The *periapical* type of film shows the crown and root of the tooth.
  (b) The *bite-wing* type of film shows the crowns of maxillary and mandibular teeth.
  (d) The *cephalometric* type of film superimposes the upper and lower jaws; it does not show a wide view.
REF: pp. 81-82

36. Screen film:
a. Is sensitive to direct exposure to radiation
b. Is sensitive to fluorescent light
c. Requires more exposure time than nonscreen film
d. Is not recommended for use in dentistry

Answer: b
Correct: Screen film is sensitive to fluorescent light.
Incorrect:
  (a) Screen film *is not sensitive to direct exposure to radiation.*
  (c) Screen film *requires less exposure than nonscreen film.*
  (d) Screen film *is used for extraoral dental radiography.*
REF: pp. 82-83

37. Blue-sensitive screen film must be paired with screens that produce _____ light.
a. red
b. yellow
c. blue
d. green

Answer: c
Correct: Blue-sensitive screen film must be paired with screens that produce blue light.
Incorrect:
  (a) Blue-sensitive screen film must be paired with screens that produce *blue* light.
  (b) Blue-sensitive screen film must be paired with screens that produce *blue* light.
  (d) Blue-sensitive screen film must be paired with screens that produce *blue* light.
REF: p. 83

38. (1) An intensifying screen is a device that transfers x-ray energy into visible light; (2) the visible light, in turn, exposes the screen film.
a. Both statements are true.
b. Both statements are false.
c. The first statement is true; the second is false.
d. The first statement is false; the second is true.

Answer: a
Correct: An intensifying screen is a device that transfers x-ray energy into visible light; the visible light, in turn, exposes the screen film.
Incorrect:
  (b) An intensifying screen is a device that transfers x-ray energy into visible light; the visible light, in turn, exposes the screen film.
  (c) An intensifying screen is a device that transfers x-ray energy into visible light; the visible light, in turn, exposes the screen film.
  (d) An intensifying screen is a device that transfers x-ray energy into visible light; the visible light, in turn, exposes the screen film.
REF: p. 83

39. An intensifying screen is a smooth plastic sheet coated with minute fluorescent crystals known as:
a. Nuclei of crystallization
b. Germinal centers
c. Sensitivity specks
d. Phosphors

Answer: d
Correct: An intensifying screen is a smooth plastic sheet coated with minute fluorescent crystals known as phosphors.
Incorrect:
  (a) An intensifying screen is a smooth plastic sheet coated with minute fluorescent crystals known as *phosphors.*
  (b) An intensifying screen is a smooth plastic sheet coated with minute fluorescent crystals known as *phosphors.*

(c) Sensitivity specks are in the film; an intensifying screen is a smooth plastic sheet coated with minute fluorescent crystals known as *phosphors*.

REF: p. 83

40. Rare earth screens:
   a. Have phosphors that emit blue light
   b. Have phosphors that emit green light
   c. Are less efficient than calcium tungstate intensifying screens
   d. Are slower than calcium tungstate intensifying screens

Answer: b

Correct: Rare earth screens have phosphors that emit green light.

Incorrect:
   (a) Rare earth screens have phosphors that emit *green* light.
   (c) Rare earth screens are *more* efficient than calcium tungstate intensifying screens.
   (d) Rare earth screens are *faster* than calcium tungstate intensifying screens.

REF: p. 84

41. Lack of contact between screen and film results in:
   a. An overexposed film
   b. An underexposed film
   c. A light leak
   d. A loss of image sharpness

Answer: d

Correct: Lack of contact between screen and film results in a loss of image sharpness.

Incorrect:
   (a) Excessive exposure time, kVp, or milliamperage would result in an overexposed film.
   (b) Insufficient exposure time, kVp, or milliamperage would result in an underexposed film.
   (c) An opening in the screen would cause a light leak.

REF: p. 84

42. Duplicating film:
   a. Is not exposed to x-rays
   b. Has an emulsion on both sides
   c. Has an emulsion on one side only
   d. Both a and c

Answer: d

Correct: Duplicating film is not exposed to x-rays and has an emulsion on one side only.

Incorrect:
   (a) Duplicating film is not exposed to x-rays and has an emulsion on one side only.
   (b) Duplicating film is not exposed to x-rays and has an emulsion on one side only.
   (c) Duplicating film is not exposed to x-rays and has an emulsion on one side only.

REF: p. 84

43. Film is best stored in an area that is:
   a. Hot
   b. Humid
   c. Cool and dry
   d. Exposed to radiation

Answer: c

Correct: Film is best stored in an area that is cool and dry.

Incorrect:
   (a) Film is best stored in an area that is *cool and dry*.
   (b) Film is best stored in an area that is *cool and dry*.
   (d) Film is best stored in an area that is *cool and dry*.

REF: p. 85

44. The optimum temperature for film storage ranges from _____ to _____ degrees Fahrenheit.
   a. 30; 50
   b. 50; 70
   c. 70; 90
   d. 90; 110

Answer: b

Correct: The optimum temperature for film storage ranges from 50 to 70 degrees Fahrenheit.

Incorrect:
   (a) The optimum temperature for film storage ranges from *50 to 70* degrees Fahrenheit.
   (c) The optimum temperature for film storage ranges from *50 to 70* degrees Fahrenheit.
   (d) The optimum temperature for film storage ranges from *50 to 70* degrees Fahrenheit.

REF: p. 85

CHAPTER 8   DENTAL X-RAY IMAGE CHARACTERISTICS

MULTIPLE CHOICE

1. Which of the following areas would appear the most radiolucent on a dental radiograph?
   a. Composite
   b. Amalgam
   c. Air space
   d. Enamel

Answer: c

Correct: An air space would appear the most radiolucent on a dental radiograph.

Incorrect:
   (a) An air space would appear more radiolucent than composite on a dental radiograph.
   (b) An air space would appear more radiolucent than amalgam on a dental radiograph.
   (d) An air space would appear more radiolucent than enamel on a dental radiograph.

REF: p. 90

2. Radiographic density is defined as:
   a. A radiopaque radiograph

b. A radiolucent radiograph
c. The overall blackness or darkness of a radiograph
d. The difference in degrees of blackness between adjacent areas on a dental radiograph

Answer: c
Correct: Radiographic density is defined as the overall blackness or darkness of a radiograph.
Incorrect:
(a) *Radiopaque* refers to that portion of a processed radiograph that appears light or white.
(b) *Radiolucent* refers to that portion of a processed radiograph that is dark or black.
(d) *Radiographic contrast* is the difference in degrees of blackness between adjacent areas on a dental radiograph.
REF: p. 91

3. Radiolucent refers to that portion of a processed radiograph that is:
   a. Black
   b. White
   c. Gray
   d. Coated with an emulsion

Answer: a
Correct: Radiolucent refers to that portion of a processed radiograph that is black.
Incorrect:
(b) *Radiopaque* refers to the portion of a processed radiograph that is white.
(c) This is not the correct choice because radiolucent refers to the *black* portion of a radiograph, not gray.
(d) This is not the correct choice because the entire film is covered with emulsion on both sides.
REF: p. 90

4. Radiopaque refers to that portion of a processed radiograph that is:
   a. Black
   b. White
   c. Gray
   d. Within the plastic base

Answer: b
Correct: Radiopaque refers to that portion of a processed radiograph that is white.
Incorrect:
(a) *Radiolucent* refers to the portion of a processed radiograph that is black.
(c) This is not the correct choice because radiopaque refers to the *white* portion of a radiograph, not gray.
(d) Radiopaque refers to that portion of a processed radiograph that is *white*.
REF: p. 90

5. If the milliamperage is increased, the film density _____, and the film appears _____.
   a. increases; lighter
   b. increases; darker
   c. decreases; darker
   d. decreases; lighter

Answer: b
Correct: If the milliamperage is increased, the film density increases, and the film appears darker.
Incorrect:
(a) If the milliamperage is increased, the film density increases, and the film appears *darker*.
(c) If the milliamperage is increased, the film density *increases*, and the film appears darker.
(d) If the milliamperage is increased, the film density *increases*, and the film appears *darker*.
REF: p. 91

6. If the operating kilovoltage is increased, the film density _____ because the average energy of the x-rays is raised.
   a. increases
   b. decreases
   c. remains the same
   d. is divided by two

Answer: a
Correct: If the operating kilovoltage is increased, the film density increases because the average energy of the x-rays is raised.
Incorrect:
(b) If the operating kilovoltage is increased, the film density *increases* because the average energy of the x-rays is raised.
(c) If the operating kilovoltage is increased, the film density *increases* because the average energy of the x-rays is raised.
(d) If the operating kilovoltage is increased, the film density *increases* because the average energy of the x-rays is raised.
REF: p. 91

7. Which of the following changes will result in a radiograph with reduced density?
   a. Increasing the exposure time
   b. Increasing the subject thickness
   c. Increasing the milliamperage
   d. Increasing the operating kilovoltage peak

Answer: b
Correct: Increasing the subject thickness will result in a radiograph with reduced density.

(a) Increasing the exposure time will result in a radiograph with increased density.

(c) Increasing the milliamperage will result in a radiograph with increased density.

(d) Increasing the operating kilovoltage peak will result in a radiograph with increased density.

REF: p. 92

8. A radiograph that has _____ is said to have low contrast.
   a. a very dark overall appearance
   b. a very light overall appearance
   c. many shades of gray
   d. very dark areas and very light areas

Answer: c

Correct: A radiograph that has many shades of gray is said to have low contrast.

Incorrect:

(a) A radiograph that has *a very dark overall appearance* is said to have *high density*.

(b) A radiograph that has *a very light overall appearance* is said to have *low density*.

(d) A radiograph that has *very dark areas and very light areas* is said to have *high contrast*.

REF: p. 92

9. A radiograph that has _____ is said to have high contrast.
   a. a very dark overall appearance
   b. a very light overall appearance
   c. many shades of gray
   d. very dark areas and very light areas

Answer: d

Correct: A radiograph that has very dark areas and very light areas is said to have high contrast.

Incorrect:

(a) A radiograph that has *a very dark overall appearance* is said to have *high density*.

(b) A radiograph that has *a very light overall appearance* is said to have *low density*.

(c) A radiograph that has *many shades of gray* is said to have *low contrast*.

REF: p. 92

10. An increase in _____ temperature will result in a film with increased contrast.
    a. development
    b. water bath
    c. fixer
    d. room

Answer: a

Correct: An increase in development temperature will result in a film with increased contrast.

Incorrect:

(a) An increase in *water bath* temperature will not result in a film with increased contrast.

(c) An increase in *fixer* temperature will not result in a film with increased contrast.

(d) An increase in *room* temperature will not result in a film with increased contrast.

REF: p. 92

11. When a high operating kilovoltage peak (>90kVp) is used, (low/high) subject contrast and (many shades of gray/areas of black and white) are seen on the radiograph.
    a. low subject contrast; many shades of gray
    b. low subject contrast; areas of black and white
    c. high subject contrast; many shades of gray
    d. high subject contrast; areas of black and white

Answer: a

Correct: When a high operating kilovoltage peak (>90kVp) is used, low subject contrast and many shades of gray are seen on the radiograph.

Incorrect:

(b) When a high operating kilovoltage peak (>90kVp) is used, low subject contrast and *many shades of gray* are seen on the radiograph.

(c) When a high operating kilovoltage peak (>90kVp) is used *low subject contrast* and many shades of gray are seen on the radiograph.

(d) When a high operating kilovoltage peak (>90kVp) is used, *low subject contrast* and *many shades of gray* are seen on the radiograph.

REF: p. 92

12. The range of useful densities seen on a dental radiograph is termed the:
    a. Film contrast
    b. Subject contrast
    c. Scale of contrast
    d. Kilovoltage peak

Answer: c

Correct: The range of useful densities seen on a dental radiograph is termed the scale of contrast.

Incorrect:

(a) *Film contrast* refers to the characteristics of the film that influence radiographic contrast.

(b) *Subject contrast* refers to the characteristics of the subject that influence radiographic contrast.

(d) *Kilovoltage peak* refers to the maximal kilovoltage potential.

REF: p. 92

13. A stepwedge will reveal that radiographs taken at a lower kVp will have _____ than radiographs taken at a higher kVp.
    a. more shades of gray
    b. higher contrast
    c. lower contrast
    d. Both a and c

Answer: b

Correct: A stepwedge will reveal that radiographs taken at a lower kVp will have higher contrast than radiographs taken at a higher kVp.

Incorrect:

   (a) A stepwedge will reveal that radiographs taken at a *higher* kVp will have *more shades of gray* than radiographs taken at a *lower* kVp.

   (c) A stepwedge will reveal that radiographs taken at a lower kVp will have *higher contrast* than radiographs taken at a higher kVp.

   (d) A stepwedge will reveal that radiographs taken at a *lower* kVp will have *fewer shades of gray* than radiographs taken at a *higher contrast*.

REF: p. 93

14. The typical stepwedge is constructed of:
   a. Aluminum
   b. Steel
   c. Wood
   d. Copper

Answer: a

Correct: The typical stepwedge is constructed of aluminum.

Incorrect:

   (b) The typical stepwedge is constructed of *aluminum*.

   (c) The typical stepwedge is constructed of *aluminum*.

   (d) The typical stepwedge is constructed of *aluminum*.

REF: p. 92

15. A stepwedge will reveal that radiographs taken at a higher kVp will have _____ versus radiographs taken at a lower kVp.
   a. long-scale contrast
   b. high contrast
   c. only two densities
   d. many areas of black and white

Answer: a

Correct: A stepwedge will reveal that radiographs taken at a higher kVp will have long-scale contrast versus radiographs taken at a lower kVp.

Incorrect:

   (b) A stepwedge will reveal that radiographs taken at a *lower* kVp will have *high* contrast versus radiographs taken at a lower kVp.

   (c) A stepwedge will reveal that radiographs taken at a *higher* kVp will have *many densities* versus radiographs taken at a *lower* kVp.

   (d) A stepwedge will reveal that radiographs taken at a *higher* kVp will have *fewer areas of black and white* versus radiographs taken at a lower kVp.

REF: p. 93

16. The geometric characteristic of _____ refers to the capability of the x-ray film to reproduce the distinct outlines of an object.
   a. magnification
   b. distortion
   c. sharpness
   d. parallax

Answer: c

Correct: The geometric characteristic of sharpness refers to the capability of the x-ray film to reproduce the distinct outlines of an object.

Incorrect:

   (a) *Magnification* refers to a radiographic image that appears larger than the actual size of the object it represents.

   (b) *Distortion* is a variation in the true size and shape of the object.

   (d) The geometric characteristic of *sharpness* refers to the capability of the x-ray film to reproduce the distinct outlines of an object.

REF: p. 94

17. Which of the following influencing factors would degrade film sharpness?
(1) Smaller silver halide crystal size
(2) Larger silver halide crystal size
(3) Smaller focal spot
(4) Larger focal spot
   a. 1 and 3
   b. 1 and 4
   c. 2 and 3
   d. 2 and 4

Answer: d

Correct: A larger silver halide crystal size and a larger focal spot would degrade film sharpness.

Incorrect:

   (a) A *smaller* silver halide crystal size and a *smaller* focal spot would *enhance* film sharpness.

   (b) A *larger* silver halide crystal size would degrade film sharpness.

   (c) A *larger* focal spot would degrade film sharpness.

REF: p. 95

18. Which of the following factors would improve image sharpness?
   a. Larger focal spot
   b. Larger crystal size in the film
   c. Smaller crystal size in the film
   d. Patient movement during x-ray film exposure

Answer: c

Correct: Smaller crystal size in the film would improve image sharpness.

REF: p. 95

19. Which of the following choices would result in increased magnification of the radiographic image?
    a. Increased target-film distance
    b. Decreased object-film distance
    c. Increased object-film distance
    d. Both a and b

Answer: c

Correct: An increased object-film distance would result in increased magnification of the radiographic image.

Incorrect:
(a) A larger focal spot would *degrade* image sharpness.
(b) A larger crystal size in the film would *degrade* image sharpness.
(d) Patient movement during film exposure would *degrade* image sharpness.

REF: p. 96

20. A longer position-indicating device (PID) results in:
    a. An increased target-film distance
    b. A more divergent x-ray beam
    c. More image magnification than when a shorter PID is used
    d. An increased object-film distance

Answer: a

Correct: A longer PID results in an increased target-film distance.

Incorrect:
(b) A longer PID results in a *less* divergent x-ray beam.
(c) A longer PID results in *less* image magnification than when a shorter PID is used.
(d) A longer PID results in a *decreased* object-film distance.

REF: p. 96

21. To minimize dimensional distortion, the object and film must be _____ one another.
    a. perpendicular to
    b. parallel to
    c. at a 45-degree angle to
    d. more than the length of the PID apart from

Answer: b

Correct: To minimize dimensional distortion, the object and film must be parallel to one another.

REF: p. 97

22. The x-ray beam must be perpendicular to the tooth and film in order to minimize:
    a. Sharpness
    b. Grain size
    c. Focal spot size
    d. Dimensional distortion

Answer: d

Correct: The x-ray beam must be perpendicular to the tooth and film in order to minimize dimensional distortion.

Incorrect:
(a) The x-ray beam must be perpendicular to the tooth and film in order to minimize *dimensional distortion.*
(b) The x-ray beam must be perpendicular to the tooth and film in order to minimize *dimensional distortion.*
(c) The x-ray beam must be perpendicular to the tooth and film in order to minimize *dimensional distortion.*

REF: p. 97

CHAPTER 9   DENTAL X-RAY FILM PROCESSING

MULTIPLE CHOICE

1. The latent image is:
   a. Visible to the naked eye
   b. The image on the radiographic film after processing
   c. The image on the radiographic film before processing but after exposure
   d. The image on the radiographic film before the exposure

Answer: c

Correct: The latent image is the image on the radiographic film before processing but after exposure.

Incorrect:
(a) The latent image is *the image on the radiographic film before processing but after exposure.*
(b) The latent image is *the image on the radiographic film before processing but after exposure.*
(d) The latent image is *the image on the radiographic film before processing but after exposure.*

REF: p. 102

2. During processing, a chemical reaction occurs, and the halide portion of the _____ silver halide crystal is removed.
   a. unexposed, unenergized
   b. exposed, unenergized
   c. unexposed, energized
   d. exposed, energized

Answer: d
Correct: During processing, a chemical reaction occurs, and the halide portion of the exposed, energized silver halide crystal is removed.
Incorrect:
   (a) During processing, a chemical reaction occurs, and the halide portion of the *exposed, energized* silver halide crystal is removed.
   (b) During processing, a chemical reaction occurs, and the halide portion of the exposed, *energized* silver halide crystal is removed.
   (c) During processing, a chemical reaction occurs, and the halide portion of the *exposed*, energized silver halide crystal is removed.
REF: p. 102

3. The black metallic silver remains on the film as a result of a _____ reaction.
   a. addition
   b. oxidation
   c. reduction
   d. subtraction

Answer: c
Correct: The black metallic silver remains on the film as a result of a reduction reaction.
Incorrect:
   (a) The black metallic silver remains on the film as a result of a *reduction* reaction.
   (b) The black metallic silver remains on the film as a result of a *reduction* reaction.
   (d) The black metallic silver remains on the film as a result of a *reduction* reaction.
REF: p. 102

4. Which type of silver halide crystals are removed from the film?
   a. Unexposed, unenergized
   b. Exposed, unenergized
   c. Unexposed, energized
   d. Exposed, energized

Answer: a
Correct: The unexposed, unenergized silver halide crystals are removed from the film.
Incorrect:
   (b) The *unexposed*, unenergized silver halide crystals are removed from the film.

   (c) The unexposed, *unenergized* silver halide crystals are removed from the film.
   (d) The *unexposed, unenergized* silver halide crystals are removed from the film.
REF: p. 102

5. The developer initiates a chemical reaction that reduces the exposed silver halide crystals into black metallic silver, but it leaves the unexposed silver halide crystals unaffected.
   a. Both statements are true.
   b. Both statements are false.
   c. The first statement is true; the second is false.
   d. The first statement is false; the second is true.

Answer: a
Correct: The developer initiates a chemical reaction that reduces the exposed silver halide crystals into black metallic silver, but it leaves the unexposed silver halide crystals unaffected.
Incorrect:
   (b) The developer initiates a chemical reaction that reduces the exposed silver halide crystals into black metallic silver, but it leaves the unexposed silver halide crystals unaffected.
   (c) The developer initiates a chemical reaction that reduces the exposed silver halide crystals into black metallic silver, but it leaves the unexposed silver halide crystals unaffected.
   (d) The developer initiates a chemical reaction that reduces the exposed silver halide crystals into black metallic silver, but it leaves the unexposed silver halide crystals unaffected.
REF: p. 103

6. Which of the following possibilities is the correct processing order for manual tanks?
   a. Rinsing, development, fixation
   b. Development, fixation, rinsing
   c. Rinsing, fixation, development
   d. Development, rinsing, fixation

Answer: d
Correct: The correct processing order for manual tanks is developing, rinsing, fixing.
   (*Note:* Some automatic processors do not have a rinse between developing and fixing. They compensate by increasing the concentration of the fixer.)
Incorrect:
   (a) The correct processing order for manual tanks is *developing, rinsing, fixing*.
   (b) The correct processing order for manual tanks is *developing, rinsing, fixing*.
   (c) The correct processing order for manual tanks is *developing, rinsing, fixing*.
REF: p. 104

7. The first step in film processing is:
   a. Washing
   b. Rinsing
   c. Development
   d. Fixation

Answer: c
Correct: The first step in film processing is development.
Incorrect:
   (a) *Washing* occurs following development.
   (b) *Rinsing* occurs following development.
   (d) *Fixation* occurs after rinsing.
REF: p. 104

8. The purpose of _____ is to chemically reduce the exposed, energized silver halide crystals into black metallic silver.
   a. developer
   b. fixer
   c. rinsing
   d. washing

Answer: a
Correct: The purpose of developer is to chemically reduce the exposed, energized silver halide crystals into black metallic silver.

Incorrect:
   (b) The purpose of *fixer* is to remove the unexposed, energized silver halide crystals from the film emulsion.
   (c) The purpose of *rinsing* is to remove the developer from the film and stop the development process.
   (d) The purpose of *washing* is to remove all chemicals from the emulsion.
REF: p. 104

9. The film emulsion is softened during which of the following stages of the development process?
   a. Development
   b. Rinsing
   c. Fixation
   d. Washing

Answer: a
Correct: The film emulsion is softened during the development stage of processing.
Incorrect:
   (b) The film emulsion is softened during the *development* stage of processing.
   (c) The film emulsion is softened during the *development* stage of processing.
   (d) The film emulsion is softened during the *development* stage of processing.
REF: p. 104

10. The film emulsion is hardened during which of the following stages of the development process?
   a. Development

   b. Rinsing
   c. Fixation
   d. Washing

Answer: c
Correct: The film emulsion is hardened during the fixation stage of processing.
Incorrect:
   (a) The film emulsion is hardened during the *fixation* stage of processing.
   (b) The film emulsion is hardened during the *fixation* stage of processing.
   (d) The film emulsion is hardened during the *fixation* stage of processing.
REF: p. 104

11. All excess chemicals are removed from the emulsion during:
   a. Development
   b. Rinsing
   c. Fixation
   d. Washing

Answer: d
Correct: All excess chemicals are removed from the emulsion during washing.
Incorrect:
   (a) All excess chemicals are removed from the emulsion during *washing*.
   (b) All excess chemicals are removed from the emulsion during *washing*.
   (d) All excess chemicals are removed from the emulsion during *washing*.
REF: p. 104

12. Concentrated powder and liquid film processing solutions are mixed with _____ before use.
   a. ammonia
   b. vinegar
   c. tap water
   d. distilled water

Answer: d
Correct: Concentrated powder and liquid film processing solutions are mixed with distilled water before use.
Incorrect:
   (a) Concentrated powder and liquid film processing solutions are mixed with *distilled water* before use.
   (b) Concentrated powder and liquid film processing solutions are mixed with *distilled water* before use.
   (c) Concentrated powder and liquid film processing solutions are mixed with *distilled water* before use.
REF: p. 104

13. To maintain freshness, film processing solutions must be replenished:
   a. Hourly

b. Daily

c. Weekly

d. Monthly

Answer: b

Correct: To maintain freshness, film processing solutions must be replenished daily.

Incorrect:

(a) To maintain freshness, film processing solutions must be replenished *daily*.

(c) To maintain freshness, film processing solutions must be replenished *daily*.

(d) To maintain freshness, film processing solutions must be replenished *daily*.

REF: p. 104

14. To maintain freshness, film processing solutions must be changed every _____.

a. day

b. week

c. 2 weeks

d. 3 to 4 weeks

Answer: d

Correct: To maintain freshness, film processing solutions must be changed every 3 to 4 weeks.

Incorrect:

(a) To maintain freshness, film processing solutions must be changed every *3 to 4 weeks*.

(b) To maintain freshness, film processing solutions must be changed every *3 to 4 weeks*.

(c) To maintain freshness, film processing solutions must be changed every *3 to 4 weeks*.

REF: p. 104

15. Normal use of processing chemistry is defined as _____ intraoral films per day.

a. 18

b. 30

c. 50

d. 60

Answer: b

Correct: Normal use of processing chemistry is defined as 30 intraoral films per day

Incorrect:

(a) Normal use of processing chemistry is defined as *30* intraoral films per day.

(c) Normal use of processing chemistry is defined as *30* intraoral films per day.

(d) Normal use of processing chemistry is defined as *30* intraoral films per day.

REF: p. 104

16. _____ generates the black tones and the sharp contrast of the radiographic image.

a. Sodium sulfite

b. Sodium carbonate

c. Hydroquinone

d. Elon

Answer: c

Correct: Hydroquinone generates the black tones and the sharp contrast of the radiographic image.

Incorrect:

(a) Sodium sulfite is the preservative in developer.

(b) Sodium carbonate activates the developing agents.

(d) *Elon* generates the *many shades of gray* and the sharp contrast of the radiographic image.

REF: p. 104

17. The optimal temperature for the developer solution is _____ degrees Fahrenheit.

a. 64

b. 68

c. 72

d. 76

Answer: b

Correct: The optimal temperature for the developer solution is 68 degrees Fahrenheit.

Incorrect:

(a) The optimal temperature for the developer solution is *68* degrees Fahrenheit.

(c) The optimal temperature for the developer solution is *68* degrees Fahrenheit.

(d) The optimal temperature for the developer solution is *68* degrees Fahrenheit.

REF: p. 104

18. Elon generates the _____ seen on a dental radiograph.

a. black tones

b. sharp contrast

c. many shades of gray

d. softening of the emulsion

Answer: c

Correct: Elon generates the many shades of gray seen on a dental radiograph.

Incorrect:

(a) *Hydroquinone* generates the *blacktones* seen on a dental radiograph.

(b) *Hydroquinon* generates the *sharp contrast* seen on a dental radiograph.

(d) Sodium carbonate generates the *softening of the emulsion* on a dental radiograph.

REF: p. 104

19. Elon is:

a. Not temperature sensitive

b. Temperature sensitive

c. Also known as metol

d. Both a and c

Answer: d

Correct: Elon is not temperature sensitive and is also known as metol.

Incorrect:

(a) Elon is not temperature sensitive and is *also known as metol.*

(b) Elon is *not* temperature sensitive.

(c) Elon is *not temperature sensitive* and is also known as metol.

REF: p. 104

20. The preservative used in developer solution is:
   a. Hydroquinone
   b. Sodium sulfite
   c. Sodium carbonate
   d. Potassium bromide

Answer: b

Correct: The preservative used in developer solution is sodium sulfite.

Incorrect:

(a) *Hydroquinone* is a *developing agent* used in developer solution.

(c) *Sodium carbonate* is the *accelerator* used in developer solution.

(d) *Potassium bromide* is the *restrainer* used in developer solution.

REF: p. 105

21. If films were processed below 60 degrees Fahrenheit:
   a. Hydroquinone and elon would both be inactive.
   b. Hydroquinone would be inactive, but elon would be active.
   c. Hydroquinone would be active, but elon would be inactive.
   d. Hydroquinone and elon would both be active.

Answer: b

Correct: If films were processed below 60 degrees Fahrenheit, hydroquinone would be inactive, but elon would be active.

Incorrect:

(a) If films were processed below 60 degrees Fahrenheit, hydroquinone would be inactive, *but elon would be active.*

(c) If films were processed below 60 degrees Fahrenheit, *hydroquinone would be inactive, but elon would be active.*

(d) If films were processed below 60 degrees Fahrenheit, hydroquinone would be inactive, *but elon would be active.*

REF: p. 104

22. The purpose of the preservative is to prevent the developer solution from oxidizing in the presence of:
   a. Silver halide
   b. Silver bromide

   c. Air
   d. Moisture

Answer: c

Correct: The purpose of the preservative is to prevent the developer solution from oxidizing in the presence of air.

Incorrect:

(a) The purpose of the preservative is to prevent the developer solution from oxidizing in the presence of *air.*

(b) The purpose of the preservative is to prevent the developer solution from oxidizing in the presence of *air.*

(d) The purpose of the preservative is to prevent the developer solution from oxidizing in the presence of *air.*

REF: p. 105

23. Which of the following chemicals is the accelerator in developer solution?
   a. Hydroquinone
   b. Elon
   c. Sodium sulfite
   d. Sodium carbonate

Answer: d

Correct: The accelerator in developer solution is sodium carbonate.

Incorrect:

(a) *Hydroquinone* is a *developing agent* used in developer solution.

(b) *Elon* is a *developing agent* used in developer solution.

(c) *Sodium sulfite* is the *preservative* used in developer solution.

REF: p. 105

24. Which of the following chemicals in developer solution softens the gelatin of the emulsion?
   a. Hydroquinone
   b. Elon
   c. Sodium sulfite
   d. Sodium carbonate

Answer: d

Correct: The gelatin of the emulsion is softened by sodium carbonate.

Incorrect:

(a) The gelatin of the emulsion is softened by *sodium carbonate.*

(b) The gelatin of the emulsion is softened by *sodium carbonate.*

(c) The gelatin of the emulsion is softened by *sodium carbonate.*

REF: p. 105

25. The developing agents are active only in a/an _____ environment.
a. basic (alkaline)
b. high pH
c. acidic
d. Both a and b

Answer: d
Correct: The developing agents are active only in a basic environment; high pH would be a basic environment.
Incorrect:
(a) The developing agents are active only in a *basic* environment; high pH would be a basic environment.
(b) The developing agents are active only in a *basic* environment; high pH would be a basic environment.
(c) The developing agents are active only in a *basic* environment; high pH would be a basic environment.
REF: p. 105

26. Potassium bromide functions as which of the following components of developer solution?
a. Developing agent
b. Preservative
c. Accelerator
d. Restrainer

Answer: d
Correct: Potassium bromide functions as the restrainer in developer solution.
Incorrect:
(a) Potassium bromide functions as the *restrainer* in developer solution.
(b) Potassium bromide functions as the *restrainer* in developer solution.
(c) Potassium bromide functions as the *restrainer* in developer solution.
REF: p. 105

27. The restrainer stops the development of:
a. Unexposed crystals only
b. Exposed crystals only
c. Unexposed crystals more than exposed crystals
d. Exposed crystals more than unexposed crystals

Answer: c
Correct: The restrainer stops the development of unexposed crystals more than exposed crystals.
Incorrect:
(a) The restrainer stops the development of *unexposed crystals more than exposed crystals.*
(b) The restrainer stops the development of *unexposed crystals more than exposed crystals.*
(d) The restrainer stops the development of *unexposed crystals more than exposed crystals.*
REF: p. 105

28. Which of the following is a component of fixer solution, but not developer solution?
a. Potassium bromide
b. Potassium alum
c. Hydroquinone
d. Sodium carbonate

Answer: b
Correct: Potassium alum is a component of fixer solution, but not developer solution.
Incorrect:
(a) *Potassium bromide* is a component of developer solution.
(c) *Hydroquinone* is a component of developer solution.
(d) *Sodium carbonate* is a component of developer solution.
REF: pp. 104-106

29. Which component of fixer solution is commonly known as "hypo"?
a. Sodium thiosulfate
b. Sodium sulfite
c. Potassium alum
d. Acetic acid

Answer: a
Correct: Sodium thiosulfate is the component of fixer solution that is commonly known as "hypo."
Incorrect:
(b) *Sodium thiosulfate* is the component of fixer solution that is commonly known as "hypo."
(c) *Sodium thiosulfate* is the component of fixer solution that is commonly known as "hypo."
(d) *Sodium thiosulfate* is the component of fixer solution that is commonly known as "hypo."
REF: p. 105

30. The purpose of the fixing agent is to remove all _____ from the film emulsion.
a. unexposed silver halide crystals
b. exposed silver halide crystals
c. unexposed and exposed silver halide crystals
d. of the emulsion

Answer: a
Correct: The purpose of the fixing agent is to remove all unexposed silver halide crystals from the film emulsion.
Incorrect:
(b) The purpose of the fixing agent is to remove all *unexposed silver halide crystals* from the film emulsion.
(c) The purpose of the fixing agent is to remove all *unexposed silver halide crystals* from the film emulsion.
(d) The purpose of the fixing agent is to remove all *unexposed silver halide crystals* from the film emulsion.
REF: p. 105

31. Sodium sulfite is the _____ used in fixer solution.
   a. fixing agent
   b. preservative
   c. hardening agent
   d. acidifier

Answer: b
Correct: Sodium sulfite is the preservative used in fixer solution.
Incorrect:
   (a) Sodium sulfite is the *preservative* used in fixer solution; the fixing agent is sodium thiosulfate.
   (c) Sodium sulfite is the *preservative* used in fixer solution; the hardening agent is potassium alum.
   (d) Sodium sulfite is the *preservative* used in fixer solution; the acidifier is acetic acid or sulfuric acid.
REF: p. 106

32. The hardening agent used in fixer solution is:
   a. Potassium bromide
   b. Potassium alum
   c. Acetic acid
   d. Sulfuric acid

Answer: b
Correct: The hardening agent used in fixer solution is potassium alum.
Incorrect:
   (a) The hardening agent used in fixer solution is *potassium alum;* potassium bromide is the restrainer used in developer solution.
   (c) The hardening agent used in fixer solution is *potassium alum;* acetic acid is an acidifier used in fixer solution.
   (d) The hardening agent used in fixer solution is *potassium alum;* sulfuric acid is an acidifier used in fixer solution.
REF: p. 106

33. The purpose of the hardening agent is to harden and shrink the:
   a. Exposed silver halide crystals
   b. Unexposed silver halide crystals
   c. Gelatin in the film emulsion
   d. Plastic film base

Answer: c
Correct: The purpose of the hardening agent is to harden and shrink the gelatin in the film emulsion.
Incorrect:
   (a) The purpose of the hardening agent is to harden and shrink the *gelatin in the film emulsion.*
   (b) The purpose of the hardening agent is to harden and shrink the *gelatin in the film emulsion.*
   (d) The purpose of the hardening agent is to harden and shrink the *gelatin in the film emulsion.*
REF: p. 106

34. Developer solution has (a/an) _____ pH, and fixer solution has (a/an) _____ pH.
   a. acidic; acidic
   b. acidic; basic
   c. basic; acidic
   d. basic; basic

Answer: c
Correct: Developer solution has a basic pH, and fixer solution has an acidic pH.
Incorrect:
   (a) Developer solution has a *basic* pH, and fixer solution has an acidic pH.
   (b) Developer solution has a *basic* pH, and fixer solution has an *acidic* pH.
   (d) Developer solution has a basic pH, and fixer solution has an *acidic* pH.
REF: pp. 104-105

35. The acidifier used in fixer solution is:
   a. Ammonium thiosulfate
   b. Potassium alum
   c. Acetic acid
   d. Sodium sulfite

Answer: c
Correct: The acidifier used in fixer solution is acetic acid.
Incorrect:
   (a) The *fixing* agent used in fixer solution is *ammonium thiosulfate.*
   (b) The *hardening agent* used in fixer solution is *potassium alum.*
   (d) The *preservative* used in fixer solution is *sodium sulfite.*
REF: p. 106

36. Any leaks of white light in the darkroom cause film:
   a. To be entirely clear on processing
   b. To become more sensitive to processing chemistry
   c. Film fog
   d. To exhibit decreased contrast between light and dark areas

Answer: c
Correct: Any leaks of white light in the darkroom cause film fog.
Incorrect:
   (a) Any leaks of white light in the darkroom cause film *fog.*
   (b) Any leaks of white light in the darkroom cause film *fog.*
   (d) Any leaks of white light in the darkroom cause film *fog.*
REF: p. 106

37. A fogged film appears:
   a. To lack contrast
   b. To have accentuated contrast
   c. Dull gray
   d. Both a and c

Answer: d

Correct: A fogged film appears to lack contrast and appears dull gray.

Incorrect:
(a) A fogged film appears to lack contrast and appears *dull gray*.
(b) A fogged film appears *to lack contrast* and appears *dull gray*.
(c) A fogged film appears *to lack contrast* and appears dull gray.

REF: p. 106

38. Safelighting is a _____-intensity light composed of _____ wavelengths of the visible light spectrum.
   a. low; long
   b. low; short
   c. high; long
   d. high; short

Answer: a

Correct: Safelighting is a low-intensity light composed of long wavelengths of the visible light spectrum.

Incorrect:
(b) Safelighting is a low-intensity light composed of *long* wavelengths of the visible light spectrum.
(c) Safelighting is a *low*-intensity light composed of long wavelengths of the visible light spectrum.
(d) Safelighting is a *low*-intensity light composed of *long* wavelengths of the visible light spectrum.

REF: p. 106

39. Safelighting is in the _____ portion of the visible light spectrum.
   a. red-orange
   b. orange-yellow
   c. yellow-green
   d. green-blue

Answer: a

Correct: Safelighting is in the red-orange portion of the visible light spectrum.

Incorrect:
(b) Safelighting is in the *red-orange* portion of the visible light spectrum.
(c) Safelighting is in the *red-orange* portion of the visible light spectrum.
(d) Safelighting is in the *red-orange* portion of the visible light spectrum.

REF: p. 106

40. A safelight must be placed a minimum of _____ feet away from the film.
   a. 2
   b. 3
   c. 4
   d. 6

Answer: c

Correct: A safelight must be placed a minimum of 4 feet away from the film.

Incorrect:
(a) A safelight must be placed a minimum of *4* feet away from the film.
(b) A safelight must be placed a minimum of *4* feet away from the film.
(d) A safelight must be placed a minimum of *4* feet away from the film.

REF: p. 106

41. Films that are exposed to safelight illumination for more than 2 or 3 minutes will appear:
   a. Lighter overall than they otherwise would appear
   b. Fogged
   c. To have higher contrast than they otherwise would appear
   d. Unchanged

Answer: b

Correct: Films that are exposed to safelight illumination for more than 2 or 3 minutes will appear fogged.

Incorrect:
(a) Films that are exposed to safelight illumination for more than 2 or 3 minutes will appear *darker* overall.
(c) Films that are exposed to safelight illumination for more than 2 or 3 minutes will appear *to have lower contrast*.
(d) Films that are exposed to safelight illumination for more than 2 or 3 minutes will appear *fogged*.

REF: p. 106

42. Static electricity may cause film artifacts when:
   a. Humidity levels are too high.
   b. Humidity levels are too low.
   c. Room temperature is too high.
   d. Both a and c.

Answer: b

Correct: Static electricity may cause film artifacts when humidity levels are too low.

Incorrect:
(a) Static electricity may cause film artifacts when humidity levels are too *low*.
(c) Static electricity may cause film artifacts when *humidity levels are too low*.
(d) Static electricity may cause film artifacts when *humidity levels are too low*.

REF: p. 107

43. A mixing valve is used with manual tanks to:
   a. Control the temperature of the water bath in the master tank.
   b. Dilute concentrated liquid developer and fixer.
   c. Reconstitute powder developer and fixer.
   d. Agitate and remove bubbles from the delicate emulsion.

Answer: a

Correct: A mixing valve is used with manual tanks to control the temperature of the water bath in the master tank.

92

(b) A mixing valve is used with manual tanks to *control the temperature of the water bath in the master tank.*

(c) A mixing valve is used with manual tanks to *control the temperature of the water bath in the master tank.*

(d) A mixing valve is used with manual tanks to *control the temperature of the water bath in the master tank.*

REF: p. 107

44. Which of the following statements is *true* of manual processing tanks?
    a. Developer and fixer are placed in the master tank.
    b. There are two master tanks and one insert tank.
    c. The two insert tanks fit in the master tank.
    d. Water is placed in the insert tank.

Answer: c
Correct: The two insert tanks fit in the master tank.
Incorrect:
(a) *The two insert tanks fit in the master tank;* developer and fixer are placed in the *insert* tanks.

(b) *The two insert tanks fit in the master tank;* there are *two* insert tanks and *one* master tank.

(d) *The two insert tanks fit in the master tank;* water is placed in the *master* tank.

REF: p. 108

45. Developer solution is typically placed in the:
    a. Master tank on the left
    b. Master tank on the right
    c. Insert tank on the left
    d. Insert tank on the right

Answer: c
Correct: Developer solution is typically placed in the insert tank on the left.
Incorrect:
(a) Developer solution is typically placed in the *insert tank on the left;* there is only one master tank.

(b) Developer solution is typically placed in the *insert tank on the left;* there is only one master tank.

(d) Developer solution is typically placed in the *insert tank on the left.*

REF: p. 108

46. The master tank is filled with:
    a. Developer
    b. Fixer
    c. Cold water
    d. Temperature-controlled water

Answer: d
Correct: The master tank is filled with temperature-controlled water.

(a) The master tank is filled with *temperature-controlled water;* the temperature is controlled by the mixing valve.

(b) The master tank is filled with *temperature-controlled water;* the temperature is controlled by the mixing valve.

(c) The master tank is filled with *temperature-controlled water;* the temperature is controlled by the mixing valve.

REF: p. 108

47. In addition to protecting developing films from exposure to light, the light-tight lid of the processing tank protects the solutions from:
    a. Oxidation and evaporation
    b. Imbibing water
    c. Raising the humidity level in the room to levels that would negatively affect processing
    d. Contaminating the water in the master tank

Answer: a
Correct: In addition to protecting developing films from exposure to light, the light-tight lid of the processing tank protects the solutions from oxidation and evaporation.
Incorrect:
(b) In addition to protecting developing films from exposure to light, the light-tight lid of the processing tank protects the solutions from *oxidation and evaporation.*

(c) In addition to protecting developing films from exposure to light, the light-tight lid of the processing tank protects the solutions from *oxidation and evaporation.*

(d) In addition to protecting developing films from exposure to light, the light-tight lid of the processing tank protects the solutions from *oxidation and evaporation.*

REF: p. 108

48. The temperatures of the developer and fixer solutions are controlled by the:
    a. Ambient room temperature
    b. Aquarium-type heaters in the insert tanks
    c. Use of a mixing valve
    d. Chemical reaction that occurs when they are mixed

Answer: c
Correct: The temperatures of the developer and fixer solutions are controlled by the use of a mixing valve.
Incorrect:
(a) The temperatures of the developer and fixer solutions are controlled by the *use of a mixing valve.*

(b) The temperatures of the developer and fixer solutions are controlled by the *use of a mixing valve;* aquarium-type heaters are not used in the insert tanks.

(d) The temperatures of the developer and fixer solutions are controlled by the *use of a mixing valve;* developer and fixer solutions are not deliberately mixed.

REF: p. 108

49. Which of the following statements is *true* of automatic film processors?
    a. All automatic film processors are capable of processing a number of different sizes of x-ray film.
    b. All automatic film processors may be used in a room with white light.
    c. Only automatic film processors with daylight loaders may be used in a room with white light.
    d. Both a and c.

Answer: c
Correct: Only automatic film processors with daylight loaders may be used in a room with white light
Incorrect:
    (a) Not all automatic film processors are capable of processing a number of different sizes of x-ray film; some are limited to certain sizes of x-ray film.
    (b) Not all automatic film processors may be used in a room with white light; *only automatic film processors with daylight loaders* may be used in a room with white light.
    (d) Not all automatic film processors are capable of processing a number of different sizes of x-ray film; some are limited to certain sizes of x-ray film. Only automatic film processors with daylight loaders may be used in a room with white light.

REF: p. 108

50. A thermometer may be clipped to the side of the _____ for manual processing.
    a. developer tank
    b. fixer tank
    c. master tank
    d. both insert tanks

Answer: a
Correct: A thermometer may be clipped to the side of the developer tank for manual processing.
Incorrect:
    (b) A thermometer may be clipped to the side of the *developer tank* for manual processing.
    (c) A thermometer may be clipped to the side of the *developer tank* for manual processing.
    (d) A thermometer may be clipped to the side of the *developer tank* for manual processing.

REF: p. 109

51. A timer is used to indicate time intervals during which of the following steps of manual processing?
    (1) Developer solution
    (2) Rinse water
    (3) Fixer solution

(4) Wash water
    a. 1, 2, 3, 4
    b. 2, 3, 4
    c. 2, 4
    d. 4 only

Answer: a
Correct: A timer is used to indicate time intervals during developer solution, rinse water, fixer solution, and wash water steps of manual processing.
Incorrect:
    (b) A timer is used to indicate time intervals during developer solution, *rinse water, fixer solution, and wash water* steps of manual processing, not leaving the films in developer solution for a sufficient length of time will result in light films and conversely, leaving the films in developer solution for an excessive amount of time will result in dark films
    (c) A timer is used to indicate time intervals during *developer solution*, rinse water, fixer solution, and *wash water* steps of manual processing.
    (d) A timer is used to indicate time intervals during *developer solution, rinse water, fixer solution,* and wash water steps of manual processing.

REF: p. 109

52. Film hangers are a device used to:
    a. Hold films during processing
    b. Mount films
    c. View films
    d. Open film packets

Answer: a
Correct: Film hangers are a device used to hold films during processing.
Incorrect:
    (b) This is not the correct choice because films are mounted manually.
    (c) This is not the correct choice because films are viewed on a viewbox.
    (d) This is not the correct choice because packets are opened manually.

REF: pp. 109-110

53. The purpose of a stirring rod is to:
    a. Scrape bubbles from the surface of the films when they are in solution.
    b. Mix the chemicals and equalize the temperature of the solutions.
    c. Mix developer and fixer together in the master tank.
    d. Recover the thermometer from the bottom of the master tank.

Answer: b
Correct: The purpose of a stirring rod is to mix the chemicals and equalize the temperature of the solutions.

(a) The purpose of a stirring rod is to *mix the chemicals and equalize the temperature of the solutions;* scraping the surface of the films will damage the emulsion.

(c) The purpose of a stirring rod is to *mix the chemicals and equalize the temperature of the solutions;* the developer and fixer are placed in the insert tanks and are never mixed.

(d) The purpose of a stirring rod is to *mix the chemicals and equalize the temperature of the solutions;* the thermometer is placed in the developer tank.

REF: p. 110

54. Developer solution should be changed _____ fixer solution.
   a. twice as often as
   b. more often than
   c. less often than
   d. at the same time as

Answer: d

Correct: Developer solution should be changed at the same time as fixer solution.

Incorrect:

(a) Developer solution should be changed *at the same time as* fixer solution.

(b) Developer solution should be changed *at the same time as* fixer solution.

(c) Developer solution should be changed *at the same time as* fixer solution.

REF: p. 112

55. The developer solution becomes depleted from evaporation and the removal of small amounts from the tank on the film hanger and films. With time and use, the developer solution decreases in volume but increases in strength.
   a. Both statements are true.
   b. Both statements are false.
   c. The first statement is true; the second is false.
   d. The first statement is false; the second is true.

Answer: c

Correct: The developer solution becomes depleted from evaporation and the removal of small amounts from the tank on the film hanger and films. With time and use, the developer solution decreases not only in volume but in strength as well.

Incorrect:

(a) The developer solution becomes depleted from evaporation and the removal of small amounts from the tank on the film hanger and films. With time and use, the developer solution decreases *not only in volume but in strength as well.*

(b) *The developer solution becomes depleted from evaporation and the removal of small amounts from the tank on the film hanger and films. With*

time and use, the developer solution decreases *not only in volume but in strength as well.*

(d) *The developer solution becomes depleted from evaporation and the removal of small amounts from the tank on the film hanger and films.* With time and use, the developer solution decreases *not only in volume but in strength as well.*

REF: p. 112

56. An exhausted developer produces a radiograph with:
   a. Reduced density and increased contrast
   b. Reduced density and reduced contrast
   c. Increased density and increased contrast
   d. Increased density and reduced contrast

Answer: b

Correct: An exhausted developer produces a radiograph with reduced density and reduced contrast.

Incorrect:

(a) An exhausted developer produces a radiograph with reduced density and *reduced contrast.*

(c) An exhausted developer produces a radiograph with *reduced density and reduced contrast.*

(d) An exhausted developer produces a radiograph with *reduced density* and reduced contrast.

REF: p. 112

57. Exhausted fixer produces a radiograph:
   a. With adequate "clearing" of the film
   b. With proper hardening of the film emulsion
   c. That will turn a yellow-brown color because exhausted fixer does not stop the chemical reaction
   d. That will require longer exposure time to achieve comparable contrast and density

Answer: c

Correct: Exhausted fixer produces a radiograph that will turn a yellow-brown color because exhausted fixer does not stop the chemical reaction.

Incorrect:

(a) Exhausted fixer produces a radiograph *that will turn a yellow-brown color because exhausted fixer does not stop the chemical reaction.*

(b) Exhausted fixer produces a radiograph *that will turn a yellow-brown color because exhausted fixer does not stop the chemical reaction.*

(d) Exhausted fixer produces a radiograph *that will turn a yellow-brown color because exhausted fixer does not stop the chemical reaction.*

REF: p. 112

58. To maintain adequate freshness, strength, and solution levels, both developer and fixer solutions must be replenished:
   a. Daily
   b. Weekly
   c. Biweekly
   d. Monthly

Answer: a

Correct: To maintain adequate freshness, strength, and solution levels, both developer and fixer solutions must be replenished daily.

Incorrect:

(b) To maintain adequate freshness, strength, and solution levels, both developer and fixer solutions must be replenished *daily.*

(c) To maintain adequate freshness, strength, and solution levels, both developer and fixer solutions must be replenished *daily.*

(d) To maintain adequate freshness, strength, and solution levels, both developer and fixer solutions must be replenished *daily.*

REF: p. 112

59. The master and insert tanks must be cleaned:
   a. Daily
   b. Each time the solutions are changed
   c. Once every 6 months
   d. Yearly

Answer: b

Correct: The master and insert tanks must be cleaned each time the solutions are changed.

Incorrect:

(a) The master and insert tanks must be cleaned *each time the solutions are changed.*

(c) The master and insert tanks must be cleaned *each time the solutions are changed.*

(d) The master and insert tanks must be cleaned *each time the solutions are changed.*

REF: p. 112

60. Deposits form on the inside walls of the insert tanks because of an interaction between mineral salts in water and _____ in the processing solutions.
   a. sodium thiosulfate
   b. carbonate
   c. acetic acid
   d. hydroquinone

Answer: b

Correct: Deposits form on the inside walls of the insert tanks because of an interaction between mineral salts in water and carbonate in the processing solutions.

Incorrect:

(a) Deposits form on the inside walls of the insert tanks because of an interaction between mineral salts in water and *carbonate* in the processing solutions.

(c) Deposits form on the inside walls of the insert tanks because of an interaction between mineral salts in water and *carbonate* in the processing solutions.

(d) Deposits form on the inside walls of the insert tanks because of an interaction between mineral salts in water and *carbonate* in the processing solutions.

REF: p. 112

61. Which of the following would be the best choice for cleaning the master and insert tanks?
   a. Plain tap water
   b. A solution of hydrochloric acid and water
   c. A powder-type abrasive cleanser
   d. A liquid-type abrasive cleanser

Answer: b

Correct: A solution of hydrochloric acid and water would be the best choice for cleaning the master and insert tanks.

Incorrect:

(a) *A solution of hydrochloric acid and water* would be the best choice for cleaning the master and insert tanks.

(c) Abrasive type cleansers may react unfavorably with the processing solutions.

(d) Abrasive type cleansers may react unfavorably with the processing solutions.

REF: p. 112

62. The major advantage of automatic film processing versus manual film processing is:
   a. Less processing time is required.
   b. Time is manually controlled.
   c. Water temperature is manually controlled.
   d. More sophisticated equipment is used.

Answer: a

Correct: The major advantage of automatic film processing versus manual film processing is less processing time is required.

Incorrect:

(b) Time is automatically controlled.

(c) Water temperature is automatically controlled.

(d) More sophisticated equipment is not necessarily advantageous.

REF: p. 113

63. Which of the following statements is *true* of automatic processing?
   a. Wrapped films are fed into the film feed slot.
   b. The developing chemistry may be used interchangeably between automatic and manual film processing.
   c. Developer solution for automatic processing is heated to the same temperature as developer solution for manual processing.
   d. The film is transported directly from the developer solution into the fixer without a rinsing step.

Answer: d

Correct: In automatic processing, the film is transported directly from the developer solution into the fixer without a rinsing step.

Incorrect:

(a) In automatic processing, *the film is transported directly from the developer solution into the fixer without a rinsing step; unwrapped* films are fed into the film feed slot.

(b) In automatic processing, *the film is transported directly from the developer solution into the fixer without a rinsing step;* the developing chemistry may *not* be used interchangeably between automatic and manual film processing.

(c) In automatic processing, *the film is transported directly from the developer solution into the fixer without a rinsing step;* developer solution for automatic processing is heated *to a higher temperature* than developer solution for manual processing.

REF: p. 113

64. An extraoral cleaning film is used to:
    a. Wipe the rollers off when the processor is disassembled.
    b. Clean residual gelatin or dirt from the rollers.
    c. Disinfect the daylight loader of the automatic processor.
    d. Clean the master tank of a manual processor.

Answer: b

Correct: An extraoral cleaning film is used to clean residual gelatin or dirt from the rollers.

Incorrect:

(a) An extraoral cleaning film is used to *clean residual gelatin or dirt from the rollers.*

(c) An extraoral cleaning film is used to *clean residual gelatin or dirt from the rollers.*

(d) An extraoral cleaning film is used to *clean residual gelatin or dirt from the rollers.*

REF: p. 114

65. Duplicating film:
    a. Is placed inside the patient's mouth
    b. Is the same as intraoral film
    c. Is gray on both sides of the film packet
    d. Requires the use of a film duplicator

Answer: d

Correct: Duplicating film requires the use of a film duplicator.

Incorrect:

(a) Duplicating film *requires the use of a film duplicator;* it is *never* placed inside the patient's mouth.

(b) Duplicating film *requires the use of a film duplicator;* it is *not* the same as intraoral film.

(c) Duplicating film *requires the use of a film duplicator;* it is *white* on both sides of the film packet.

REF: p. 115

66. Underdeveloped films may result from:
    a. Excess development time
    b. Overconcentrated developer solution

c. High developer temperature
d. Low developer temperature

Answer: d

Correct: An underdeveloped film may result from low developer temperature.

Incorrect:

(a) An underdeveloped film may result from *low developer temperature,* or from inadequate development time.

(b) An underdeveloped film may result from *low developer temperature,* or from depleted or contaminated developer solution.

(c) An underdeveloped film may result from *low developer temperature.*

REF: p. 116

67. Overdeveloped films may result from:
    a. Inadequate development time
    b. Overconcentrated developer solution
    c. Low developer temperature
    d. Depleted or contaminated developer solution

Answer: b

Correct: Overdeveloped films may result from overconcentrated developer solution.

Incorrect:

(a) Overdeveloped films may result from *overconcentrated developer solution* or from *excess* development time.

(c) Overdeveloped films may result from *overconcentrated developer solution* or from *high* developer temperature.

(d) Overdeveloped films may result from *overconcentrated developer solution* or from *concentrated* (overactive) developer solution.

REF: p. 117

68. Reticulation means the film appears:
    a. To have white spots
    b. To have dark spots
    c. Cracked
    d. As thin, black branching lines

Answer: c

Correct: Reticulation means the film appears cracked.

Incorrect:

(a) Reticulation means the film appears *cracked;* white spots would be fixer spots.

(b) Reticulation means the film appears *cracked;* dark spots would be developer spots.

(d) Reticulation means the film appears *cracked;* static electricity would appear as thin, black branching lines.

REF: p. 117

69. Insufficient fixation time or insufficient rinsing would lead to:
   a. Overdeveloped film
   b. Reticulation of emulsion
   c. Yellow-brown films
   d. Fixer cutoff

Answer: c
Correct: Insufficient fixation time or insufficient rinsing would lead to yellow-brown films.
Incorrect:
   (a) Insufficient fixation time or insufficient rinsing would lead to *yellow-brown films*.
   (b) Insufficient fixation time or insufficient rinsing would lead to *yellow-brown films*.
   (d) Insufficient fixation time or insufficient rinsing would lead to *yellow-brown films*.
REF: p. 119

70. Developer cutoff appears as a:
   a. Straight white border on the film
   b. Straight black border on the film
   c. Curved white border on the film
   d. Curved black border on the film

Answer: a
Correct: Developer cutoff appears as a straight white border on the film.
Incorrect:
   (b) *Fixer cutoff* appears as a straight black border on the film.
   (c) Developer cutoff appears as a *straight white border on the film*.
   (d) *Cone cutting* creates a curved black border on the film.
REF: p. 118

CHAPTER 10   QUALITY ASSURANCE IN THE DENTAL OFFICE

MULTIPLE CHOICE
1. A calibration test for accurate kilovoltage and milliamperage readings would most likely be performed to ensure that the dental _____ is functioning properly.
   a. x-ray machine
   b. film
   c. film processing
   d. darkroom

Answer: a
Correct: A calibration test for accurate kilovoltage and milliamperage readings would most likely be performed to ensure that the dental x-ray machine is functioning properly.
Incorrect:
   (b) A calibration test for accurate kilovoltage and milliamperage readings would most likely be performed to ensure that the dental *x-ray machine* is functioning properly.
   (c) A calibration test for accurate kilovoltage and milliamperage readings would most likely be performed to ensure that the dental *x-ray machine* is functioning properly.
   (d) A calibration test for accurate kilovoltage and milliamperage readings would most likely be performed to ensure that the dental *x-ray machine* is functioning properly.
REF: p. 129

2. According to the test for dental x-ray film, if the processed film appears clear with a slight blue tint, the film:
   a. Has expired
   b. Is fresh and has been properly stored and protected
   c. Has been improperly stored
   d. Has been exposed to radiation

Answer: b
Correct: According to the test for dental x-ray film, if the processed film appears clear with a slight blue tint, the film is fresh and has been properly stored and protected.
Incorrect:
   (a) According to the test for dental x-ray film, if the processed film appears clear with a slight blue tint, the film *is fresh and has been properly stored and protected*.
   (c) According to the test for dental x-ray film, if the processed film appears clear with a slight blue tint, the film *is fresh and has been properly stored and protected*.
   (d) According to the test for dental x-ray film, if the processed film appears clear with a slight blue tint, the film *is fresh and has been properly stored and protected*.
REF: p. 130

3. Extraoral intensifying screens that appear visibly scratched should:
   a. Be cleaned with commercially available cleaner
   b. Have antistatic solution applied
   c. Be replaced
   d. Be polished and then reused

Answer: c
Correct: Extraoral intensifying screens that appear visibly scratched should be replaced.
Incorrect:
   (a) Extraoral intensifying screens that appear visibly scratched should *be replaced*.
   (b) Extraoral intensifying screens that appear visibly scratched should *be replaced*.
   (d) Extraoral intensifying screens that appear visibly scratched should *be replaced*.
REF: p. 130

4. Extraoral intensifying screens should be cleaned:
   a. Daily
   b. Weekly
   c. Monthly
   d. Yearly

Answer: c
Correct: Extraoral intensifying screens should be cleaned monthly.
Incorrect:
   (a) Extraoral intensifying screens should be cleaned *monthly*.
   (b) Extraoral intensifying screens should be cleaned *monthly*.
   (d) Extraoral intensifying screens should be cleaned *monthly*.
REF: p. 130

5. A film-screen contact test is used to test the:
   a. Output of the x-ray machine
   b. Quality of intraoral films
   c. Cassette holder for extraoral films
   d. Freshness of extraoral film

Answer: c
Correct: A film-screen contact test is used to test the cassette holder for extraoral films.
Incorrect:
   (a) An x-ray output is used to test the output of the x-ray machine.
   (b) A fresh film is used to test the quality of intraoral film.
   (d) A fresh film is used to test the freshness of extraoral film.
REF: p. 130

6. To conduct a film-screen contact test, the wire mesh test object is placed:
   a. On top of the loaded cassette
   b. On the side of the film closest to the tubehead within the loaded cassette
   c. On the side of the film farthest from the tubehead within the loaded cassette
   d. Over the end of the PID

Answer: a
Correct: To conduct a film-screen contact test, the wire mesh test object is placed on top of the loaded cassette.
Incorrect:
   (b) To conduct a film-screen contact test, the wire mesh test object is placed *on top of the loaded cassette*.
   (c) To conduct a film-screen contact test, the wire mesh test object is placed *on top of the loaded cassette*.
   (d) To conduct a film-screen contact test, the wire mesh test object is placed *on top of the loaded cassette*.
REF: p. 130

7. The results of the film-screen contact test should be viewed on a viewbox in a:
   a. Dimly lit room at a distance of 1 foot
   b. Brightly lit room at a distance of 1 foot
   c. Dimly lit room at a distance of 6 feet
   d. Brightly lit room at a distance of 6 feet

Answer: c
Correct: The results of the film-screen contact test should be viewed in a dimly lit room at a distance of 6 feet.
Incorrect:
   (a) This is not the correct choice because viewing at 1 foot would be too close.
   (b) This is not the correct choice because viewing in a brightly lit room degrades contrast, and 1 foot is too close.
   (d) This is not the correct choice because viewing in a brightly lit room degrades contrast.
REF: p. 130

8. To conduct the film-screen contact test, the position-indicating device (PID) should have a _____-inch target-film distance.
   a. 6
   b. 12
   c. 40
   d. 72

Answer: c
Correct: To conduct the film-screen contact test, the PID should have a 40-inch target-film distance.
Incorrect:
   (a) To conduct the film-screen contact test, the PID should have a *40*-inch target-film distance.
   (b) To conduct the film-screen contact test, the PID should have a *40*-inch target-film distance.
   (d) To conduct the film-screen contact test, the PID should have a *40*-inch target-film distance.
REF: p. 130

9. Which of the following statements is *true* of the evaluation of the film-screen contact test?
   a. Areas of poor film-screen contact appear darker than good contact areas.
   b. Areas of poor film-screen contact appear lighter than good contact areas.
   c. If the wire mesh image on the film exhibits varying densities, good film-screen contact has taken place.
   d. Both a and c.

Answer: a
Correct: Areas of poor film-screen contact appear darker than good contact areas.
Incorrect:
   (b) Areas of poor film-screen contact appear *darker* than good contact areas.
   (c) If the wire mesh image on the film exhibits *a uniform density*, good film-screen contact has taken place.

(d) Areas of poor film-screen contact appear darker than good contact areas; however, if the wire mesh image on the film exhibits *a uniform density*, good film-screen contact has taken place.

REF: p. 130

10. The viewbox should emit a uniform and subdued light when it is functioning properly. Permanently discolored plexiglass surfaces and blackened fluorescent light bulbs must be replaced.
    a. Both statements are true.
    b. Both statements are false.
    c. The first statement is true; the second is false.
    d. The first statement is false; the second is true.

Answer: a
Correct: The viewbox should emit a uniform and subdued light when it is functioning properly. Permanently discolored plexiglass surfaces and blackened fluorescent light bulbs must be replaced.
Incorrect:
    (b) The viewbox should emit a uniform and subdued light when it is functioning properly. Permanently discolored plexiglass surfaces and blackened fluorescent light bulbs must be replaced.
    (c) The viewbox should emit a uniform and subdued light when it is functioning properly. Permanently discolored plexiglass surfaces and blackened fluorescent light bulbs must be replaced.
    (d) The viewbox should emit a uniform and subdued light when it is functioning properly. Permanently discolored plexiglass surfaces and blackened fluorescent light bulbs must be replaced.

REF: p. 131

11. During the light leak test for the darkroom:
    a. A flashlight should be used to check for light leaks.
    b. The overhead lights should be off, but the safelight should be on.
    c. All lights within the darkroom should be off.
    d. Light a match within the darkroom and see if any light is visible from the outside.

Answer: c
Correct: During the light leak test for the darkroom, all lights within the darkroom should be off.
Incorrect:
    (a) During the light leak test for the darkroom, *all lights within the darkroom should be off;* a flashlight should *not* be used to check for light leaks.
    (b) During the light leak test for the darkroom, *all lights within the darkroom should be off.*
    (d) During the light leak test for the darkroom, *all lights within the darkroom should be off; do not* light a match within the darkroom and see if any light is visible from the outside.

REF: p. 131

12. Safelighting can be checked with the _____ test.
    a. wire mesh
    b. fogging
    c. coin
    d. stepwedge

Answer: c
Correct: Safelighting can be checked with the coin test.
Incorrect:
    (a) Safelighting can be checked with the *coin* test; the wire mesh test was used for the cassette.
    (b) Safelighting can be checked with the *coin* test; fogging was part of the fresh film test.
    (d) Safelighting can be checked with the *coin* test; the stepwedge was used for contrast.

REF: p. 131

13. To perform the coin test, the film and coin are exposed to _____.
    a. the safelight
    b. the darkroom ceiling or white light
    c. the light with the darkroom door open
    d. no light at all

Answer: a
Correct: To perform the coin test, the film and coin are exposed to the safelight.
Incorrect:
    (b) To perform the coin test, the film and coin are exposed to *the safelight.*
    (c) To perform the coin test, the film and coin are exposed to *the safelight.*
    (d) To perform the coin test, the film and coin are exposed to *the safelight.*

REF: p. 131

14. To conduct the coin test, the film and coin are exposed for:
    a. 10 seconds
    b. 3 or 4 minutes
    c. 15 minutes
    d. An entire workday

Answer: b
Correct: To conduct the coin test, the film and coin are exposed for 3 or 4 minutes.
Incorrect:
    (a) To conduct the coin test, the film and coin are exposed for *3 or 4 minutes.*
    (c) To conduct the coin test, the film and coin are exposed for *3 or 4 minutes.*
    (d) To conduct the coin test, the film and coin are exposed for *3 or 4 minutes.*

REF: p. 131

15. If the image of the coin appears on the processed radiograph after the coin test:
    a. The safelighting is correct.
    b. The safelighting is not safe to use with that type of film.

c. Conduct the test again with the darkroom door closed rather than open.
d. Conduct the test again with the safelight off rather than on.

Answer: b
Correct: If the image of the coin appears on the processed radiograph after the coin test, the safelighting is not safe to use with that type of film.
Incorrect:
(a) If the image of the coin appears on the processed radiograph after the coin test, *the safelighting is not safe to use with that type of film.*
(c) If the image of the coin appears on the processed radiograph after the coin test, *the safelighting is not safe to use with that type of film;* the darkroom door should have been closed to conduct the test the first time.
(d) If the image of the coin appears on the processed radiograph after the coin test, *the safelighting is not safe to use with that type of film;* the safelight should be *on* to conduct the test.
REF: p. 131

16. To test the automatic film processor, _____ in the automatic processor.
a. unwrap one film, expose it to light, and then process the film
b. unwrap one film, do not expose it to light, and then process the film
c. unwrap two unexposed films, expose one to light, and then process the exposed film
d. unwrap two unexposed films, expose one to light, and then process both films

Answer: d
Correct: To test the automatic film processor, unwrap two unexposed films, expose one to light, and then process both films in the automatic processor.
Incorrect:
(a) To test the automatic film processor, *unwrap two unexposed films, expose one to light, and then process both films* in the automatic processor.
(b) To test the automatic film processor, *unwrap two unexposed films, expose one to light, and then process both films* in the automatic processor.
(c) To test the automatic film processor, unwrap two unexposed films, expose one to light, *and then process both films* in the automatic processor.
REF: p. 132

17. The results of the automatic processor test films will be that _____ if the processor is functioning properly.
a. the unexposed film appears clear and dry and the film exposed to light appears black and dry
b. the unexposed film appears clear and wet and the film exposed to light appears black and wet

c. the unexposed film appears black and dry and the film exposed to light appears clear and dry
d. the unexposed film appears black and wet and the film exposed to light appears clear and wet

Answer: a
Correct: The results of the automatic processor test films will be that the unexposed film appears clear and dry and the film exposed to light appears black and dry if the processor is functioning properly.
Incorrect:
(b) The results of the automatic processor test films will be that the unexposed film appears *clear and dry* and the film exposed to light appears *black and dry* if the processor is functioning properly.
(c) The results of the automatic processor test films will be that the unexposed film appears *clear and dry* and the film exposed to light appears *black and dry* if the processor is functioning properly.
(d) The results of the automatic processor test films will be that the unexposed film appears *clear and dry* and the film exposed to light appears *black and dry* if the processor is functioning properly.
REF: p. 132

18. A reference radiograph is used to evaluate:
a. The viewbox
b. Darkroom lighting
c. Safelighting
d. Developer strength

Answer: d
Correct: A reference radiograph is used to evaluate developer strength.
Incorrect:
(a) A reference radiograph is used to evaluate *developer strength.*
(b) A reference radiograph is used to evaluate *developer strength.*
(c) A reference radiograph is used to evaluate *developer strength.*
REF: p. 132

19. To create a reference radiograph, which of the following must be fresh?
(1) Film
(2) Developer
(3) Fixer
a. 1, 2, 3
b. 1, 2
c. 2, 3
d. 1 only

Answer: a
Correct: To create a reference radiograph, the film, developer, and fixer must all be fresh.

Incorrect:

   (b) To create a reference radiograph, the film, developer, and *fixer* must all be fresh.
   (c) To create a reference radiograph, the *film,* developer, and fixer must all be fresh.
   (d) To create a reference radiograph, the film, *developer, and fixer* must all be fresh.

REF: p. 132

20. A reference radiograph is compared with a radiograph taken each day for matched:
   a. Milliamperage
   b. kVp
   c. Color
   d. Density

Answer: d

Correct: A reference radiograph is compared with a radiograph taken each day for matched density.

Incorrect:

   (a) A reference radiograph is compared with a radiograph taken each day for matched *density;* milliamperage is a property of the tubehead and should be consistent for both films.
   (b) A reference radiograph is compared with a radiograph taken each day for matched *density;* kVp is a property of the tubehead and should be consistent for both films.
   (c) A reference radiograph is compared with a radiograph taken each day for matched *density;* radiographs are black and white, not color.

REF: p. 132

21. If the densities seen on the daily radiographs appear darker than those seen on the reference radiographs, the developer solution is (1) weak, (2) too concentrated, (3) cold, and/or (4) too warm.
   a. 1 and 3
   b. 1 and 4
   c. 2 and 3
   d. 2 and 4

Answer: d

Correct: If the densities seen on the daily radiographs appear darker than those seen on the reference radiographs, the developer solution is either too concentrated or too warm.

Incorrect:

   (a) If the densities seen on the daily radiographs appear darker than those seen on the reference radiographs, the developer solution is either *too concentrated or too warm.*
   (b) If the densities seen on the daily radiographs appear darker than those seen on the reference radiographs, the developer solution is either *too concentrated or too warm.*
   (c) If the densities seen on the daily radiographs appear darker than those seen on the reference radiographs, the developer solution is either *too concentrated or too warm.*

REF: p. 133

22. The stepwedge technique for evaluating developer strength relies on exposing one exposed stepwedge film:
   a. Each day
   b. Each week
   c. Every time 20 films have been processed
   d. Every time 40 films have been processed

Answer: a

Correct: The stepwedge technique for evaluating developer strength relies on exposing one exposed stepwedge film each day.

Incorrect:

   (b) The stepwedge technique for evaluating developer strength relies on exposing one exposed stepwedge film *each day.*
   (c) The stepwedge technique for evaluating developer strength relies on exposing one exposed stepwedge film *each day.*
   (d) The stepwedge technique for evaluating developer strength relies on exposing one exposed stepwedge film *each day.*

REF: p. 133

23. When the stepwedge technique is used to evaluate developer strength, if the density on the daily radiograph differs from that on the standard radiograph by more than _____ steps, the developer solution is depleted.
   a. two
   b. three
   c. five
   d. seven

Answer: a

Correct: When the stepwedge technique is used to evaluate developer strength, if the density on the daily radiograph differs from that on the standard radiograph by more than two steps, the developer solution is depleted.

Incorrect:

   (b) When the stepwedge technique is used to evaluate developer strength, if the density on the daily radiograph differs from that on the standard radiograph by more than *two* steps, the developer solution is depleted.
   (c) When the stepwedge technique is used to evaluate developer strength, if the density on the daily radiograph differs from that on the standard radiograph by more than *two* steps, the developer solution is depleted.
   (d) When the stepwedge technique is used to evaluate developer strength, if the density on the daily radiograph differs from that on the standard radiograph by more than *two* steps, the developer solution is depleted.

REF: p. 133

24. The clearing test is used to monitor:
   a. Developer strength
   b. Fixer strength
   c. Water bath temperature
   d. Processing speed

Answer: b
Correct: The clearing test is used to monitor fixer strength.
Incorrect:
   (a) The clearing test is used to monitor *fixer strength*.
   (c) The clearing test is used to monitor *fixer strength*.
   (d) The clearing test is used to monitor *fixer strength*.
REF: p. 134

25. If the film clears in _____ minutes, the chemistry is of adequate strength.
   a. 2
   b. 6
   c. 8
   d. 14

Answer: a
Correct: If the film clears in 2 minutes, the chemistry is of adequate strength.
Incorrect:
   (b) If the film clears in *2* minutes, the chemistry is of adequate strength.
   (c) If the film clears in *2* minutes, the chemistry is of adequate strength.
   (d) If the film clears in *2* minutes, the chemistry is of adequate strength.
REF: p. 134

CHAPTER 11   DENTAL RADIOGRAPHS AND THE DENTAL RADIOGRAPHER

MULTIPLE CHOICE

1. Radiographs are a(n) _____ comprehensive patient care.
   a. adjunct to
   b. necessary component of
   c. option for
   d. supplement to

Answer: b
Correct: Radiographs are a necessary component of comprehensive patient care.
Incorrect:
   (a) Radiographs are a *necessary component of* comprehensive patient care.
   (c) Radiographs are a *necessary component of* comprehensive patient care.
   (d) Radiographs are a *necessary component of* comprehensive patient care.
REF: p. 141

2. The dental radiographer requires which of the following to perform dental radiographic procedures?
   a. Sufficient knowledge
   b. Technical skills
   c. Sufficient knowledge and technical skills
   d. Neither sufficient knowledge nor technical skills

Answer: c
Correct: The dental radiographer requires sufficient knowledge and technical skills to perform dental radiographic procedures.
Incorrect:
   (a) The dental radiographer requires sufficient knowledge *and technical skills* to perform dental radiographic procedures.
   (b) The dental radiographer requires *sufficient knowledge and* technical skills to perform dental radiographic procedures.
   (d) The dental radiographer requires *sufficient knowledge and technical skills* to perform dental radiographic procedures.
REF: p. 141

3. An oral examination limits the practitioner to knowledge of what is seen clinically. Dental radiographs allow the practitioner to see many conditions that are not apparent clinically.
   a. Both statements are true.
   b. Both statements are false.
   c. The first statement is true; the second is false.
   d. The first statement is false; the second is true.

Answer: a
Correct: An oral examination limits the practitioner to knowledge of what is seen clinically. Dental radiographs allow the practitioner to see many conditions that are not apparent clinically.
Incorrect:
   (b) An oral examination limits the practitioner to knowledge of what is seen clinically. Dental radiographs allow the practitioner to see many conditions that are not apparent clinically.
   (c) An oral examination limits the practitioner to knowledge of what is seen clinically. Dental radiographs allow the practitioner to see many conditions that are not apparent clinically.
   (d) An oral examination limits the practitioner to knowledge of what is seen clinically. Dental radiographs allow the practitioner to see many conditions that are not apparent clinically.
REF: p. 141

4. Radiographs enable the dental professional to see _____ conditions that may otherwise go undetected.
   a. rare
   b. occasional common
   c. occasional
   d. many

Answer: d
Correct: Radiographs enable the dental professional to see many conditions that may otherwise go undetected.

(a) Radiographs enable the dental professional to see *many* conditions that may otherwise go undetected.

(b) Radiographs enable the dental professional to see *many* conditions that may otherwise go unde-tected.

(c) Radiographs enable the dental professional to see *many* conditions that may otherwise go undetected.

REF: p. 141

5. According to the text, "_____ is one of the most important uses of dental radiographs."
   a. habitual rote frequency
   b. detection
   c. maintaining a routine
   d. insurance verification

Answer: b

Correct: According to the text, "detection is one of the most important uses of dental radiographs."

Incorrect:

(a) According to the text, "*detection* is one of the most important uses of dental radiographs," not habitual rote frequency.

(c) According to the text, "*detection* is one of the most important uses of dental radiographs," not maintaining a routine.

(d) According to the text, "*detection* is one of the most important uses of dental radiographs," not insurance verification.

REF: p. 141

6. Through the use of dental radiographs, the dental radiographer can detect _____ that cannot be detected clinically.
   (1) diseases
   (2) lesions
   (3) conditions of teeth and bones
      a. 1, 2, 3
      b. 1, 2
      c. 2, 3
      d. 3 only

Answer: a

Correct: Through the use of dental radiographs, the dental radiographer can detect diseases, lesions, and conditions of teeth and bones that cannot be detected clinically.

Incorrect:

(b) Through the use of dental radiographs, the dental radiographer can detect diseases, lesions, and *conditions of teeth and bones* that cannot be detected clinically.

(c) Through the use of dental radiographs, the dental radiographer can detect *diseases,* lesions, and conditions of teeth and bones that cannot be detected clinically.

(d) Through the use of dental radiographs, the dental radiographer can detect *diseases, lesions,* and conditions of teeth and bones that cannot be detected clinically.

REF: p. 141

7. When radiographs are properly prescribed, exposed, and processed, the benefit of disease detection _____ the risk of small doses of x-radia-tion.
   a. does not outweigh
   b. is considered equal
   c. slightly outweighs
   d. far outweighs

Answer: d

Correct: When radiographs are properly prescribed, exposed, and processed, the benefit of disease detection far outweighs the risk of small doses of x-radiation.

Incorrect:

(a) When radiographs are properly prescribed, exposed, and processed, the benefit of disease detection *far outweighs* the risk of small doses of x-radiation.

(b) When radiographs are properly prescribed, exposed, and processed, the benefit of disease detection *far outweighs* the risk of small doses of x-radiation.

(c) When radiographs are properly prescribed, exposed, and processed, the benefit of disease detection *far outweighs* the risk of small doses of x-radiation.

REF: p. 141

8. A _____ may be a dental radiographer.
   (1) dental hygienist
   (2) dental assistant
   (3) dentist
      a. 1, 2, 3
      b. 1, 2
      c. 1, 3
      d. 3 only

Answer: a

Correct: A dental hygienist, dental assistant, or dentist may be a dental radiographer.

Incorrect:

(b) A dental hygienist, dental assistant, or *dentist* may be a dental radiographer.

(c) A dental hygienist, *dental assistant,* or dentist may be a dental radiographer.

(d) A *dental hygienist, dental assistant,* or dentist may be a dental radiographer.

REF: p. 142

9. Assigned responsibilities of dental auxiliaries in regard to dental radiography may include the:
   a. Mounting and identification of dental radiographs
   b. Implementation and monitoring of quality control procedures
   c. Education of patients about dental radiography
   d. Choices a, b, and c

Answer: d

Correct: Assigned responsibilities of dental auxiliaries in regard to dental radiography may include the mounting and identification of dental radiographs, implementation and monitoring of quality control procedures, and education of patients about dental radiography.

Incorrect:

(a) Assigned responsibilities of dental auxiliaries in regard to dental radiography may include the mounting and identification of dental radiographs, *implementation and monitoring of quality control procedures, and education of patients about dental radiography;* all are permitted depending on the state dental practice act.

(b) Assigned responsibilities of dental auxiliaries in regard to dental radiography may include the *mounting and identification of dental radiographs,* implementation and monitoring of quality control procedures, *and education of patients about dental radiography;* all are permitted depending on the state dental practice act.

(c) Assigned responsibilities of dental auxiliaries in regard to dental radiography may include the *mounting and identification of dental radiographs, implementation and monitoring of quality control procedures,* and education of patients about dental radiography; all are permitted depending on the state dental practice act.

REF: p. 142

10. Retakes resulting in unnecessary patient exposure to x-radiation must be avoided:
    a. Whenever it is convenient because the dose is so low
    b. Only if the patient is uncomfortable with exposure
    c. Only if older (pre-1975) equipment is used
    d. At all times

Answer: d

Correct: Retakes resulting in unnecessary patient exposure to x-radiation must be avoided at all times.

Incorrect:

(a) Retakes resulting in unnecessary patient exposure to x-radiation must be avoided *at all times.*

(b) Retakes resulting in unnecessary patient exposure to x-radiation must be avoided *at all times.*

(c) Retakes resulting in unnecessary patient exposure to x-radiation must be avoided *at all times.*

REF: p. 142

11. To avoid occupational exposure to x-radiation, the dental radiographer must always:
    (*Note:* All are true, but one is the most critical and encompasses the others.)
    a. Maintain an adequate distance
    b. Have proper positioning
    c. Have proper shielding
    d. Avoid the primary beam

Answer: d

Correct: To avoid occupational exposure to x-radiation, the dental radiographer must always avoid the primary beam.

Incorrect:

(a) To avoid occupational exposure to x-radiation, the dental radiographer must always *avoid the primary beam.*

(c) To avoid occupational exposure to x-radiation, the dental radiographer must always *avoid the primary beam.*

(d) To avoid occupational exposure to x-radiation, the dental radiographer must always *avoid the primary beam.*

REF: p. 142

CHAPTER 12   PATIENT RELATIONS AND THE DENTAL RADIOGRAPHER

MULTIPLE CHOICE

1. Which of the following would be an example of the use of interpersonal skills rather than technical skills with patients?
    a. Proper maintenance of processing equipment
    b. Discussing the rationale for use of dental radiographs
    c. Correct film positioning
    d. Preventing light leaks in the darkroom

Answer: b

Correct: Discussing the rationale for use of dental radiographs would be an example of the use of interpersonal skills rather than technical skills with patients.

Incorrect:

(a) Proper maintenance of processing equipment would be an example of technical skills.

(c) Correct film positioning would be an example of technical skills.

(d) Preventing light leaks in the darkroom would be an example of technical skills.

REF: p. 146

2. Communication is defined by the text as:
    a. Having a conversation
    b. Establishing a connection
    c. The process by which information is exchanged between two or more persons
    d. Two or more persons in the same location or room

Answer: c

Correct: Communication is defined by the text as the process by which information is exchanged between two or more persons.

Incorrect:
- (a) Communication is defined by the text as *the process by which information is exchanged between two or more persons.*
- (b) Communication is defined by the text as *the process by which information is exchanged between two or more persons.*
- (d) Communication is defined by the text as *the process by which information is exchanged between two or more persons.*

REF: p. 146

3. Good verbal communication skills for dental radiographers involve:
   a. Speaking in a rushed manner to convince the patient that the radiographer is working hard
   b. Using words such as "cut," "drill," and "scrape" to put the procedure in the patient's language so that the patient may understand
   c. A loud tone of voice so that the patient may hear clearly
   d. A soft tone of voice

Answer: d
Correct: Good verbal communication skills for dental radiographers involve a soft tone of voice.
Incorrect:
- (a) Good verbal communication skills for dental radiographers involve *a soft tone of voice.*
- (b) Good verbal communication skills for dental radiographers involve *a soft tone of voice.*
- (c) Good verbal communication skills for dental radiographers involve *a soft tone of voice.*

REF: p. 146

4. _____ is a nonverbal communication skill associated with interest and warmth.
   a. Leaning slightly away from the patient
   b. A slumped posture
   c. Tapping fingers
   d. An attentive posture

Answer: d
Correct: An attentive posture is a nonverbal communication skill associated with interest and warmth.
Incorrect:
- (a) *An attentive posture* is a nonverbal communication skill associated with interest and warmth.
- (b) *An attentive posture* is a nonverbal communication skill associated with interest and warmth.
- (c) *An attentive posture* is a nonverbal communication skill associated with interest and warmth.

REF: p. 146

5. When nonverbal messages are not consistent with verbal messages, the patient is more likely to:
   a. Relax
   b. Trust the dental professional
   c. Respond with apprehension
   d. Both a and b

Answer: c
Correct: When nonverbal messages are not consistent with verbal messages, the patient is more likely to respond with apprehension.
Incorrect:
- (a) When nonverbal messages are not consistent with verbal messages, the patient is more likely to *respond with apprehension.*
- (b) When nonverbal messages are not consistent with verbal messages, the patient is more likely to *respond with apprehension.*
- (d) When nonverbal messages are not consistent with verbal messages, the patient is more likely to *respond with apprehension.*

REF: p. 146

6. When listening to a patient, the dental radiographer should:
   a. Interrupt if the patient gets "off track."
   b. Correct the patient if he or she is wrong.
   c. Finish the patient's sentences to show that the radiographer is following the patient's train of thought.
   d. Give the patient undivided attention.

Answer: d
Correct: When listening to a patient, the dental radiographer should give the patient undivided attention.
Incorrect:
- (a) When listening to a patient, the dental radiographer should *give the patient undivided attention;* never interrupt the patient.
- (b) When listening to a patient, the dental radiographer should *give the patient undivided attention;* never correct the patient.
- (c) When listening to a patient, the dental radiographer should *give the patient undivided attention;* never finish the patient's sentences.

REF: p. 147

7. The term *facilitation* means:
   a. Initiating
   b. The act of making easier
   c. The act of continuing
   d. Construction of a facility

Answer: b
Correct: The term *facilitation* means the act of making easier.
Incorrect:
- (a) The term *facilitation* means *the act of making easier.*
- (c) The term *facilitation* means *the act of making easier.*
- (d) The term *facilitation* means *the act of making easier.*

REF: p. 147

8. When a patient trusts the dental professional, the patient is:
   a. Less likely to provide information
   b. Less likely to cooperate during treatment
   c. More likely to comply with prescribed treatment
   d. Less likely to return for further treatment

Answer: c
Correct: When a patient trusts the dental professional, the patient is more likely to comply with prescribed treatment.
Incorrect:
   (a) When a patient trusts the dental professional, the patient is *more likely to comply with prescribed treatment.*
   (b) When a patient trusts the dental professional, the patient is *more likely to comply with prescribed treatment.*
   (d) When a patient trusts the dental professional, the patient is *more likely to comply with prescribed treatment.*
REF: p. 147

9. Inviting a patient to ask questions:
   a. Wastes time
   b. Discourages communication
   c. Enhances communication
   d. Intimidates the patient

Answer: c
Correct: Inviting a patient to ask questions enhances communication.
Incorrect:
   (a) Inviting a patient to ask questions *enhances communication.*
   (b) Inviting a patient to ask questions *enhances communication.*
   (d) Inviting a patient to ask questions *enhances communication.*
REF: p. 147

10. The patient's first impression of the dental team most often involves the:
   a. Dentist
   b. Dental hygienist
   c. Dental auxiliary
   d. Entrance to the building

Answer: c
Correct: The patient's first impression of the dental team most often involves the dental auxiliary.
Incorrect:
   (a) The patient's first impression of the dental team most often involves the *dental auxiliary.*
   (b) The patient's first impression of the dental team most often involves the *dental auxiliary.*
   (d) The patient's first impression of the dental team most often involves the *dental auxiliary.*
REF: p. 147

CHAPTER 13   PATIENT EDUCATION AND THE DENTAL RADIOGRAPHER

MULTIPLE CHOICE
1. Patient education is likely to result in decreased:
   a. Acceptance of prescribed treatment
   b. Fears of x-ray exposure
   c. Cooperation
   d. Motivation for regular dental visits

Answer: b
Correct: Patient education is likely to result in decreased fears of x-ray exposure.
Incorrect:
   (a) Patient education is likely to result in decreased *fears of x-ray exposure;* it is likely to result in increased acceptance of prescribed treatment.
   (c) Patient education is likely to result in decreased *fears of x-ray exposure;* it is likely to result in increased cooperation.
   (d) Patient education is likely to result in decreased *fears of x-ray exposure;* it is likely to result in increased motivation for regular dental visits.
REF: p. 151

2. A patient who is knowledgeable about the importance of dental radiographs is:
   a. Less likely to realize the benefit of dental radiographs
   b. Less likely to follow prevention plans
   c. More likely to accept prescribed treatment
   d. Both a and c

Answer: c
Correct: A patient who is knowledgeable about the importance of dental radiographs is more likely to accept prescribed treatment.
Incorrect:
   (a) A patient who is knowledgeable about the importance of dental radiographs is *likely to realize the benefits* of dental radiographs.
   (b) A patient who is knowledgeable about the importance of dental radiographs is *likely to follow prevention plans.*
   (d) A patient who is knowledgeable about the importance of dental radiographs is *likely to realize the benefits* of dental radiographs.
REF: p. 151

3. The dental radiographer can use _____ to educate the dental patient.
   a. an oral presentation
   b. printed literature
   c. a combination of oral presentation and printed literature
   d. neither oral presentation nor printed literature

Answer: c
Correct: The dental radiographer can use a combination of oral presentation and printed literature to educate the dental patient.

107

Incorrect:
   (a) The dental radiographer can use *a combination of oral presentation and printed literature* to educate the dental patient.
   (b) The dental radiographer can use *a combination of oral presentation and printed literature* to educate the dental patient.
   (d) The dental radiographer can use *a combination of oral presentation and printed literature* to educate the dental patient.
REF: p. 151

4. Which of the following types of questions must be answered only by the dentist?
   a. The need for dental radiographs
   b. X-ray exposure
   c. Questions about diagnosis
   d. The safety of dental x-rays

Answer: c
Correct: Questions about diagnosis must be answered only by the dentist.
Incorrect:
   (a) *Questions about the need for dental radiographs* may be answered by auxiliaries.
   (b) *Questions about x-ray exposure* may be answered by auxiliaries.
   (d) *Questions about the safety of dental x-rays* must be answered by auxiliaries.
REF: p. 151

5. To answer questions about the necessity of dental x-ray films, tell the patient:
   a. They are an option, not a necessity.
   b. There are many diseases and conditions that cannot be detected simply by looking into the mouth.
   c. All diseases and conditions produce signs and symptoms that render x-ray films unnecessary.
   d. Tooth decay, gum disease, cysts, and tumors all can be detected eventually simply by looking in the mouth.

Answer: b
Correct: To answer questions about the necessity of dental x-ray films, tell the patient there are many diseases and conditions that cannot be detected simply by looking into the mouth.
Incorrect:
   (a) To answer questions about the necessity of dental x-ray films, tell the patient *there are many diseases and conditions that cannot be detected simply by looking into the mouth;* they are a *necessity,* not an option.
   (c) To answer questions about the necessity of dental x-ray films, tell the patient *there are many diseases and conditions that cannot be detected simply by looking into the mouth;* many diseases and conditions produce *no* signs or symptoms.

   (d) To answer questions about the necessity of dental x-ray films, tell the patient *there are many diseases and conditions that cannot be detected simply by looking into the mouth.*
REF: p. 152

6. There is _____ interval between x-ray examinations.
   a. no set time
   b. a set 6-month
   c. a set 12-month
   d. a set 24-month

Answer: a
Correct: There is no set time interval between x-ray examinations.
Incorrect:
   (b) There is *no set time* interval between x-ray examinations
   (c) There is *no set time* interval between x-ray examinations.
   (d) There is *no set time* interval between x-ray examinations.
REF: p. 152

7. Decisions about the number, type, and frequency of dental x-rays are determined by the _____ based on the patient's individual needs.
   a. insurance company
   b. dental assistant
   c. dental hygienist
   d. dentist

Answer: d
Correct: Decisions about the number, type, and frequency of dental x-rays are determined by the dentist based on the patient's individual needs.
Incorrect:
   (a) Decisions about the number, type, and frequency of dental x-rays are determined by the *dentist* based on the patient's individual needs.
   (b) Decisions about the number, type, and frequency of dental x-rays are determined by the *dentist* based on the patient's individual needs.
   (c) Decisions about the number, type, and frequency of dental x-rays are determined by the *dentist* based on the patient's individual needs.
REF: p. 152

8. A patient with gum disease will require:
   a. Less frequent radiographic examinations than a patient without such disease.
   b. Less frequent radiographic examinations than a patient without such disease if pocket depth readings are regularly recorded.
   c. Radiographic examinations at regular intervals regardless of circumstances.
   d. More frequent radiographic examinations than a patient without such disease.

Answer: d

Correct: A patient with gum disease will require more frequent radiographic examinations than a patient without such disease.

Incorrect:
(a) A patient with gum disease will require *more frequent radiographic examinations than a patient without such disease.*
(b) A patient with gum disease will require *more frequent radiographic examinations than a patient without such disease.*
(c) A patient with gum disease will require *more frequent radiographic examinations than a patient without such disease.*

REF: p. 152

9. The time interval between radiographic examinations for children should be based on:
   a. Their age
   b. The individual needs of the child
   c. A 6-month interval for bite-wing films
   d. A 12-month interval for bite-wing films

Answer: b

Correct: The time interval between radiographic examinations for children should be based on the individual needs of the child.

Incorrect:
(a) The time interval between radiographic examinations for children should be based on *the individual needs of the child;* there is no set time interval between x-ray examinations.
(c) The time interval between radiographic examinations for children should be based on *the individual needs of the child;* there is no set time interval between x-ray examinations.
(d) The time interval between radiographic examinations for children should be based on *the individual needs of the child;* there is no set time interval between x-ray examinations.

REF: p. 152

10. Radiographs from a previous dentist may be used, provided they are:
    a. Recent
    b. Of acceptable diagnostic quality
    c. Original films
    d. Both a and b

Answer: d

Correct: Radiographs from a previous dentist may be used, provided they are recent and of acceptable diagnostic quality.

Incorrect:
(a) Radiographs from a previous dentist may be used, provided they are recent *and of acceptable diagnostic quality.*
(b) Radiographs from a previous dentist may be used, provided they are *recent and* of acceptable diagnostic quality.

(c) Radiographs from a previous dentist may be used, provided they are *recent and of acceptable diagnostic quality.*

REF: p. 152

11. With faster F-speed film, a single intraoral film results in a surface skin exposure of _____ milliroentgens.
    a. 1.25
    b. 12.5
    c. 125
    d. 1250

Answer: c

Correct: With faster F-speed film, a single intraoral film results in a surface skin exposure of 125 milliroentgens.

Incorrect:
(a) With faster F-speed film, a single intraoral film results in a surface skin exposure of *125* milliroentgens.
(b) With faster F-speed film, a single intraoral film results in a surface skin exposure of *125* milliroentgens.
(d) With faster F-speed film, a single intraoral film results in a surface skin exposure of *125* milliroentgens.

REF: p. 153

12. For dental x-rays to produce permanent skin damage, such as skin cancer, exposures in the range of _____ roentgens are needed.
    a. 10
    b. hundreds of
    c. thousands of
    d. millions of

Answer: c

Correct: For dental x-rays to produce permanent skin damage, such as skin cancer, exposures in the range of thousands of roentgens are needed.

Incorrect:
(a) For dental x-rays to produce permanent skin damage, such as skin cancer, exposures in the range of *thousands of* roentgens are needed.
(b) For dental x-rays to produce permanent skin damage, such as skin cancer, exposures in the range of *thousands of* roentgens are needed.
(d) For dental x-rays to produce permanent skin damage, such as skin cancer, exposures in the range of *thousands of* roentgens are needed.

REF: p. 153

13. Exposures in the range of thousands of roentgens are _____ in dental radiography.
    a. often exceeded
    b. exceeded with full mouth series
    c. rarely exceeded
    d. inconceivable

109

Answer: d
Correct: Exposures in the range of thousands of roentgens are inconceivable in dental radiography.
Incorrect:
  (a) Exposures in the range of thousands of roentgens are *inconceivable* in dental radiography.
  (b) Exposures in the range of thousands of roentgens are *inconceivable* in dental radiography.
  (c) Exposures in the range of thousands of roentgens are *inconceivable* in dental radiography.
REF: p. 153

14. According to the "Guidelines for Prescribing Dental Radiographs," dental x-ray procedures _____ because of pregnancy.
  a. must be avoided
  b. should be minimized
  c. should be limited to emergency care
  d. do not need to be altered

Answer: d
Correct: According to the "Guidelines for Prescribing Dental Radiographs," dental x-ray procedures do not need to be altered because of pregnancy.
Incorrect:
  (a) According to the "Guidelines for Prescribing Dental Radiographs," dental x-ray procedures *do not need to be altered* because of pregnancy.
  (b) According to the "Guidelines for Prescribing Dental Radiographs," dental x-ray procedures *do not need to be altered* because of pregnancy.
  (c) According to the "Guidelines for Prescribing Dental Radiographs," dental x-ray procedures *do not need to be altered* because of pregnancy.
REF: p. 153

15. How many recorded cases are there of a patient developing cancer from diagnostic x-rays?
  a. Zero
  b. Less than 50
  c. Between 50 and 100
  d. More than 100

Answer: a
Correct: There are zero recorded cases of a patient developing cancer from diagnostic x-rays.
Incorrect:
  (b) There are *zero* recorded cases of a patient developing cancer from diagnostic x-rays.
  (c) There are *zero* recorded cases of a patient developing cancer from diagnostic x-rays.
  (d) There are *zero* recorded cases of a patient developing cancer from diagnostic x-rays.
REF: p. 153

16. A panoramic radiograph can be substituted for a complete series of dental radiographs. A panoramic radiograph does not clearly reveal changes in teeth, such as tooth decay, or the details of the supporting bone.

  a. Both statements are true.
  b. Both statements are false.
  c. The first statement is true; the second statement is false.
  d. The first statement is false; the second statement is true.

Answer: d
Correct: A panoramic radiograph *cannot* be substituted for a complete series of dental radiographs. A panoramic radiograph does not clearly reveal changes in teeth, such as tooth decay, or the details of the supporting bone.
Incorrect:
  (a) A panoramic radiograph *cannot* be substituted for a complete series of dental radiographs. A panoramic radiograph does not clearly reveal changes in teeth, such as tooth decay, or the details of the supporting bone.
  (b) A panoramic radiograph *cannot* be substituted for a complete series of dental radiographs. A panoramic radiograph does not clearly reveal changes in teeth, such as tooth decay, or the details of the supporting bone.
  (c) A panoramic radiograph *cannot* be substituted for a complete series of dental radiographs. A panoramic radiograph does not clearly reveal changes in teeth, such as tooth decay, or the details of the supporting bone.
REF: p. 153

17. Original dental radiographs are the property of:
  a. The dentist
  b. The patient
  c. Both patient and dentist
  d. The government

Answer: a
Correct: Original dental radiographs are the property of the dentist.
Incorrect:
  (b) Original dental radiographs are the property of *the dentist.*
  (c) Original dental radiographs are the property of *the dentist.*
  (d) Original dental radiographs are the property of *the dentist.*
REF: p. 153

CHAPTER 14 LEGAL ISSUES AND THE DENTAL RADIOGRAPHER

MULTIPLE CHOICE
  1. The Consumer-Patient Radiation Health and Safety Act:
     (1) Outlines requirements for the safe use of dental x-ray equipment.
     (2) Establishes guidelines for the proper maintenance of x-ray equipment.

(3) Requires persons who take dental radiographs to be properly trained and certified.
  a. 1, 2, 3
  b. 1, 2
  c. 2, 3
  d. 1, 3

Answer: a

Correct: The Consumer-Patient Radiation Health and Safety Act outlines requirements for the safe use of dental x-ray equipment, establishes guidelines for the proper maintenance of x-ray equipment, and requires persons who take dental radiographs to be properly trained and certified.

Incorrect:
  (b) The Consumer-Patient Radiation Health and Safety Act outlines requirements for the safe use of dental x-ray equipment, establishes guidelines for the proper maintenance of x-ray equipment, *and requires persons who take dental radiographs to be properly trained and certified.*
  (c) The Consumer-Patient Radiation Health and Safety Act *outlines requirements for the safe use of dental x-ray equipment,* establishes guidelines for the proper maintenance of x-ray equipment, and requires persons who take dental radiographs to be properly trained and certified.
  (d) The Consumer-Patient Radiation Health and Safety Act outlines requirements for the safe use of dental x-ray equipment, *establishes guidelines for the proper maintenance of x-ray equipment,* and requires persons who take dental radiographs to be properly trained and certified.

REF: p. 157

2. The Consumer-Patient Radiation Health and Safety Act is a _____ law.
  a. federal
  b. state
  c. county
  d. city

Answer: a

Correct: The Consumer-Patient Radiation Health and Safety Act is a federal law.

Incorrect:
  (b) The Consumer-Patient Radiation Health and Safety Act is a *federal* law.
  (c) The Consumer-Patient Radiation Health and Safety Act is a *federal* law.
  (d) The Consumer-Patient Radiation Health and Safety Act is a *federal* law.

REF: p. 157

3. The process of informing the patient about the particulars of exposing dental radiographs is termed:
  a. A treatment alternative
  b. Disclosure
  c. Self-determination
  d. Behavior modification

Answer: b

Correct: The process of informing the patient about the particulars of exposing dental radiographs is termed disclosure.

Incorrect:
  (a) The process of informing the patient about the particulars of exposing dental radiographs is termed *disclosure.*
  (c) The process of informing the patient about the particulars of exposing dental radiographs is termed *disclosure.*
  (d) The process of informing the patient about the particulars of exposing dental radiographs is termed *disclosure.*

REF: p. 157

4. Informed consent:
  a. Must be in language that the patient can readily understand
  b. Does not require that patients have their questions answered before x-ray exposure
  c. Is waived if the patient is a minor
  d. Does not require that patients receive enough information to make informed choices

Answer: a

Correct: Informed consent must be in language that the patient can readily understand.

Incorrect:
  (b) *Informed consent must be in language that the patient can readily understand;* it *does* require that patients have their questions answered before x-ray exposure.
  (c) *Informed consent must be in language that the patient can readily understand;* it must be obtained from a legal guardian if the patient is a minor.
  (d) *Informed consent must be in language that the patient can readily understand;* it *does* require that patients receive enough information to make informed choices.

REF: p. 158

5. If the patient is a minor, informed consent:
  a. Is waived
  b. May still be obtained from the patient
  c. Must be obtained from the parent
  d. Must be obtained from a legal guardian

Answer: d

Correct: If the patient is a minor, informed consent must be obtained from a legal guardian.

Incorrect:
  (a) If the patient is a minor, informed consent *is not waived.*
  (b) If the patient is a minor, informed consent *must be obtained from a legal guardian.*
  (c) If the patient is a minor, informed consent *must be obtained from a legal guardian.*

REF: p. 158

6. Generally, there are _____ elements to informed consent.
   a. two
   b. three
   c. four
   d. six

Answer: c
Correct: Generally, there are four elements to informed consent: the purpose of the procedure, benefits, risks, and the opportunity for the patient to ask questions.
Incorrect:
   (a) Generally, there are *four* elements to informed consent: the purpose of the procedure, benefits, risks, and the opportunity for the patient to ask questions.
   (b) Generally, there are *four* elements to informed consent: the purpose of the procedure, benefits, risks, and the opportunity for the patient to ask questions.
   (d) Generally, there are *four* elements to informed consent: the purpose of the procedure, benefits, risks, and the opportunity for the patient to ask questions.
REF: p. 158

7. If informed consent is not obtained from a patient before the exposure of dental radiographs, a patient may legally claim:
   a. Negligence
   b. Malpractice
   c. Malpractice or negligence
   d. Disclosure

Answer: c
Correct: If informed consent is not obtained from a patient before the exposure of dental radiographs, a patient may legally claim malpractice or negligence.
Incorrect:
   (a) If informed consent is not obtained from a patient before the exposure of dental radiographs, a patient may legally claim *malpractice or* negligence.
   (b) If informed consent is not obtained from a patient before the exposure of dental radiographs, a patient may legally claim malpractice *or negligence.*
   (d) If informed consent is not obtained from a patient before the exposure of dental radiographs, a patient may legally claim *malpractice or negligence.*
REF: p. 158

8. Lack of informed consent may be shown by the following:
   a. Consent from an individual under the influence of drugs or alcohol
   b. Consent from an individual with legal right to give it
   c. Consent from an individual under duress
   d. Both a and c

Answer: d
Correct: Lack of informed consent may be shown by consent from an individual under the influence of drugs or alcohol or consent from an individual under duress.
Incorrect:
   (a) Lack of informed consent may be shown by consent from an individual under the influence of drugs or alcohol *or consent from an individual under duress.*
   (b) Lack of informed consent may be shown by *consent from an individual under the influence of drugs or alcohol or consent from an individual under duress.*
   (c) Lack of informed consent may be shown by *consent from an individual under the influence of drugs or alcohol or* consent from an individual under duress.
REF: p. 158

9. The trend in dental negligence or malpractice actions has historically been to sue the supervising dentist alone. However, cases exist in which the dentist and the dental auxiliary have both been sued for the actions of the dental auxiliary.
   a. Both statements are true.
   b. Both statements are false.
   c. The first statement is true; the second statement is false.
   d. The first statement is false; the second statement is true.

Answer: a
Correct: The trend in dental negligence or malpractice actions has historically been to sue the supervising dentist alone. However, cases exist in which the dentist and the dental auxiliary have both been sued for the actions of the dental auxiliary.
Incorrect:
   (b) The trend in dental negligence or malpractice actions has historically been to sue the supervising dentist alone. However, cases exist in which the dentist and the dental auxiliary have both been sued for the actions of the dental auxiliary.
   (c) The trend in dental negligence or malpractice actions has historically been to sue the supervising dentist alone. *However, cases exist in which the dentist and the dental auxiliary have both been sued for the actions of the dental auxiliary.*
   (d) *The trend in dental negligence or malpractice actions has historically been to sue the supervising dentist alone.* However, cases exist in which the dentist and the dental auxiliary have both been sued for the actions of the dental auxiliary.
REF: p. 158

10. The standard of care can be defined as the quality of care that is provided by dental practitioners in _____ locality under the _____ conditions.
   a. any; similar or very different
   b. a similar; same or similar
   c. any; same or similar
   d. a similar; similar or very different

Answer: b

Correct: The standard of care can be defined as the quality of care that is provided by dental practitioners in a similar locality under the same or similar conditions.

Incorrect:
   (a) The standard of care can be defined as the quality of care that is provided by dental practitioners in *a similar* locality under the *same or similar* conditions.
   (c) The standard of care can be defined as the quality of care that is provided by dental practitioners in a *similar* locality under the same or similar conditions.
   (d) The standard of care can be defined as the quality of care that is provided by dental practitioners in a similar locality under *the same or similar* conditions.

REF: p. 158

11. Which of the following statements is *true* of the statute of limitations?
   (1) It often begins when the patient discovers or should have discovered that an injury has occurred as a result of dental negligence.
   (2) It is the time period during which a patient may bring a malpractice action.
   (3) It may not begin until years after the dental negligence occurred.
      a. 1, 2, 3
      b. 1, 3
      c. 1, 2
      d. 2, 3

Answer: a

Correct: The statute of limitations (1) often begins when the patient discovers or should have discovered that an injury has occurred as a result of dental negligence, (2) is the time period during which a patient may bring a malpractice action, and (3) may not begin until years after the dental negligence occurred.

Incorrect:
   (b) The statute of limitations often begins when the patient discovers or should have discovered that an injury has occurred as a result of dental negligence, *is the time period during which a patient may bring a malpractice action,* and may not begin until years after the dental negligence occurred.
   (c) The statute of limitations often begins when the patient discovers or should have discovered that

an injury has occurred as a result of dental negligence, is the time period during which a patient may bring a malpractice action, *and may not begin until years after the dental negligence occurred.*

   (d) The statute of limitations *often begins when the patient discovers or should have discovered that an injury has occurred as a result of dental negligence,* is the time period during which a patient may bring a malpractice action, and may not begin until years after the dental negligence occurred.

REF: p. 158

12. Which of the following statements is *true* of radiographs and the patient's dental record?
   a. Radiographs may be discarded when outdated.
   b. It is advised to keep patient radiographs in a file separate from patient charts.
   c. The dental record must include documentation of the number and type of radiographs exposed.
   d. Dental radiographs are an optional rather than integral part of the dental record.

Answer: c

Correct: The dental record must include documentation of the number and type of radiographs exposed.

Incorrect:
   (a) *The dental record must include documentation of the number and type of radiographs exposed;* radiographs should *not* be discarded when outdated.
   (b) *The dental record must include documentation of the number and type of radiographs exposed;* it is *not* advised to keep patient radiographs in a file separate from patient charts.
   (d) *The dental record must include documentation of the number and type of radiographs exposed;* dental radiographs are an *integral* part of the dental record.

REF: p. 159

13. Erroneous entries in the dental record should:
   a. Be erased
   b. Be blocked out
   c. Be covered with white-out
   d. Never be erased or blocked out

Answer: d

Correct: Erroneous entries in the dental record should never be erased or blocked out.

Incorrect:
   (a) Erroneous entries in the dental record should *never be erased or blocked out.*
   (b) Erroneous entries in the dental record should *never be erased or blocked out.*
   (c) Erroneous entries in the dental record should *never be erased or blocked out.*

REF: p. 159

113

14. It is appropriate for any dental professional to discuss a patient's care with:
  (1) Another patient
  (2) Office staff members who are not involved in the treatment of the patient
  (3) Another dentist involved in the patient's care
  (4) A physician with whom care is shared
    a. 1, 2, 3, 4
    b. 1, 2, 3
    c. 1, 2
    d. 3, 4

Answer: d
Correct: It is appropriate for any dental professional to discuss a patient's care with another dentist involved in the patient's care or a physician with whom care is shared.
Incorrect:
  (a) It is appropriate for any dental professional to discuss a patient's care with *another dentist involved in the patient's care or a physician with whom care is shared;* it is *not* appropriate to discuss patient care with another patient or office staff members who are not involved in the treatment of the patient.
  (b) It is appropriate for any dental professional to discuss a patient's care *with another dentist involved in the patient's care;* it is *not* appropriate to discuss patient care with another patient or office staff members who are not involved in the treatment of the patient.
  (c) It is appropriate for any dental professional to discuss a patient's care with *another dentist involved in the patient's care or a physician with whom care is shared;* it is *not* appropriate to discuss patient care with another patient or office staff members who are not involved in the treatment of the patient.
REF: p. 159

15. Radiographs are the property of the dentist:
  a. Unless they were paid for by the patient
  b. Unless they were paid for by the insurance company
  c. Only if the patient has signed a waiver
  d. Period

Answer: d
Correct: Radiographs are the property of the dentist, period.
Incorrect:
  (a) Radiographs are the property of the dentist, *period.*
  (b) Radiographs are the property of the dentist, *period.*
  (c) Radiographs are the property of the dentist, *period.*
REF: p. 159

16. When radiographs are forwarded to a subsequent dentist:
  a. The original films should be forwarded.
  b. Duplicate films should be forwarded unless the patient signs a release for original films.
  c. The original films should be copied and then forwarded; retain the duplicate.
  d. The original films should not be forwarded.

Answer: d
Correct: When radiographs are forwarded to a subsequent dentist, the original films should not be forwarded.
Incorrect:
  (a) When radiographs are forwarded to a subsequent dentist, the original films should *not* be forwarded.
  (b) When radiographs are forwarded to a subsequent dentist, *the original films should not be forwarded.*
  (c) When radiographs are forwarded to a subsequent dentist, the original films should *not* be forwarded.
REF: p. 159

CHAPTER 15   INFECTION CONTROL AND THE DENTAL RADIOGRAPHER

MULTIPLE CHOICE
  1. Infectious diseases may be transmitted from:
  (1) A patient to the dental professional
  (2) The dental professional to a patient
  (3) One patient to another patient
    a. 1, 2, 3
    b. 1, 3
    c. 2, 3
    d. 1, 2

Answer: a
Correct: Infectious diseases may be transmitted from a patient to the dental professional, from the dental professional to a patient, and from one patient to another patient.
Incorrect:
  (b) Infectious diseases may be transmitted from a patient to the dental professional, *from the dental professional to a patient,* and from one patient to another patient.
  (c) Infectious diseases may be transmitted *from a patient to the dental professional,* from the dental professional to a patient, and from one patient to another patient.
  (d) Infectious diseases may be transmitted from a patient to the dental professional, from the dental professional to a patient, and *from one patient to another patient.*
REF: p. 163

2. Pathogens are:
   a. Any microorganisms
   b. Bacteria but not viruses
   c. Viruses but not bacteria
   d. Microorganisms capable of causing disease

Answer: d
Correct: Pathogens are microorganisms capable of causing disease.
Incorrect:
   (a) Pathogens are *microorganisms capable of causing disease.*
   (b) Pathogens are *microorganisms capable of causing disease.*
   (c) Pathogens are *microorganisms capable of causing disease.*
REF: p. 163

3. Which of the following viruses may be present in oral secretions?
   (1) Cytomegalovirus
   (2) Hepatitis B virus
   (3) Herpes simplex virus
   (4) Human immunodeficiency virus
   a. 1, 2, 3, 4
   b. 2, 3, 4
   c. 1, 2, 3
   d. 2, 4

Answer: a
Correct: Cytomegalovirus, hepatitis B virus, herpes simplex virus, and human immunodeficiency virus all may be present in oral secretions.
Incorrect:
   (b) *Cytomegalovirus,* hepatitis B virus, herpes simplex virus, and human immunodeficiency virus *all* may be present in oral secretions.
   (c) Cytomegalovirus, hepatitis B virus, herpes simplex virus, and *human immunodeficiency virus all* may be present in oral secretions.
   (d) *Cytomegalovirus,* hepatitis B virus, *herpes simplex virus,* and human immunodeficiency virus *all* may be present in oral secretions.
REF: p. 163

4. _____ is defined as the absence of pathogens, or disease-causing microorganisms.
   a. Antiseptic
   b. Antibiotic
   c. Antiinfective
   d. Asepsis

Answer: d
Correct: Asepsis is defined as the absence of pathogens, or disease-causing microorganisms.
Incorrect:
   (a) *Asepsis* is defined as the absence of pathogens, or disease-causing microorganisms.
   (b) *Asepsis* is defined as the absence of pathogens, or disease-causing microorganisms.

   (c) *Asepsis* is defined as the absence of pathogens, or disease-causing microorganisms.
REF: p. 163

5. Antiseptic is:
   a. The absence of pathogens, or disease-causing microorganisms
   b. A substance that inhibits the growth of bacteria
   c. The use of a chemical or physical procedure to inhibit or destroy pathogens
   d. The act of sterilizing

Answer: b
Correct: Antiseptic is a substance that inhibits the growth of bacteria.
Incorrect:
   (a) Antiseptic is *a substance that inhibits the growth of bacteria;* asepsis is the absence of pathogens, or disease-causing microorganisms.
   (c) Antiseptic is *a substance that inhibits the growth of bacteria;* disinfect is the use of a chemical or physical procedure to inhibit or destroy pathogens.
   (d) Antiseptic is *a substance that inhibits the growth of bacteria;* sterilization is the act of sterilizing.
REF: p. 163

6. Highly resistant bacterial and mycotic (fungal) spores are not killed during disinfection procedures; however, highly resistant bacterial and mycotic spores are killed during sterilization.
   a. Both statements are true.
   b. Both statements are false.
   c. The first statement is true; the second statement is false.
   d. The first statement is false; the second statement is true.

Answer: a
Correct: Highly resistant bacterial and mycotic (fungal) spores are not killed during disinfection procedures; however, highly resistant bacterial and mycotic spores are killed during sterilization.
Incorrect:
   (b) Highly resistant bacterial and mycotic (fungal) spores are not killed during disinfection procedures; however, highly resistant bacterial and mycotic spores are killed during sterilization.
   (c) Highly resistant bacterial and mycotic (fungal) spores are not killed during disinfection procedures; *however, highly resistant bacterial and mycotic spores are killed during sterilization.*
   (d) *Highly resistant bacterial and mycotic (fungal) spores are not killed during disinfection procedures;* however, highly resistant bacterial and mycotic spores are killed during sterilization.
REF: p. 163

115

7. Recommendations concerning gloves would fall under which of the following categories of infection control practices that directly relate to dental radiography procedures?
   a. Protective attire and barrier techniques
   b. Handwashing and care of hands
   c. Sterilization or disinfection of instruments
   d. Cleaning and disinfection of dental unit and environmental surfaces

Answer: a
Correct: Recommendations concerning gloves would fall under protective attire and barrier techniques.
Incorrect:
   (b) Recommendations concerning gloves would fall under *protective attire and barrier techniques.*
   (c) Recommendations concerning gloves would fall under *protective attire and barrier techniques.*
   (d) Recommendations concerning gloves would fall under *protective attire and barrier techniques.*
REF: p. 164

8. Protective clothing:
   a. Must prevent skin exposure when contact with blood or other bodily fluids is anticipated
   b. Must prevent mucous membrane exposure when contact with blood or other bodily fluids is anticipated
   c. Should be worn home and laundered daily
   d. Both a and b

Answer: d
Correct: Protective clothing must prevent skin and mucous membrane exposure when contact with blood or other bodily fluids is anticipated.
Incorrect:
   (a) Protective clothing must prevent skin *and mucous membrane* exposure when contact with blood or other bodily fluids is anticipated.
   (b) Protective clothing must prevent *skin and* mucous membrane exposure when contact with blood or other bodily fluids is anticipated.
   (c) Protective clothing *must prevent skin and mucous membrane exposure when contact with blood or other bodily fluids is anticipated;* it should not be worn home and laundered daily.
REF: p. 164

9. _____ when using medical latex or vinyl gloves.
   a. Gloves may be rewashed between patients and reused until damaged
   b. Nonsterile gloves are recommended for examinations and nonsurgical procedures
   c. Hands should not be washed before gloving
   d. Hands should not be washed between patients

Answer: b
Correct: Nonsterile gloves are recommended for examinations and nonsurgical procedures when using medical latex or vinyl gloves.

Incorrect:
   (a) *Nonsterile gloves are recommended for examinations and nonsurgical procedures* when using medical latex or vinyl gloves; gloves should *never* be rewashed between patients or reused until damaged.
   (c) *Nonsterile gloves are recommended for examinations and nonsurgical procedures* when using medical latex or vinyl gloves; hands *must* be washed before gloves are worn.
   (d) *Nonsterile gloves are recommended for examinations and nonsurgical procedures* when using medical latex or vinyl gloves; dental professionals must *always* wash their hands and reglove between patients.
REF: p. 164

10. All dental professionals must use surgical masks and protective eyewear to protect the eyes and face:
    a. Only during surgical procedures
    b. Whenever the high-speed handpiece is used
    c. Whenever spatter and aerosolized sprays of blood and saliva are likely
    d. If desired

Answer: c
Correct: All dental professionals must use surgical masks and protective eyewear to protect the eyes and face whenever spatter and aerosolized sprays of blood and saliva are likely.
Incorrect:
   (a) All dental professionals must use surgical masks and protective eyewear to protect the eyes and face *whenever spatter and aerosolized sprays of blood and saliva are likely.*
   (b) All dental professionals must use surgical masks and protective eyewear to protect the eyes and face *whenever spatter and aerosolized sprays of blood and saliva are likely.*
   (d) All dental professionals must use surgical masks and protective eyewear to protect the eyes and face *whenever spatter and aerosolized sprays of blood and saliva are likely.*
REF: p. 164

11. Critical instruments are defined as instruments:
    a. That are used to penetrate soft tissue or bone
    b. That contact but do not penetrate soft tissue
    c. That contact but do not penetrate bone
    d. Or devices that do not come in contact with mucous membranes

Answer: a
Correct: Critical instruments are defined as instruments that are used to penetrate soft tissue or bone.
Incorrect:
   (b) Critical instruments are defined as instruments *that are used to penetrate soft tissue or bone.*
   (c) Critical instruments are defined as instruments *that are used to penetrate soft tissue or bone.*

(d) Critical instruments are defined as instruments *that are used to penetrate soft tissue or bone.*

REF: p. 165

12. In dental radiography, no _____ are used.
    (1) critical instruments
    (2) semicritical instruments
    (3) noncritical instruments
        a. 1, 2, 3
        b. 1, 2
        c. 3 only
        d. 1 only

Answer: d
Correct: In dental radiography, no critical instruments are used.
Incorrect:
    (a) In dental radiography, no *critical instruments* are used.
    (b) In dental radiography, no *critical instruments* are used.
    (c) In dental radiography, no *critical instruments* are used.

REF: p. 165

13. Which of the following are considered to be semicritical instruments?
    a. The exposure button
    b. The x-ray control panel
    c. The lead apron
    d. X-ray film–holding devices

Answer: d
Correct: X-ray film–holding devices are considered to be semicritical instruments.
Incorrect:
    (a) The *exposure button* is considered to be a noncritical instrument.
    (b) The *x-ray control panel* is considered to be a noncritical instrument.
    (c) The *lead apron* is considered to be a noncritical instrument.

REF: p. 165

14. Which of the following statements is *true* concerning cleaning and disinfection of the dental unit and environmental surfaces?
    a. An intermediate-level disinfectant is recommended.
    b. A low-level disinfectant is recommended.
    c. EPA-registered chemical germicides labeled as both hospital disinfectants and tuberculocidals are classified as low-level disinfectants.
    d. Both a and c.

Answer: a
Correct: An intermediate-level disinfectant is recommended for cleaning and disinfection of the dental unit and environmental surfaces.

Incorrect:
    (b) An *intermediate-level disinfectant* is recommended for cleaning and disinfection of the dental unit and environmental surfaces.
    (c) EPA-registered chemical germicides labeled as both hospital disinfectants and tuberculocidals are classified as *intermediate-level disinfectants.*
    (d) An intermediate-level disinfectant is recommended for cleaning and disinfection of the dental unit and environmental surfaces; EPA-registered chemical germicides labeled as both hospital disinfectants and tuberculocidals are classified as *intermediate-level disinfectants.*

REF: p. 165

15. Before dental x-ray films are exposed, the treatment area must be prepared using:
    a. Antiseptic
    b. Aseptic technique
    c. Sterilization of critical instruments
    d. Low-level disinfectant

Answer: b
Correct: Before dental x-ray films are exposed, the treatment area must be prepared using aseptic technique.
Incorrect:
    (a) Before dental x-ray films are exposed, the treatment area must be prepared using *aseptic technique.*
    (c) Before dental x-ray films are exposed, the treatment area must be prepared using *aseptic technique.*
    (d) Before dental x-ray films are exposed, the treatment area must be prepared using *aseptic technique.*

REF: p. 166

16. Covering exposed surfaces with disposable materials _____ adequate protection _____ the need for surface cleaning and disinfection between patients.
    a. provides; while eliminating
    b. provides; but does not eliminate
    c. does not provide; but does eliminate
    d. neither provides; nor eliminates

Answer: a
Correct: Covering exposed surfaces with disposable materials provides adequate protection while eliminating the need for surface cleaning and disinfection between patients.
Incorrect:
    (b) Covering exposed surfaces with disposable materials provides adequate protection *while eliminating* the need for surface cleaning and disinfection between patients.
    (c) Covering exposed surfaces with disposable materials *provides* adequate protection while eliminating the need for surface cleaning and disinfection between patients.

117

Test Bank

(d) Covering exposed surfaces with disposable materials *provides* adequate protection *while eliminating* the need for surface cleaning and disinfection between patients.

REF: p. 166

17. Which of the following surfaces on the x-ray machine must be covered or disinfected?
    (1) Control panel
    (2) Exposure button
    (3) Tubehead
    (4) Position-indicating device (PID)
       a. 1, 2, 3, 4
       b. 1, 2, 3
       c. 2, 3, 4
       d. 2 only

Answer: a
Correct: The control panel, exposure button, tubehead, and PID must all be covered or disinfected.
Incorrect:
    (b) The control panel, exposure button, tubehead, *and PID* must all be covered or disinfected.
    (c) The *control panel,* exposure button, tubehead, and PID must all be covered or disinfected.
    (d) The *control panel,* exposure button, *tubehead, and PID* must all be covered or disinfected.
REF: p. 166

18. Commercially available barrier envelopes:
    a. Minimize contamination before exposure of the film
    b. Minimize contamination after exposure of the film
    c. Are made of a material that blocks the passage of photons
    d. Are made of a material that blocks the passage of electrons

Answer: b
Correct: Commercially available barrier envelopes minimize contamination after exposure of the film.
Incorrect:
    (a) Commercially available barrier envelopes minimize contamination *after* exposure of the film.
    (c) Commercially available barrier envelopes *minimize contamination after exposure of the film;* they are *not* made of a material that blocks the passage of photons.
    (d) Commercially available barrier envelopes *minimize contamination after exposure of the film;* they are *not* made of a material that blocks the passage of electrons.
REF: p. 167

19. Preparation of supplies and equipment involves sterilizing which of the following items?
    a. Film
    b. Film-holding devices

c. Lead apron
d. PID

Answer: b
Correct: Film-holding devices are sterilized during the preparation of supplies and equipment.
Incorrect:
    (a) *Film-holding devices* are sterilized during the preparation of supplies and equipment; the film is not sterilized, but it is disinfected.
    (c) *Film-holding devices* are sterilized during the preparation of supplies and equipment; the lead apron is not sterilized, but it is disinfected.
    (d) *Film-holding devices* are sterilized during the preparation of supplies and equipment; the PID is not sterilized, but it is disinfected.
REF: p. 167

20. After seating the patient, the radiographer must complete which of the following procedures before washing the hands and putting on gloves?
    (1) Chair adjustment
    (2) Headrest adjustment
    (3) Placing the lead apron
       a. 1, 2, 3
       b. 1, 2
       c. 2, 3
       d. 3 only

Answer: a
Correct: The radiographer must complete the chair adjustment, headrest adjustment, and placing the lead apron before washing the hands and putting on gloves.
Incorrect:
    (b) The radiographer must complete the chair adjustment, headrest adjustment, *and placing the lead apron* before washing the hands and putting on gloves.
    (c) The radiographer must complete the *chair adjustment,* headrest adjustment, and placing the lead apron before washing the hands and putting on gloves.
    (d) The radiographer must complete the *chair adjustment, headrest adjustment,* and placing the lead apron before washing the hands and putting on gloves.
REF: p. 167

21. Which of the following items should be removed by the patient during preparation for radiographic procedures?
    (1) Eyeglasses
    (2) Dentures
    (3) Chewing gum
       a. 1, 2, 3
       b. 2, 3
       c. 1, 3
       d. 2 only

Answer: a

Correct: Eyeglasses, dentures, and chewing gum should be removed by the patient during preparation for radiographic procedures.

Incorrect:
(b) *Eyeglasses,* dentures, and chewing gum should be removed by the patient during preparation for radiographic procedures.
(c) Eyeglasses, *dentures,* and chewing gum should be removed by the patient during preparation for radiographic procedures.
(d) *Eyeglasses,* dentures, *and chewing gum* should be removed by the patient during preparation for radiographic procedures.

REF: p. 167

22. Preparation of the dental radiographer should include:
    a. Removing film-holding devices before handwashing.
    b. Removing film-holding devices after handwashing but before placing gloves.
    c. Mandatory use of a surgical mask and protective eyewear.
    d. Optional use of a surgical mask and protective eyewear.

Answer: d

Correct: Preparation of the dental radiographer should include optional use of a surgical mask and protective eyewear.

Incorrect:
(a) Preparation of the dental radiographer should include *optional use of a surgical mask and protective eyewear;* film-holding devices must be removed from sterilized packages with gloved hands in the presence of the patient.
(b) Preparation of the dental radiographer should include *optional use of a surgical mask and protective eyewear;* film-holding devices must be removed from sterilized packages with gloved hands in the presence of the patient.
(c) Preparation of the dental radiographer should include *optional* use of a surgical mask and protective eyewear.

REF: p. 167

23. Exposed films should _____ dried and then placed in a _____ for transport to the darkroom for processing.
    a. not be; gloved hand
    b. be; gloved hand
    c. not be; disposable container
    d. be; disposable container

Answer: d

Correct: Exposed films should be dried and then placed in a disposable container for transport to the darkroom for processing.

Incorrect:
(a) Exposed films should *be* dried and then placed in a *disposable container* for transport to the darkroom for processing.
(b) Exposed films should be dried and then placed in a *disposable container* for transport to the darkroom for processing.
(c) Exposed films should *be* dried and then placed in a disposable container for transport to the darkroom for processing.

REF: p. 168

24. When handling film with barrier envelopes, the barrier envelopes are opened with _____ hands and the films unwrapped with _____ hands.
    a. gloved; gloved
    b. gloved; nongloved
    c. nongloved; gloved
    d. nongloved; nongloved

Answer: b

Correct: When handling film with barrier envelopes, the barrier envelopes are opened with gloved hands and the films unwrapped with nongloved hands.

Incorrect:
(a) When handling film with barrier envelopes, the barrier envelopes are opened with gloved hands and the films unwrapped with *nongloved* hands.
(c) When handling film with barrier envelopes, the barrier envelopes are opened with *gloved* hands and the films unwrapped with *nongloved* hands.
(d) When handling film with barrier envelopes, the barrier envelopes are opened with *gloved* hands and the films unwrapped with nongloved hands.

REF: p. 168

25. When handling film with barrier envelopes, the films are unwrapped with _____ hands, and when handling film without barrier envelopes, the films are unwrapped with _____ hands.
    a. gloved; gloved
    b. gloved; nongloved
    c. nongloved; gloved
    d. nongloved; nongloved

Answer: c

Correct: When handling film with barrier envelopes, the films are unwrapped with nongloved hands, and when handling film without barrier envelopes, the films are unwrapped with gloved hands

Incorrect:
(a) When handling film with barrier envelopes, the films are unwrapped with *nongloved* hands, and when handling film without barrier envelopes, the films are unwrapped with gloved hands.
(b) When handling film with barrier envelopes, the films are unwrapped with *nongloved* hands, and

119

when handling film without barrier envelopes, the films are unwrapped with *gloved* hands.

(d) When handling film with barrier envelopes, the films are unwrapped with nongloved hands, and when handling film without barrier envelopes, the films are unwrapped with *gloved* hands.

REF: p. 168

CHAPTER 16 INTRODUCTION TO RADIOGRAPHIC EXAMINATIONS

MULTIPLE CHOICE

1. The _____ intraoral radiographic examination is used to examine the entire tooth (crown and root) and supporting bone.
   a. periapical
   b. interproximal
   c. occlusal
   d. panoramic

Answer: a

Correct: The periapical intraoral radiographic examination is used to examine the entire tooth (crown and root) and supporting bone.

Incorrect:
   (b) The *periapical* intraoral radiographic examination is used to examine the entire tooth (crown and root) and supporting bone; the interproximal examination does not show the entire root.
   (c) The *periapical* intraoral radiographic examination is used to examine the entire tooth (crown and root) and supporting bone.
   (d) The *periapical* intraoral radiographic examination is used to examine the entire tooth (crown and root) and supporting bone; the panoramic examination is an *extraoral* film.

REF: p. 177

2. There are _____ methods for obtaining periapical radiographs.
   a. two
   b. three
   c. five
   d. ten

Answer: a

Correct: There are two methods for obtaining periapical radiographs.

Incorrect:
   (b) There are *two* methods for obtaining periapical radiographs.
   (c) There are *two* methods for obtaining periapical radiographs.
   (d) There are *two* methods for obtaining periapical radiographs.

REF: p. 177

3. Which of the following methods is/are used for obtaining periapical radiographs?
   a. Paralleling
   b. Bisecting
   c. Interproximal
   d. Both a and b

Answer: d

Correct: Paralleling and bisecting are methods for obtaining periapical radiographs.

Incorrect:
   (a) Paralleling *and bisecting* are methods for obtaining periapical radiographs.
   (b) *Paralleling and* bisecting are methods for obtaining periapical radiographs.
   (c) *Paralleling and bisecting* are methods for obtaining periapical radiographs; interproximal films are bite-wing films, not periapical films.

REF: p. 177

4. Which technique examines the crowns of both maxillary and mandibular teeth on a single film?
   a. Periapical paralleling technique
   b. Periapical bisecting technique
   c. Occlusal technique
   d. Interproximal examination

Answer: d

Correct: The interproximal examination examines the crowns of both maxillary and mandibular teeth on a single film.

Incorrect:
   (a) The periapical paralleling technique examines the crowns of both the maxillary and mandibular teeth, but not on a single film.
   (b) The periapical bisecting technique examines the crowns of the maxillary or mandibular teeth.
   (c) The periapical bisecting technique examines the crowns of the maxillary or mandibular teeth.

REF: p. 177

5. The bite-wing film is used in the:
   a. Periapical paralleling technique
   b. Periapical bisecting technique
   c. Occlusal technique
   d. Interproximal examination

Answer: d

Correct: The bite-wing film is used in the interproximal examination.

Incorrect:
   (a) A periapical film is used in the paralleling or bisecting technique.
   (b) A periapical film is used in the paralleling or bisecting technique.
   (c) An occlusal film is used in the occlusal technique.

REF: p. 177

6. *CMRS* stands for:
   a. Complete mouth restorative series
   b. Complete mouth radiographic series
   c. Complete mouth restorative service
   d. Complete mouth radiographic service

Answer: b
Correct: *CMRS* stands for complete mouth radiographic series.
Incorrect:
   (a) *CMRS* stands for complete mouth *radiographic* series.
   (c) CMRS stands for complete mouth *radiographic series*.
   (d) CMRS stands for complete mouth radiographic *series*.
REF: p. 177

7. The CMRS is defined as a series of intraoral dental radiographs that shows:
   a. All the dentulous tooth-bearing areas of the upper and lower jaws
   b. All the edentulous tooth-bearing areas of the upper and lower jaws
   c. All the dentulous or edentulous tooth-bearing areas of the upper and lower jaws
   d. All the dentulous tooth-bearing areas of the upper and lower jaws that can be verified clinically

Answer: c
Correct: The CMRS is defined as a series of intraoral dental radiographs that shows all the dentulous or edentulous tooth-bearing areas of the upper and lower jaws.
Incorrect:
   (a) The CMRS is defined as a series of intraoral dental radiographs that shows all the dentulous *or edentulous* tooth-bearing areas of the upper and lower jaws.
   (b) The CMRS is defined as a series of intraoral dental radiographs that shows all the *dentulous or* edentulous tooth-bearing areas of the upper and lower jaws.
   (d) The CMRS is defined as a series of intraoral dental radiographs that shows all the dentulous *or edentulous* tooth-bearing areas of the upper and lower jaws.
REF: p. 177

8. A total of _____ to _____ films may be included in the CMRS.
   a. 4; 7
   b. 7; 14
   c. 14; 19
   d. 19; 21

Answer: c
Correct: A total of 14 to 19 films may be included in the CMRS.

Incorrect:
   (a) A total of *14 to 19* films may be included in the CMRS.
   (b) A total of *14 to 19* films may be included in the CMRS.
   (d) A total of *14 to 19* films may be included in the CMRS.
REF: p. 178

9. In a patient without teeth, _____ periapical films are usually sufficient to cover the edentulous areas.
   a. 4
   b. 7
   c. 14
   d. 18

Answer: c
Correct: In a patient without teeth, 14 periapical films are usually sufficient to cover the edentulous areas.
Incorrect:
   (a) In a patient without teeth, *14* periapical films are usually sufficient to cover the edentulous areas.
   (b) In a patient without teeth, *14* periapical films are usually sufficient to cover the edentulous areas.
   (d) In a patient without teeth, *14* periapical films are usually sufficient to cover the edentulous areas.
REF: p. 178

10. Which of the following is an extraoral technique for radiographic examination?
   a. Panoramic
   b. Interproximal
   c. Periapical
   d. Occlusal

Answer: a
Correct: The panoramic film is an extraoral technique for radiographic examination.
Incorrect:
   (b) The *interproximal* film is an intraoral technique for radiographic examination.
   (c) The *periapical* film is an intraoral technique for radiographic examination.
   (d) The *occlusal* film is an intraoral technique for radiographic examination.
REF: p. 178

11. Periapical radiographs must show the entire crowns and roots of the teeth being examined as well as _____ to _____ mm beyond the root apices.
   a. 0.1; 0.5
   b. 1.0; 2.0
   c. 2.0; 3.0
   d. 4.0; 5.0

Answer: c
Correct: Periapical radiographs must show the entire crowns and roots of the teeth being examined as well as 2.0 to 3.0 mm beyond the root apices.

121

(a) Periapical radiographs must show the entire crowns and roots of the teeth being examined as well as *2.0 to 3.0* mm beyond the root apices.

(b) Periapical radiographs must show the entire crowns and roots of the teeth being examined as well as *2.0 to 3.0* mm beyond the root apices.

(d) Periapical radiographs must show the entire crowns and roots of the teeth being examined as well as *2.0 to 3.0* mm beyond the root apices.

REF: p. 178

CHAPTER 17 PARALLELING TECHNIQUE

MULTIPLE CHOICE

1. *Parallel* is defined as:
a. To cut across or through
b. Intersecting at or forming a right angle
c. Moving or lying in the same plane, always separated by the same distance and not intersecting
d. An angle of 90 degrees formed by two lines perpendicular to each other

Answer: c

Correct: *Parallel* is defined as moving or lying in the same plane, always separated by the same distance and not intersecting.

Incorrect:
(a) *Intersecting* is defined as *to cut across or through.*
(b) *Perpendicular* is defined as *intersecting at or forming a right angle.*
(d) *Right angle* is defined as *an angle of 90 degrees formed by two lines perpendicular to each other.*

REF: p. 182

2. According to the basic principles of the paralleling technique, the film is placed in the mouth _____ to the long axis of the tooth being radiographed, and the central ray of the x-ray beam is directed _____ to the film and long axis of the tooth.
a. parallel; perpendicular
b. parallel; parallel
c. perpendicular; parallel
d. perpendicular; perpendicular

Answer: a

Correct: According to the basic principles of the paralleling technique, the film is placed in the mouth parallel to the long axis of the tooth being radiographed, and the central ray of the x-ray beam is directed perpendicular to the film and long axis of the tooth.

Incorrect:
(b) According to the basic principles of the paralleling technique, the film is placed in the mouth parallel to the long axis of the tooth being radiographed, and the central ray of the x-ray

beam is directed *perpendicular* to the film and long axis of the tooth.

(c) According to the basic principles of the paralleling technique, the film is placed in the mouth *parallel* to the long axis of the tooth being radiographed, and the central ray of the x-ray beam is directed *perpendicular* to the film and long axis of the tooth.

(d) According to the basic principles of the paralleling technique, the film is placed in the mouth *parallel* to the long axis of the tooth being radiographed, and the central ray of the x-ray beam is directed perpendicular to the film and long axis of the tooth.

REF: p. 183

3. To achieve parallelism between the film and the tooth, the _____ distance must be increased to keep the film parallel with the long axis of the tooth.
a. target-object
b. object-film
c. target-film
d. operator-patient

Answer: b

Correct: To achieve parallelism between the film and the tooth, the object-film distance must be increased to keep the film parallel with the long axis of the tooth.

Incorrect:
(a) To achieve parallelism between the film and the tooth, the *object-film* distance must be increased to keep the film parallel with the long axis of the tooth.

(c) To achieve parallelism between the film and the tooth, the *object-film* distance must be increased to keep the film parallel with the long axis of the tooth.

(d) To achieve parallelism between the film and the tooth, the *object-film* distance must be increased to keep the film parallel with the long axis of the tooth.

REF: p. 183

4. An increased _____ distance results in increased image magnification.
a. target-object
b. object-film
c. target-film
d. operator-patient

Answer: b

Correct: An increased object-film distance results in increased image magnification.

Incorrect:
(a) An increased *object-film* distance results in increased image magnification.

(c) An increased *object-film* distance results in increased image magnification.

(d) An increased *object-film* distance results in increased image magnification.
REF: p. 183

5. An increased _____ distance can compensate for image magnification.
   a. target-object
   b. object-film
   c. target-film
   d. operator-patient

Answer: c
Correct: An increased target-film distance can compensate for image magnification.
Incorrect:
   (a) An increased *target-film* distance can compensate for image magnification.
   (b) An increased *target-film* distance can compensate for image magnification.
   (d) An increased *target-film* distance can compensate for image magnification.
REF: p. 183

6. Which of the following is a disposable film holder designed for one-time use only?
   a. Rinn XCP instruments
   b. Precision film holders
   c. Stabe bite-block
   d. EEZEE-Grip film holder

Answer: c
Correct: The Stabe bite-block is a disposable film holder designed for one-time use only.
Incorrect:
   (a) Rinn XCP instruments are autoclaved between patients.
   (b) Precision film holders are autoclaved between patients.
   (d) The EEZEE-Grip film holder is autoclaved between patients.
REF: p. 184

7. Reusable film holders must be _____ after each use.
   a. rinsed with tap water
   b. wiped with disinfectant
   c. placed in an immersion disinfectant
   d. sterilized

Answer: d
Correct: Reusable film holders must be sterilized after each use.
Incorrect:
   (a) Rinsing with tap water is insufficient; reusable film holders must be sterilized after each use.
   (b) Wiping with disinfectant is inadequate; reusable film holders must be sterilized after each use.
   (c) Placing in an immersion disinfectant is insufficient; reusable film holders must be sterilized after each use.
REF: p. 184

8. Which of the following film holders include aiming rings that aid in the alignment of the position-indicating device (PID) with the film?
   a. Hemostat with bite-block
   b. Stabe bite-block
   c. EEZEE-Grip film holder
   d. Rinn XCP instruments

Answer: d
Correct: Rinn XCP instruments include aiming rings that aid in the alignment of the PID with the film.
Incorrect:
   (a) *Rinn XCP instruments* include aiming rings that aid in the alignment of the PID with the film.
   (b) *Rinn XCP instruments* include aiming rings that aid in the alignment of the PID with the film.
   (c) *Rinn XCP instruments* include aiming rings that aid in the alignment of the PID with the film.
REF: p. 184

9. The authors recommend using size _____ film for anterior teeth and size _____ film for posterior teeth.
   a. 1; 1
   b. 2; 2
   c. 1; 2
   d. 2; 1

Answer: c
Correct: The authors recommend using size 1 film for anterior teeth and size 2 film for posterior teeth.
Incorrect:
   (a) The authors recommend using size 1 film for anterior teeth and size *2* film for posterior teeth.
   (b) The authors recommend using size *1* film for anterior teeth and size 2 film for posterior teeth.
   (d) The authors recommend using size *1* film for anterior teeth and size *2* film for posterior teeth.
REF: p. 185

10. According to the text, size 1 film is always positioned with the long portion of the film in a _____ direction, and size 2 film is always positioned with the long portion of the film in a _____ direction.
   a. vertical; vertical
   b. horizontal; horizontal
   c. vertical; horizontal
   d. horizontal; vertical

Answer: c
Correct: According to the text, size 1 film is always positioned with the long portion of the film in a vertical direction, and size 2 film is always positioned with the long portion of the film in a horizontal direction.
Incorrect:
   (a) According to the text, size 1 film is always positioned with the long portion of the film in a vertical direction, and size 2 film is always

123

Test Bank

positioned with the long portion of the film in a *horizontal* direction.

(b) According to the text, size 1 film is always positioned with the long portion of the film in a *vertical* direction, and size 2 film is always positioned with the long portion of the film in a horizontal direction.

(d) According to the text, size 1 film is always positioned with the long portion of the film in a *vertical* direction, and size 2 film is always positioned with the long portion of the film in a *horizontal* direction.

REF: p. 185

11. Anterior film placements are less likely to cause the patient to gag. Once the gag reflex is stimulated, the patient may gag on films that could normally be tolerated.
   a. Both statements are true.
   b. Both statements are false.
   c. The first statement is true; the second statement is false.
   d. The first statement is false; the second statement is true.

Answer: a
Correct: Anterior film placements are less likely to cause the patient to gag. Once the gag reflex is stimulated, the patient may gag on films that could normally be tolerated.
Incorrect:
   (b) Anterior film placements are less likely to cause the patient to gag. Once the gag reflex is stimulated, the patient may gag on films that could normally be tolerated.
   (c) Anterior film placements are less likely to cause the patient to gag. *Once the gag reflex is stimulated, the patient may gag on films that could normally be tolerated.*
   (d) *Anterior film placements are less likely to cause the patient to gag.* Once the gag reflex is stimulated, the patient may gag on films that could normally be tolerated.

REF: p. 189

12. With size 1 film, a total of _____ anterior film placements are used in the paralleling technique.
   a. four
   b. six
   c. seven
   d. eight

Answer: c
Correct: With size 1 film, a total of seven anterior film placements are used in the paralleling technique.
Incorrect:
   (a) With size 1 film, a total of *seven* anterior film placements are used in the paralleling technique.
   (b) With size 1 film, a total of *seven* anterior film placements are used in the paralleling technique.

(d) With size 1 film, a total of *seven* anterior film placements are used in the paralleling technique.

REF: p. 189

13. With size 2 film, a total of _____ anterior film placements are used with the paralleling technique.
   a. four
   b. six
   c. seven
   d. eight

Answer: b
Correct: With size 2 film, a total of six anterior film placements are used with the paralleling technique.
Incorrect:
   (a) With size 2 film, a total of *six* anterior film placements are used with the paralleling technique.
   (c) With size 2 film, a total of *six* anterior film placements are used with the paralleling technique.
   (d) With size 2 film, a total of *six* anterior film placements are used with the paralleling technique.

REF: p. 189

14. The authors recommend an exposure sequence starting with tooth No.:
   a. 6
   b. 8
   c. 9
   d. 11

Answer: a
Correct: The authors recommend an exposure sequence starting with tooth No. 6.
Incorrect:
   (b) The authors recommend an exposure sequence starting with tooth No. *6.*
   (c) The authors recommend an exposure sequence starting with tooth No. *6.*
   (d) The authors recommend an exposure sequence starting with tooth No. *6.*

REF: p. 189

15. _____ posterior film placements are used in the paralleling technique.
   a. Four
   b. Six
   c. Seven
   d. Eight

Answer: d
Correct: Eight posterior film placements are used in the paralleling technique.
Incorrect:
   (a) *Eight* posterior film placements are used in the paralleling technique.
   (b) *Eight* posterior film placements are used in the paralleling technique.
   (c) *Eight* posterior film placements are used in the paralleling technique.

REF: pp. 189-190

16. The recommended posterior periapical sequence for the Rinn XCP instruments starts with the:
a. Maxillary left quadrant
b. Maxillary right quadrant
c. Mandibular left quadrant
d. Mandibular right quadrant

Answer: b
Correct: The recommended posterior periapical sequence for the Rinn XCP instruments starts with the maxillary right quadrant.
Incorrect:
(a) The recommended posterior periapical sequence for the Rinn XCP instruments starts with the maxillary *right* quadrant.
(c) The recommended posterior periapical sequence for the Rinn XCP instruments starts with the *maxillary right* quadrant.
(d) The recommended posterior periapical sequence for the Rinn XCP instruments starts with the *maxillary* right quadrant.
REF: p. 190

17. The second quadrant in the recommended posterior periapical sequence for the Rinn XCP instruments is the:
a. Maxillary left quadrant
b. Maxillary right quadrant
c. Mandibular left quadrant
d. Mandibular right quadrant

Answer: c
Correct: The second quadrant in the recommended posterior periapical sequence for the Rinn XCP instruments is the mandibular left quadrant.
Incorrect:
(a) The second quadrant in the recommended posterior periapical sequence for the Rinn XCP instruments is the *mandibular* left quadrant.
(b) The second quadrant in the recommended posterior periapical sequence for the Rinn XCP instruments is the *mandibular left* quadrant.
(d) The second quadrant in the recommended posterior periapical sequence for the Rinn XCP instruments is the mandibular *left* quadrant.
REF: p. 190

18. If the patient has a shallow palate, a lack of parallelism of greater than _____ degrees requires a modification in technique.
a. 10
b. 20
c. 30
d. 45

Answer: b
Correct: If the patient has a shallow palate, a lack of parallelism of greater than 20 degrees requires a modification in technique.

Incorrect:
(a) If the patient has a shallow palate, a lack of parallelism of greater than *20* degrees requires a modification in technique.
(c) If the patient has a shallow palate, a lack of parallelism of greater than *20* degrees requires a modification in technique.
(d) If the patient has a shallow palate, a lack of parallelism of greater than *20* degrees requires a modification in technique.
REF: p. 193

19. When the patient has a shallow palate requiring a modification in technique:
a. Two cotton rolls can be placed, one on each side of the bite-block.
b. The patient can be asked to tilt the head to one side.
c. The vertical angulation can be increased by 5 to 15 degrees more than the XCP instrument indicates.
d. Both a and c.

Answer: d
Correct: When the patient has a shallow palate requiring a modification in technique, two cotton rolls can be placed, one on each side of the bite-block, or the vertical angulation can be increased by 5 to 15 degrees more than the XCP instrument indicates.
Incorrect:
(a) When the patient has a shallow palate requiring a modification in technique, two cotton rolls can be placed, one on each side of the bite-block, *or the vertical angulation can be increased by 5 to 15 degrees more than the XCP instrument indicates.*
(b) When the patient has a shallow palate requiring a modification in technique, two cotton rolls can be placed, one on each side of the bite-block or the vertical angulation can be increased by 5 to 15 degrees more than the XCP instrument indicates.
(c) When the patient has a shallow palate requiring a modification in technique, *two cotton rolls can be placed, one on each side of the bite-block*, or the vertical angulation can be increased by 5 to 15 degrees more than the XCP instrument indicates.
REF: p. 193

20. When tori are present:
a. The patient will require a panoramic film.
b. The film should be placed on the torus and exposed.
c. The patient should be referred for surgical tori reduction before films are taken.
d. The film must be placed on the far side of the torus.

Answer: d
Correct: When tori are present, the film must be placed on the far side of the torus.

(a) When tori are present, *the film must be placed on the far side of the torus.*

(b) When tori are present, *the film must be placed on the far side of the torus.*

(c) When tori are present, *the film must be placed on the far side of the torus.*

REF: p. 208

21. When placing films in the mandibular premolar region, the film must be placed _____ the tongue. When inserting the film holder into the mouth, the film is tipped _____ the tongue.
   a. over; toward
   b. over; away
   c. under; toward
   d. under; away

Answer: c
Correct: When placing films in the mandibular premolar region, the film must be placed under the tongue. When inserting the film holder into the mouth, the film is tipped toward the tongue.
Incorrect:
(a) When placing films in the mandibular premolar region, the film must be placed *under* the tongue. When inserting the film holder into the mouth, the film is tipped toward the tongue.

(b) When placing films in the mandibular premolar region, the film must be placed *under* the tongue. When inserting the film holder into the mouth, the film is tipped *toward* the tongue.

(d) When placing films in the mandibular premolar region, the film must be placed under the tongue. When inserting the film holder into the mouth, the film is tipped *toward* the tongue.

REF: p. 210

22. The paralleling technique _____ on fixed vertical angulations and produces a radiographic image _____ dimensional distortion.
   a. does not rely; without
   b. relies; without
   c. does not rely; with
   d. relies; without

Answer: a
Correct: The paralleling technique does not rely on fixed vertical angulations and produces a radiographic image without dimensional distortion.
Incorrect:
(b) The paralleling technique *does not rely* on fixed vertical angulations and produces a radiographic image without dimensional distortion.

(c) The paralleling technique *does not rely* on fixed vertical angulations and produces a radiographic image without dimensional distortion.

(d) The paralleling technique *does not rely* on fixed vertical angulations and produces a radiographic image without dimensional distortion.

REF: p. 210

23. The authors recommend that each film be placed in the bite-block with the dot:
   a. Down
   b. Up
   c. Distal
   d. In the slot

Answer: d
Correct: The authors recommend that each film be placed in the bite-block with the dot in the slot.
Incorrect:
(a) The authors recommend that each film be placed in the bite-block with the dot *in the slot.*

(b) The authors recommend that each film be placed in the bite-block with the dot *in the slot.*

(c) The authors recommend that each film be placed in the bite-block with the dot *in the slot.*

REF: p. 211

24. The lingual cusp of the first premolar usually obscures the distal contact of the canine on the _____ exposure.
   a. maxillary canine
   b. maxillary incisor
   c. mandibular canine
   d. mandibular incisor

Answer: a
Correct: The lingual cusp of the first premolar usually obscures the distal contact of the canine on the maxillary canine exposure.
Incorrect:
(b) The lingual cusp of the first premolar usually obscures the distal contact of the canine on the *maxillary canine* exposure.

(c) The lingual cusp of the first premolar usually obscures the distal contact of the canine on the *maxillary canine* exposure.

(d) The lingual cusp of the first premolar usually obscures the distal contact of the canine on the *maxillary canine* exposure.

REF: p. 191

25. The entire crowns and roots of one lateral and one central incisor, including the apices of the teeth and surrounding structures, must be seen on the _____ radiograph.
   a. maxillary canine
   b. maxillary incisor
   c. mandibular canine
   d. mandibular incisor

Answer: b
Correct: The entire crowns and roots of one lateral and one central incisor, including the apices of the teeth and surrounding structures, must be seen on the maxillary incisor radiograph.
Incorrect:
  (a) The entire crowns and roots of one lateral and one central incisor, including the apices of the teeth and surrounding structures, must be seen on the maxillary *incisor* radiograph.
  (c) The entire crowns and roots of one lateral and one central incisor, including the apices of the teeth and surrounding structures, must be seen on the *maxillary incisor* radiograph.
  (d) The entire crowns and roots of one lateral and one central incisor, including the apices of the teeth and surrounding structures, must be seen on the *maxillary* incisor radiograph.
REF: p. 191

26. All crowns and roots of the first, second, and third molars, including the apices, alveolar crests, contact areas, surrounding bone, and tuberosity region, must be seen on the _____ radiograph.
  a. maxillary premolar
  b. maxillary molar
  c. mandibular premolar
  d. mandibular molar

Answer: b
Correct: All crowns and roots of the first, second, and third molars, including the apices, alveolar crests, contact areas, surrounding bone, and tuberosity region, must be seen on the maxillary molar radiograph.
Incorrect:
  (a) All crowns and roots of the first, second, and third molars, including the apices, alveolar crests, contact areas, surrounding bone, and tuberosity region, must be seen on the maxillary *molar* radiograph.
  (c) All crowns and roots of the first, second, and third molars, including the apices, alveolar crests, contact areas, surrounding bone, and tuberosity region, must be seen on the *maxillary molar* radiograph.
  (d) All crowns and roots of the first, second, and third molars, including the apices, alveolar crests, contact areas, surrounding bone, and tuberosity region, must be seen on the *maxillary* molar radiograph.
REF: p. 191

CHAPTER 18   BISECTING TECHNIQUE

MULTIPLE CHOICE
1. The rule of isometry states that two triangles are equal if they have _____ equal angles and share a common side.
  a. one
  b. two

  c. three
  d. four

Answer: b
Correct: The rule of isometry states that two triangles are equal if they have two equal angles and share a common side.
Incorrect:
  (a) The rule of isometry states that two triangles are equal if they have *two* equal angles and share a common side.
  (c) The rule of isometry states that two triangles are equal if they have *two* equal angles and share a common side.
  (d) The rule of isometry states that two triangles are equal if they have *two* equal angles and share a common side.
REF: pp. 217-218

2. When the bisecting technique is used, the film must be placed along the _____ surface of the tooth.
  a. buccal
  b. lingual
  c. mesial
  d. distal

Answer: b
Correct: When the bisecting technique is used, the film must be placed along the lingual surface of the tooth.
Incorrect:
  (a) When the bisecting technique is used, the film must be placed along the *lingual* surface of the tooth.
  (c) When the bisecting technique is used, the film must be placed along the *lingual* surface of the tooth.
  (d) When the bisecting technique is used, the film must be placed along the *lingual* surface of the tooth.
REF: p. 218

3. When the bisecting technique is used, which of the following angles is bisected?
  a. The angle formed by the film and the long axis of the tooth
  b. The angle formed by the central ray and the tooth
  c. The angle formed by the central ray and the film
  d. The angle that is perpendicular to the film

Answer: a
Correct: The angle formed by the film and the long axis of the tooth is the angle that is bisected when the bisecting technique is used.
Incorrect:
  (b) *The angle formed by the film and the long axis of the tooth* is the angle that is bisected when the bisecting technique is used.
  (c) *The angle formed by the film and the long axis of the tooth* is the angle that is bisected when the bisecting technique is used.

(d) *The angle formed by the film and the long axis of the tooth* is the angle that is bisected when the bisecting technique is used.

REF: p. 218

4. When the bisecting technique is used, the central ray is directed at 90 degrees to the:
   a. Film
   b. Long axis of the tooth in the same arch
   c. Long axis of the tooth in the opposing arch
   d. Imaginary bisector

Answer: d
Correct: When the bisecting technique is used, the central ray is directed at 90 degrees to the imaginary bisector.
Incorrect:
   (b) When the Stabe Bite-Block is used with the bisecting technique, *the scored front section is removed.*
   (c) When the Stabe Bite-Block is used with the bisecting technique, *the film is placed as close to the teeth as possible.*
   (d) When the Stable Bite-Block is used with the bisecting technique, *the film is placed as close to the teeth as possible*, and *the scored front section is removed.*

REF: p. 218

5. According to the authors, in the bisecting technique, film-holding instruments or the patient's finger may be used to position and stabilize the film. With the bisecting technique, using film holders is recommended because it eliminates use of the patient's finger to stabilize the film.
   a. Both statements are true.
   b. Both statements are false.
   c. The first statement is true; the second statement is false.
   d. The first statement is false; the second statement is true.

Answer: a
Correct: According to the authors, in the bisecting technique, film-holding instruments or the patient's finger may be used to position and stabilize the film. With the bisecting technique, using film holders is recommended because it eliminates use of the patient's finger to stabilize the film.
Incorrect:
   (b) According to the authors, in the bisecting technique, film-holding instruments or the patient's finger may be used to position and stabilize the film. With the bisecting technique, using film holders is recommended because it eliminates use of the patient's finger to stabilize the film.
   (c) According to the authors, in the bisecting technique, film-holding instruments or the patient's finger may be used to position and stabilize the film. *With the bisecting technique, using film*

holders is recommended because it eliminates use of the patient's finger to stabilize the film.
   (d) According to the authors, *in the bisecting technique, film-holding instruments or the patient's finger may be used to position and stabilize the film*. With the bisecting technique, using film holders is recommended because it eliminates use of the patient's finger to stabilize the film.

REF: p. 219

6. The primary benefit of using film holders with the bisecting technique is:
   a. Assisting in determining vertical angulation
   b. Helping to minimize cone cuts
   c. Reducing the patient's exposure to radiation
   d. Allowing the operator to have the film parallel to the long axis of the tooth

Answer: c
Correct: The primary benefit of using film holders with the bisecting technique is reducing the patient's exposure to radiation.
Incorrect:
   (a) The primary benefit to using film holders with the bisecting technique is *reducing the patient's exposure to radiation.*
   (b) The primary benefit of using film holders with the bisecting technique is *reducing the patient's exposure to radiation.*
   (d) The primary benefit of using film holders with the bisecting technique is *reducing the patient's exposure to radiation.*

REF: p. 219

7. Which of the following commercially available film holders can be used with the bisecting technique?
   a. Rinn BAI instruments
   b. Rinn XCP instruments
   c. Stabe bite-block
   d. Both a and c

Answer: d
Correct: The Rinn BAI instruments and the Stabe bite-block can be used with the bisecting technique.
Incorrect:
   (a) The *Stabe Bite-Block* as well as the *Rinn BAI instruments* can be used with the bisecting technique.
   (b) The *Rinn XCP instruments* are not used with the bisecting technique.
   (c) The *Rinn BAI instruments* and the *Stabe Bite-Block* can be used with the bisecting technique.

REF: p. 219

8. When the Stabe bite-block is used with the bisecting technique:
   (1) The film is placed as close to the teeth as possible.
   (2) The film is placed as parallel to the long axis of the teeth as possible.
   (3) The scored front section is removed.

(4) The scored front section is not removed.
   a. 1 and 3
   b. 1 and 4
   c. 2 and 3
   d. 2 and 4

Answer: a
Correct: When the Stabe bite-block is used with the bisecting technique, the film is placed as close to the teeth as possible, and the scored front section is removed.
Incorrect:
   (b) When the Stabe Bite-Block is used with the bisecting technique, *the scored front section is removed.*
   (c) When the Stabe Bite-Block is used with the bisecting technique, *the film is placed as close to the teeth as possible.*
   (d) When the Stabe Bite-Block is used with the bisecting technique, *the film is placed as close to the teeth as possible,* and *the scored front section is removed.*
REF: p. 219

9. When Rinn BAI instruments are used, "BAI" refers to which of the following?
   a. Bisecting, aiming, instrument
   b. Bisecting, angle, instrument
   c. Bisecting, angle, integration
   d. Both, angle, integration

Answer: b
Correct: "BAI" refers to bisecting, angle, instrument.
Incorrect:
   (a) "BAI" refers to bisecting, *angle*, instrument.
   (c) "BAI" refers to bisecting, angle, *instrument*.
   (d) "BAI" refers to *bisecting*, angle, *instrument*.
REF: p. 219

10. Which of the following commercially available film holders are recommended for use with either the paralleling or the bisecting technique?
   (1) Rinn XCP instruments
   (2) Rinn BAI instruments
   (3) Precision film holder
   (4) Stabe bite-block
   (5) EEZEE-Grip film holder
      a. 1, 2, 3, 4, 5
      b. 2, 3, 4, 5
      c. 3, 4, 5
      d. 2, 4, 5

Answer: d
Correct: Rinn BAI instruments, Stabe bite-block, and EEZEE-Grip film holder are recommended for use with either the paralleling or the bisecting technique.

Incorrect:
   (a) Rinn BAI instruments, Stabe bite-block, and EEZEE-Grip film holder are recommended for use with either the paralleling or the bisecting technique.
   (b) Rinn BAI instruments, Stabe bite-block, and EEZEE-Grip film holder are recommended for use with either the paralleling or the bisecting technique.
   (c) Rinn BAI instruments, Stabe bite-block, and EEZEE-Grip film holder are recommended for use with either the paralleling or the bisecting technique.
REF: p. 219

11. Which of the following commercially available film holders is/are recommended for one-time use only?
   a. Rinn XCP instruments
   b. Rinn BAI instruments
   c. Stabe bite-block
   d. EEZEE-Grip film holder

Answer: c
Correct: The *Stabe bite-block* is recommended for one-time use only.
Incorrect:
   (a) The *Stabe bite-block* is recommended for one-time use only.
   (b) The *Stabe bite-block* is recommended for one-time use only.
   (d) The *Stabe bite-block* is recommended for one-time use only.
REF: p. 219

12. With the finger-holding method, which of the following would be used to hold the maxillary right molar film?
   a. Left thumb
   b. Right thumb
   c. Left finger
   d. Right finger

Answer: a
Correct: The patient's left thumb would be used to hold the maxillary right molar film.
Incorrect:
   (b) The patient's *left* thumb would be used to hold the maxillary right molar film; the patient's right thumb would be used to hold the maxillary *left* molar film.
   (c) The patient's left *thumb* would be used to hold the maxillary right molar film; the patient's left finger would be used to hold the *mandibular* right molar film.
   (d) The patient's *left thumb* would be used to hold the maxillary right molar film; the patient's right finger would be used to hold the *mandibular left* molar film.
REF: p. 219

13. When the _____ is/are used, the patient may use excessive force to stabilize the film, causing the film to bend and resulting in image distortion.
   a. Rinn BAI instruments
   b. Stabe bite-block
   c. finger-holding method
   d. EEZEE-Grip film holder

Answer: c
Correct: When the finger-holding method is used, the patient may use excessive force to stabilize the film, causing the film to bend and resulting in image distortion.
Incorrect:
   (a) When the *finger-holding method* is used, the patient may use excessive force to stabilize the film, causing the film to bend and resulting in image distortion.
   (b) When the *finger-holding method* is used, the patient may use excessive force to stabilize the film, causing the film to bend and resulting in image distortion.
   (d) When the *finger-holding method* is used, the patient may use excessive force to stabilize the film, causing the film to bend and resulting in image distortion.
REF: p. 219

14. Which size film is traditionally used with the bisecting technique?
   a. #1 film for anterior teeth, #1 film for posterior teeth
   b. #1 film for anterior teeth, #2 film for posterior teeth
   c. #2 film for anterior teeth, #1 film for posterior teeth
   d. #2 film for anterior teeth and for posterior teeth

Answer: d
Correct: With the bisecting technique, #2 film is traditionally used for anterior teeth and for posterior teeth.
Incorrect:
   (a) With the bisecting technique, *#2 film* is traditionally used *for anterior teeth and for posterior teeth*; #1 film is recommended for the paralleling technique.
   (b) With the bisecting technique, *#2 film* is traditionally used *for anterior teeth* and for posterior teeth; #1 film is recommended for the paralleling technique.
   (c) With the bisecting technique, #2 film is traditionally used for anterior teeth *and for posterior teeth*; #1 film is recommended for the paralleling technique.
REF: p. 219

15. Which of the following techniques use the same principles of horizontal angulation?
   (1) Paralleling
   (2) Bisecting

   (3) Bite-wing
   a. 1, 2, 3
   b. 1, 2
   c. 2, 3
   d. 1, 3

Answer: a
Correct: Paralleling, bisecting, and bite-wing techniques all use the same principles of horizontal angulation.
Incorrect:
   (b) Paralleling, bisecting, *and bite-wing* techniques all use the same principles of horizontal angulation.
   (c) *Paralleling*, bisecting, and bite-wing techniques all use the same principles of horizontal angulation.
   (d) Paralleling, *bisecting*, and bite-wing techniques all use the same principles of horizontal angulation.
REF: p. 221

16. With the bite-wing technique, the vertical angulation is predetermined; the central ray is directed at _____ degrees to the occlusal plane
   a. +10
   b. −10
   c. +20
   d. −20

Answer: a
Correct: With the bite-wing technique, the vertical angulation is predetermined; the central ray is directed at +10 degrees to the occlusal plane.
Incorrect:
   (b) With the bite-wing technique, the vertical angulation is predetermined; the central ray is directed at *+10* degrees to the occlusal plane.
   (c) With the bite-wing technique, the vertical angulation is predetermined; the central ray is directed at *+10* degrees to the occlusal plane.
   (d) With the bite-wing technique, the vertical angulation is predetermined; the central ray is directed at *+10* degrees to the occlusal plane.
REF: p. 222

17. With the _____ technique, the vertical angulation is determined by the imaginary bisector; the central ray is directed perpendicular to the imaginary bisector.
   a. paralleling
   b. bisecting
   c. bite-wing
   d. occlusal

Answer: b
Correct: With the bisecting technique, the vertical angulation is determined by the imaginary bisector; the central ray is directed perpendicular to the imaginary bisector.

Incorrect:
- (a) With the *bisecting* technique, the vertical angulation is determined by the imaginary bisector; the central ray is directed perpendicular to the imaginary bisector.
- (c) With the *bisecting* technique, the vertical angulation is determined by the imaginary bisector; the central ray is directed perpendicular to the imaginary bisector.
- (d) With the *bisecting* technique, the vertical angulation is determined by the imaginary bisector; the central ray is directed perpendicular to the imaginary bisector.

REF: p. 221

18. Foreshortened images refer to images of the teeth that appear _____. Foreshortening of images results from _____ vertical angulation.
    a. shortened; insufficient
    b. shortened; excessive
    c. too long; insufficient
    d. too long; excessive

Answer: b
Correct: Foreshortened images refer to images of the teeth that appear shortened. Foreshortening of images results from excessive vertical angulation.

Incorrect:
- (a) Foreshortened images refer to images of the teeth that appear shortened. Foreshortening of images results from *excessive* vertical angulation.
- (c) Foreshortened images refer to images of the teeth that appear *shortened*. Foreshortening of images results from *excessive* vertical angulation.
- (d) Foreshortened images refer to images of the teeth that appear *shortened*. Foreshortening of images results from excessive vertical angulation.

REF: p. 222

19. When the bisecting technique is used, foreshortening will occur if the central ray is directed perpendicular to the:
    a. Plane of the film
    b. Imaginary bisector
    c. Long axis of the tooth on the same arch
    d. Long axis of the tooth on the opposite arch

Answer: a
Correct: When the bisecting technique is used, foreshortening will occur if the central ray is directed perpendicular to the plane of the film.

Incorrect:
- (b) When the bisecting technique is used, foreshortening will occur if the central ray is directed perpendicular to the *plane of the film.*
- (c) When the bisecting technique is used, foreshortening will occur if the central ray is directed perpendicular to the *plane of the film.*

- (d) When the bisecting technique is used, foreshortening will occur if the central ray is directed perpendicular to the *plane of the film.*

REF: p. 222

20. Elongated images refer to images of the teeth that appear _____. Elongation of images results from _____ vertical angulation.
    a. too long; excessive
    b. too long; insufficient
    c. shortened; excessive
    d. shortened; insufficient

Answer: b
Correct: Elongated images refer to images of the teeth that appear too long. Elongation of images results from insufficient vertical angulation.

Incorrect:
- (a) Elongated images refer to images of the teeth that appear too long. Elongation of images results from *insufficient* vertical angulation.
- (c) Elongated images refer to images of the teeth that appear *too long*. Elongation of images results from *insufficient* vertical angulation.
- (d) Elongated images refer to images of the teeth that appear *too long*. Elongation of images results from insufficient vertical angulation.

REF: p. 222

21. Film should be placed approximately _____ inch beyond the incisal or occlusal surfaces when using the bisecting technique.
    a. $\frac{1}{16}$
    b. $\frac{1}{8}$
    c. $\frac{1}{4}$
    d. $\frac{1}{2}$

Answer: b
Correct: Film should be placed approximately $\frac{1}{8}$ inch beyond the incisal or occlusal surfaces when using the bisecting technique.

Incorrect:
- (a) Film should be placed approximately $\frac{1}{8}$ inch beyond the incisal or occlusal surfaces when using the bisecting technique.
- (c) Film should be placed approximately $\frac{1}{8}$ inch beyond the incisal or occlusal surfaces when using the bisecting technique.
- (d) Film should be placed approximately $\frac{1}{8}$ inch beyond the incisal or occlusal surfaces when using the bisecting technique.

REF: p. 223

22. With size 2 film, a total of _____ anterior film placements are used in the bisecting technique.
    a. four
    b. six
    c. seven
    d. eight

131

Test Bank

Answer: b

Correct: With size 2 film, a total of six anterior film placements are used in the bisecting technique.

Incorrect:
- (a) With size 2 film, a total of *six* anterior film placements are used in the bisecting technique.
- (c) With size 2 film, a total of *six* anterior film placements are used in the bisecting technique.
- (d) With size 2 film, a total of *six* anterior film placements are used in thc bisecting technique.

REF: p. 224

23. The recommended anterior periapical exposure sequence for the bisecting technique starts with the:
    - a. Maxillary right canine
    - b. Maxillary left canine
    - c. Mandibular right canine
    - d. Mandibular left canine

Answer: a

Correct: The recommended anterior periapical exposure sequence for the bisecting technique starts with the maxillary right canine.

Incorrect:
- (b) The recommended anterior periapical exposure sequence for the bisecting technique starts with the maxillary *right* canine.
- (c) The recommended anterior periapical exposure sequence for the bisecting technique starts with the *maxillary* right canine.
- (d) The recommended anterior periapical exposure sequence for the bisecting technique starts with the *maxillary right* canine.

REF: p. 224

24. The recommended posterior periapical exposure sequence for the bisecting technique is to begin with the:
    - a. Maxillary right quadrant
    - b. Maxillary left quadrant
    - c. Mandibular right quadrant
    - d. Mandibular left quadrant

Answer: a

Correct: The recommended posterior periapical exposure sequence for the bisecting technique is to begin with the maxillary right quadrant.

Incorrect:
- (b) The recommended posterior periapical exposure sequence for the bisecting technique is to begin with the maxillary *right* quadrant.
- (c) The recommended posterior periapical exposure sequence for the bisecting technique is to begin with the *maxillary* right quadrant.
- (d) The recommended posterior periapical exposure sequence for the bisecting technique is to begin with the *maxillary right* quadrant.

REF: p. 225

25. According to the recommended posterior periapical exposure sequence for the bisecting technique, the second posterior quadrant exposed should be the:
    - a. Maxillary right quadrant
    - b. Maxillary left quadrant
    - c. Mandibular right quadrant
    - d. Mandibular left quadrant

Answer: c

Correct: According to the recommended posterior periapical exposure sequence for thc bisecting technique, the second posterior quadrant exposed should be the mandibular right quadrant.

Incorrect:
- (a) According to the recommended posterior periapical exposure sequence for the bisecting technique, the second posterior quadrant exposed should be the *mandibular* right quadrant.
- (b) According to the recommended posterior periapical exposure sequence for the bisecting technique, the second posterior quadrant exposed should be the *mandibular right* quadrant.
- (d) According to the recommended posterior periapical exposure sequence for the bisecting technique, the second posterior quadrant exposed should be the mandibular *right* quadrant.

REF: p. 225

26. According to the text, when exposing a complete mouth radiographic series (CMRS) using the bisecting technique, there are _____ recommended size 2 film placements?
    - a. 7
    - b. 12
    - c. 14
    - d. 19

Answer: c

Correct: According to the text, when exposing a CMRS using the bisecting technique, there are 14 recommended size 2 periapical film placements.

Incorrect:
- (a) According to the text, when exposing a CMRS using the bisecting technique, there are *14* recommended size 2 periapical film placements.
- (b) According to the text, when exposing a CMRS using the bisecting technique, there are *14* recommended size 2 periapical film placements.
- (d) According to the text, when exposing a CMRS using the bisecting technique, there are *14* recommended size 2 periapical film placements.

REF: p. 226

27. According to the text, the disadvantages of the bisecting technique outweigh the advantages. Therefore, the paralleling technique is preferred over the bisecting technique for exposure of periapical films and should be used whenever possible.
    - a. Both statements are true.
    - b. Both statements are false.

c. The first statement is true; the second statement is false.

d. The first statement is false, the second statement is true.

Answer: a

Correct: According to the text, the disadvantages of the bisecting technique outweigh the advantages. Therefore, the paralleling technique is preferred over the bisecting technique for exposure of periapical films and should be used whenever possible.

Incorrect:

(b) According to the text, the disadvantages of the bisecting technique outweigh the advantages. Therefore, the paralleling technique is preferred over the bisecting technique for exposure of periapical films and should be used whenever possible.

(c) According to the text, the disadvantages of the bisecting technique outweigh the advantages. *Therefore, the paralleling technique is preferred over the bisecting technique for exposure of periapical films and should be used whenever possible.*

(d) According to the text, *the disadvantages of the bisecting technique outweigh the advantages.* Therefore, the paralleling technique is preferred over the bisecting technique for exposure of periapical films and should be used whenever possible.

REF: p. 248

28. The primary disadvantage of the bisecting technique when contrasted with the paralleling technique is:
a. Longer exposure times
b. Dimensional distortion
c. Requirement of a film holder
d. Greater magnification

Answer: b

Correct: The primary disadvantage of the bisecting technique when contrasted with the paralleling technique is dimensional distortion.

Incorrect:

(a) The primary disadvantage of the bisecting technique when contrasted with the paralleling technique is *dimensional distortion.*

(c) The primary disadvantage of the bisecting technique when contrasted with the paralleling technique is *dimensional distortion.*

(d) The primary disadvantage of the bisecting technique when contrasted with the paralleling technique is *dimensional distortion.*

REF: p. 248

29. Horizontal angulation refers to the placement of the position-indicating device (PID) in a/an _____ plane. Vertical angulation refers to the positioning of the PID in a/an _____ plane.

a. side-to-side; side-to-side
b. side-to-side; up-and-down
c. up-and-down; side-to-side
d. up-and-down; up-and-down

Answer: b

Correct: Horizontal angulation refers to the placement of the PID in a side-to-side plane. Vertical angulation refers to the positioning of the PID in an up-and-down plane.

Incorrect:

(a) Horizontal angulation refers to the placement of the PID in a side-to-side plane. Vertical angulation refers to the positioning of the PID in an *up-and-down* plane.

(c) Horizontal angulation refers to the placement of the PID in a *side-to-side* plane. Vertical angulation refers to the positioning of the PID in an *up-and-down* plane.

(d) Horizontal angulation refers to the placement of the PID in a *side-to-side* plane. Vertical angulation refers to the positioning of the PID in an up-and-down plane.

REF: pp. 220-221

30. For the maxillary premolar exposure, the front edge of the film should be aligned with the midline of the maxillary:
a. Lateral incisor
b. Canine
c. First bicuspid
d. Second bicuspid

Answer: b

Correct: For the maxillary premolar exposure, the front edge of the film should be aligned with the midline of the maxillary canine.

Incorrect:

(a) For the maxillary premolar exposure, the front edge of the film should be aligned with the midline of the maxillary *canine.*

(c) For the maxillary premolar exposure, the front edge of the film should be aligned with the midline of the maxillary *canine.*

(d) For the maxillary premolar exposure, the front edge of the film should be aligned with the midline of the maxillary *canine.*

REF: p. 236

31. For the mandibular molar exposure, the front edge of the film should be aligned with the midline of the:
a. Canine
b. First premolar
c. Second premolar
d. First molar

Answer: c

Correct: For the mandibular molar exposure, the front edge of the film should be aligned with the midline of the second premolar.

133

Incorrect:

(a) For the mandibular molar exposure, the front edge of the film should be aligned with the midline of the *second premolar.*

(b) For the mandibular molar exposure, the front edge of the film should be aligned with the midline of the *second premolar.*

(d) For the mandibular molar exposure, the front edge of the film should be aligned with the midline of the *second premolar.*

REF: p. 242

32. With the bisecting technique, the recommended vertical angulation range for maxillary canines is _____ degrees.

    a. +20 to +30
    b. +30 to +40
    c. +40 to +50
    d. +45 to +55

Answer: d

Correct: With the bisecting technique, the recommended vertical angulation range for maxillary canines is +45 to +55 degrees.

Incorrect:

(a) With the bisecting technique, the recommended vertical angulation range for maxillary canines is *+45 to +55* degrees.

(b) With the bisecting technique, the recommended vertical angulation range for maxillary canines is *+45 to +55* degrees.

(c) With the bisecting technique, the recommended vertical angulation range for maxillary canines is *+45 to +55* degrees.

REF: p. 222

33. With the bisecting technique, the recommended vertical angulation range for mandibular molars is _____ degrees.

    a. −5 to 0
    b. + 20 to +30
    c. −20 to −30
    d. −10 to −15

Answer: a

Correct: With the bisecting technique, the recommended vertical angulation range for mandibular molars is −5 to 0 degrees.

Incorrect:

(b) With the bisecting technique, the recommended vertical angulation range for mandibular molars is *−5 to 0* degrees.

(c) With the bisecting technique, the recommended vertical angulation range for mandibular molars is *−5 to 0* degrees.

(d) With the bisecting technique, the recommended vertical angulation range for mandibular molars is *−5 to 0* degrees.

REF: p. 222

MULTIPLE CHOICE

1. The bite-wing tab is a heavy paperboard tab or loop fitted around a periapical film and used to stabilize the film during exposure. The periapical film is oriented in the bite loop so that the tab portion extends from the white side (tube side) of the film.

    a. Both statements are true.
    b. Both statements are false.
    c. The first statement is true; the second statement is false.
    d. The first statement is false; the second statement is true.

Answer: a

Correct: The bite-wing tab is a heavy paperboard tab or loop fitted around a periapical film and used to stabilize the film during exposure. The periapical film is oriented in the bite loop so that the tab portion extends from the white side (tube side) of the film.

Incorrect:

(b) The bite-wing tab is a heavy paperboard tab or loop fitted around a periapical film and used to stabilize the film during exposure. The periapical film is oriented in the bite loop so that the tab portion extends from the white side (tube side) of the film.

(c) The bite-wing tab is a heavy paperboard tab or loop fitted around a periapical film and used to stabilize the film during exposure. *The periapical film is oriented in the bite loop so that the tab portion extends from the white side (tube side) of the film.*

(d) *The bite-wing tab is a heavy paperboard tab or loop fitted around a periapical film and used to stabilize the film during exposure.* The periapical film is oriented in the bite loop so that the tab portion extends from the white side (tube side) of the film.

REF: p. 256

2. _____ sizes of bite-wing films are available.

    a. Two
    b. Three
    c. Four
    d. Six

Answer: c

Correct: Four sizes of bite-wing films are available.

Incorrect:

(a) *Four* sizes of bite-wing films are available.

(b) *Four* sizes of bite-wing films are available.

(d) *Four* sizes of bite-wing films are available.

REF: p. 256

3. Which size of bite-wing film is used to examine the posterior teeth of children with mixed dentition?

    a. Size 0
    b. Size 1
    c. Size 2
    d. Size 3

Answer: b
Correct: Size 1 bite-wing film is used to examine the posterior teeth of children with mixed dentition.
Incorrect:
  (a) *Size 1* bite-wing film is used to examine the posterior teeth of children with mixed dentition.
  (c) *Size 1* bite-wing film is used to examine the posterior teeth of children with mixed dentition.
  (d) *Size 1* bite-wing film is used to examine the posterior teeth of children with mixed dentition.
REF: p. 256

4. Which size bite-wing film may be placed in a horizontal or vertical position?
   a. Size 0
   b. Size 1
   c. Size 2
   d. Size 3

Answer: c
Correct: Size 2 bite-wing film may be placed in a horizontal or vertical position.
Incorrect:
  (a) *Size 2* bite-wing film may be placed in a horizontal or vertical position.
  (b) *Size 2* bite-wing film may be placed in a horizontal or vertical position.
  (d) *Size 2* bite-wing film may be placed in a horizontal or vertical position.
REF: p. 257

5. When vertical posterior bite-wing exposures are indicated, size _____ film is placed with the long portion of the film in a _____ direction.
   a. 1; horizontal
   b. 2; horizontal
   c. 1; vertical
   d. 2; vertical

Answer: d
Correct: When vertical posterior bite-wing exposures are indicated, size 2 film is placed with the long portion of the film in a vertical direction.
Incorrect:
  (a) When vertical posterior bite-wing exposures are indicated, size 2 film is placed with the long portion of the film in a *vertical* direction.
  (b) When vertical posterior bite-wing exposures are indicated, size 2 film is placed with the long portion of the film in a *vertical* direction.
  (c) When vertical posterior bite-wing exposures are indicated, Size 2 film is placed with the long portion of the film in a vertical direction.
REF: p. 257

6. Which size film is used only for bite-wings?
   a. Size 0
   b. Size 1
   c. Size 2
   d. Size 3

Answer: d
Correct: Size 3 film is used only for bite-wings.
Incorrect:
  (a) *Size 3* film is used only for bite-wings.
  (b) *Size 3* film is used only for bite-wings.
  (c) *Size 3* film is used only for bite-wings.
REF: p. 257

7. In the adult patient, which size film is recommended for bite-wing exposures?
   a. Size 0
   b. Size 1
   c. Size 2
   d. Size 3

Answer: c
Correct: In the adult patient, size 2 film is recommended for bite-wing exposures.
Incorrect:
  (a) In the adult patient, *size 2* film is recommended for bite-wing exposures.
  (b) In the adult patient, *size 2* film is recommended for bite-wing exposures.
  (d) In the adult patient, *size 2* film is recommended for bite-wing exposures.
REF: p. 257

8. According to the text, which size bite-wing film is *not* recommended?
   a. Size 0
   b. Size 1
   c. Size 2
   d. Size 3

Answer: d
Correct: According to the text, size 3 bite-wing film is not recommended.
Incorrect:
  (a) According to the text, *size 3* bite-wing film is not recommended.
  (b) According to the text, *size 3* bite-wing film is not recommended.
  (c) According to the text, *size 3* bite-wing film is not recommended.
REF: p. 257

9. The problem with a single bite-wing film per side for adult patients is increased:
   a. X-ray exposure
   b. Possibility of inciting the gag reflex
   c. Overlapped contacts
   d. Useful diagnostic information

Answer: c
Correct: The problem with a single bite-wing film per side for adult patients is increased overlapped contacts.
Incorrect:
  (a) The problem with a single bite-wing film per side for adult patients is increased *overlapped contacts*.

(b) The problem with a single bite-wing film per side for adult patients is increased *overlapped contacts*.

(d) The problem with a single bite-wing film per side for adult patients is increased *overlapped contacts*.

REF: p. 257

10. When determining vertical angulation, if the position-indicating device (PID) is positioned above the occlusal plane and the central ray is directed _____, the vertical angulation is termed _____.

a. upward; positive
b. downward; positive
c. upward; negative
d. downward; negative

Answer: b
Correct: When determining vertical angulation, if the PID is positioned above the occlusal plane and the central ray is directed downward, the vertical angulation is termed *positive*.
Incorrect:
(a) When determining vertical angulation, if the PID is positioned above the occlusal plane and the central ray is directed *downward*, the vertical angulation is termed *positive*.
(c) When determining vertical angulation, if the PID is positioned above the occlusal plane and the central ray is directed *downward*, the vertical angulation is termed *positive*.
(d) When determining vertical angulation, if the PID is positioned above the occlusal plane and the central ray is directed downward, the vertical angulation is termed *positive*.

REF: p. 257

11. Which of the following exposure sequences is recommended for the patient who requires both periapical and bite-wing radiographs?
(1) Bite-wing exposures
(2) Anterior periapical films
(3) Posterior periapical films
    a. 1, 2, 3
    b. 2, 1, 3
    c. 2, 3, 1
    d. 3, 1, 2

Answer: c
Correct: The recommended exposure sequence for the patient who requires both periapical and bite-wing radiographs is anterior periapical films, posterior periapical films, and bite-wing exposures.
Incorrect:
(a) The recommended exposure sequence for the patient who requires both periapical and bite-wing radiographs is *anterior periapical films, posterior periapical films, and bite-wing exposures*.

(b) The recommended exposure sequence for the patient who requires both periapical and bite-wing radiographs is *anterior periapical films, posterior periapical films, and bite-wing exposures*.

(c) The recommended exposure sequence for the patient who requires both periapical and bite-wing radiographs is *anterior periapical films, posterior periapical films, and bite-wing exposures*.

REF: p. 260

12. Vertical bite-wings are often used for patients with:
a. Mixed dentition
b. Extensive decay
c. Bone loss
d. Sealants

Answer: c
Correct: Vertical bite-wings are often used for patients with bone loss.
Incorrect:
(a) Vertical bite-wings are often used for patients with *bone loss*.
(b) Vertical bite-wings are often used for patients with *bone loss*.
(d) Vertical bite-wings are often used for patients with *bone loss*.

REF: p. 260

13. What modification in technique is recommended when the patient has an edentulous space causing a problem with bite-wing film placement?
a. Skip the bite-wing film.
b. Place a cotton roll in the area of the missing tooth or teeth.
c. Have the patient hold the film in position with a hemostat.
d. Take a periapical film with a bite-block instead.

Answer: b
Correct: Place a cotton roll in the area of the missing tooth or teeth.
Incorrect:
(a) Place a cotton roll in the area of the missing tooth or teeth.
(c) Place a cotton roll in the area of the missing tooth or teeth.
(d) Place a cotton roll in the area of the missing tooth or teeth.

REF: p. 268

14. According to the text, the identification dot in bite-wing film placement:
a. Should be oriented "dot down"
b. Should be oriented "dot distal"
c. Should be oriented "dot up"
d. Has no significance

Answer: d
Correct: According to the text, the identification dot in bite-wing film placement has no significance.

Incorrect:
- (a) According to the text, the identification dot in bite-wing film placement *has no significance*.
- (b) According to the text, the identification dot in bite-wing film placement *has no significance*.
- (c) According to the text, the identification dot in bite-wing film placement *has no significance*.

REF: p. 260

15. For the premolar bite-wing exposure, the PID is positioned far enough forward to cover both maxillary and mandibular:
    - a. Lateral incisors
    - b. Canines
    - c. First premolars
    - d. Second premolars

Answer: b
Correct: For the premolar bite-wing exposure, the PID is positioned far enough forward to cover both maxillary and mandibular canines.
Incorrect:
- (a) For the premolar bite-wing exposure, the PID is positioned far enough forward to cover both maxillary and mandibular *canines*.
- (c) For the premolar bite-wing exposure, the PID is positioned far enough forward to cover both maxillary and mandibular *canines*.
- (d) For the premolar bite-wing exposure, the PID is positioned far enough forward to cover both maxillary and mandibular *canines*.

REF: p. 261

16. For the premolar bite-wing exposure, the front edge of the film should be aligned with the midline of the:
    - a. Maxillary canine
    - b. Mandibular canine
    - c. Maxillary first premolar
    - d. Mandibular first premolar

Answer: b
Correct: For the premolar bite-wing exposure, the front edge of the film should be aligned with the midline of the mandibular canine.
Incorrect:
- (a) For the premolar bite-wing exposure, the front edge of the film should be aligned with the midline of the *mandibular* canine.
- (c) For the premolar bite-wing exposure, the front edge of the film should be aligned with the midline of the *mandibular canine*.
- (d) For the premolar bite-wing exposure, the front edge of the film should be aligned with the midline of the mandibular *canine*.

REF: p. 262

17. For the molar bite-wing exposure, the front edge of the film should be aligned with the midline of the:
    - a. Maxillary first premolar
    - b. Mandibular first premolar
    - c. Maxillary second premolar
    - d. Mandibular second premolar

Answer: d
Correct: For the molar bite-wing exposure, the front edge of the film should be aligned with the midline of the mandibular second premolar.
Incorrect:
- (a) For the molar bite-wing exposure, the front edge of the film should be aligned with the midline of the mandibular second *premolar*.
- (b) For the molar bite-wing exposure, the front edge of the film should be aligned with the midline of the mandibular *second* premolar.
- (c) For the molar bite-wing exposure, the front edge of the film should be aligned with the midline of the *mandibular second* premolar.

REF: p. 266

CHAPTER 20 EXPOSURE AND TECHNIQUE ERRORS

MULTIPLE CHOICE

1. An unexposed film appears:
    - a. Clear
    - b. Black
    - c. Dark
    - d. Light

Answer: a
Correct: An unexposed film appears clear.
Incorrect:
- (b) An unexposed film appears *clear*; an exposed film appears dark or black.
- (c) An unexposed film appears *clear*; an exposed film appears dark or black.
- (d) An unexposed film appears *clear,* not light.

REF: p. 274

2. Which of the following choices may be the cause of an unexposed film?
    - a. Excessive exposure time
    - b. Failure to turn on the x-ray machine
    - c. Excessive kilovoltage
    - d. Excessive milliamperage

Answer: b
Correct: Failure to turn on the x-ray machine may be the cause of an unexposed film.
Incorrect:
- (a) *Failure to turn on the x-ray machine* may be the cause of an unexposed film; excessive exposure time would create a film that appears dark.
- (c) *Failure to turn on the x-ray machine* may be the cause of an unexposed film; excessive kilovoltage would create a film that appears dark.
- (d) *Failure to turn on the x-ray machine* may be the cause of an unexposed film; excessive milliamperage would create a film that appears dark.

REF: p. 274

3. Which of the following films would most likely appear black?
   a. An unexposed film
   b. A film exposed to light
   c. An overexposed film
   d. An underexposed film

Answer: b
Correct: A film exposed to light would most likely appear black.
Incorrect:
   (a) *A film exposed to light* would most likely appear black; an unexposed film would be clear.
   (c) *A film exposed to light* would most likely appear black; an overexposed film would appear dark, and with sufficient exposure the darkness may approach that of a film exposed to light.
   (d) *A film exposed to light* would most likely appear black; an underexposed film would appear light.
REF: p. 274

4. The possibility of exposure of radiographic film to white light can be reduced by:
   a. Turning off the safelight and unwrapping the films in a pitch-dark room.
   b. Pre-exposing the entire package of film to radiation before opening the package.
   c. Not unwrapping the film in a room with white light.
   d. Turning off the fluorescent lighting in the treatment room before exposing radiographic films.

Answer: c
Correct: The possibility of exposure of radiographic film to white light can be reduced by not unwrapping the film in a room with white light.
Incorrect:
   (a) The possibility of exposure of radiographic film to white light can be reduced by *not unwrapping the film in a room with white light.*
   (b) The possibility of exposure of radiographic film to white light can be reduced by *not unwrapping the film in a room with white light.*
   (d) The possibility of exposure of radiographic film to white light can be reduced by *not unwrapping the film in a room with white light.*
REF: p. 274

5. An underexposed film results from:
   a. Inadequate exposure time
   b. Inadequate tissue density
   c. Excessive milliamperage
   d. Excessive kilovoltage

Answer: a
Correct: An underexposed film results from insufficient exposure time.
Incorrect:
   (b) An underexposed film results from *insufficient exposure time;* manufacturers have titrated the

properties of the film so that inadequate tissue density is not a possible factor.
   (c) An underexposed film results from *insufficient exposure time;* excessive milliamperage would create an overexposed film.
   (d) An underexposed film results from *insufficient exposure time;* excessive kilovoltage would create an overexposed film.
REF: p. 275

6. To prevent underexposure, check and increase _____ as needed.
   (1) Exposure time
   (2) Kilovoltage
   (3) Milliamperage
   a. 1, 2, 3
   b. 1, 2
   c. 2, 3
   d. 1, 3

Answer: a
Correct: To prevent underexposure, check and increase exposure time, kilovoltage, or milliamperage as needed.
Incorrect:
   (b) To prevent underexposure, check and increase exposure time, kilovoltage, *or milliamperage* as needed.
   (c) To prevent underexposure, check and increase *exposure time*, kilovoltage, or milliamperage as needed.
   (d) To prevent underexposure, check and increase exposure time, *kilovoltage*, or milliamperage as needed.
REF: p. 275

7. The cause of an excessive margin of film edge (which appears as a black band) on a nondiagnostic periapical film is:
   a. The edge of the film was not placed parallel to the incisal-occlusal surfaces of the teeth.
   b. The film was not positioned in the patient's mouth to cover the apical regions of the teeth.
   c. The film was underexposed.
   d. The central ray was not directed through the interproximal spaces.

Answer: b
Correct: The cause of an excessive margin of film edge (which appears as a black band) on a nondiagnostic periapical film is the film was not positioned in the patient's mouth to cover the apical regions of the teeth.
Incorrect:
   (a) *The film was not positioned in the patient's mouth to cover the apical regions of the teeth.* If the edge of the film is not placed parallel to the incisal-occlusal surfaces of the teeth, the margin of the film edge will be skewed.

(c) *The film was not positioned in the patient's mouth to cover the apical regions of the teeth.* If the film is underexposed, the entire film will be light.

(d) *The film was not positioned in the patient's mouth to cover the apical regions of the teeth.* If the central ray is not directed through the interproximal spaces, the teeth will be overlapped.

REF: p. 276

8. To correct a film where apices do not appear:
   a. Make certain that no more than 3/4 inch of the film edge extends beyond the incisal-occlusal surfaces of the teeth.
   b. Make certain that no more than 1/8 inch of the film edge extends beyond the incisal-occlusal surfaces of the teeth.
   c. Increase the exposure time.
   d. Direct the x-ray beam through the interproximal spaces.

Answer: b
Correct: To correct a film where apices do not appear, make certain that no more than 1/8 inch of the film edge extends beyond the incisal-occlusal surfaces of the teeth.
Incorrect:
   (a) To correct a film in which apices do not appear, *ensure that no more than 1/8 inch of the film edge extends beyond the incisal-occlusal surfaces of the teeth.* Three-quarters inch increases the chances that the apices will not appear.
   (c) To correct a film in which apices do not appear, *ensure that no more than 1/8 inch of the film edge extends beyond the incisal-occlusal surfaces of the teeth.* Increasing the exposure time will have no appreciable effect.
   (d) To correct a film in which apices do not appear, *ensure that no more than 1/8 inch of the film edge extends beyond the incisal-occlusal surfaces of the teeth.* Directing the beam through interproximal spaces will have no appreciable effect.

REF: p. 276

9. When the occlusal plane appears tipped or tilted, the error is a(n):
   a. Incorrect horizontal angulation
   b. Incorrect vertical angulation
   c. Dropped film corner
   d. Elongated image

Answer: c
Correct: When the occlusal plane appears tipped or tilted, the error is a dropped film corner.
Incorrect:
   (a) When the occlusal plane appears tipped or tilted, the error is a *dropped film corner;* incorrect horizontal angulation would create overlapped contact areas.
   (b) When the occlusal plane appears tipped or tilted, the error is a *dropped film corner;* incorrect verti-

cal angulation would produce a foreshortened or elongated image.

   (d) When the occlusal plane appears tipped or tilted, the error is a *dropped film corner;* an elongated image occurs when the vertical angulation was insufficient (too flat).

REF: p. 276

10. To prevent a dropped film corner:
    a. Change the horizontal angulation.
    b. Increase the vertical angulation.
    c. Decrease the vertical angulation.
    d. Make certain the edge of the film is placed parallel to the incisal-occlusal surfaces of the teeth.

Answer: d
Correct: To prevent a dropped film corner, make certain the edge of the film is placed parallel to the incisal-occlusal surfaces of the teeth.
Incorrect:
    (a) *Make certain the edge of the film is placed parallel to the incisal-occlusal surfaces of the teeth.* Changing the horizontal angulation will cause overlapping.
    (b) *Make certain the edge of the film is placed parallel to the incisal-occlusal surfaces of the teeth.* Increasing vertical angulation will cause foreshortening.
    (c) *Make certain the edge of the film is placed parallel to the incisal-occlusal surfaces of the teeth.* Decreasing vertical angulation will cause elongation.

REF: p. 276

11. When overlapped contacts appear on film, the cause is:
    a. Incorrect vertical angulation
    b. Incorrect horizontal angulation
    c. A dropped film corner
    d. An underexposed film

Answer: b
Correct: When overlapped contacts appear on film, the cause is incorrect horizontal angulation.
Incorrect:
    (a) When overlapped contacts appear on film, the cause is *incorrect horizontal angulation;* incorrect vertical angulation would produce a foreshortened or an elongated film.
    (c) When overlapped contacts appear on film, the cause is *incorrect horizontal angulation.*
    (d) When overlapped contacts appear on film, the cause is *incorrect horizontal angulation;* an underexposed film would be light.

REF: pp. 276-277

12. To avoid overlapped contacts on periapical film:
    a. Increase vertical angulation.
    b. Decrease vertical angulation.
    c. Direct the x-ray beam through the interproximal regions.

d. Make certain that no more than ⅛ inch of the film edge extends beyond the incisal-occlusal surfaces of the teeth.

Answer: c
Correct: To avoid overlapped contacts on periapical film, direct the x-ray beam through the interproximal regions.
Incorrect:
(a) *Direct the x-ray beam through the interproximal regions.* Increasing vertical angulation will not have an appreciable effect.
(b) *Direct the x-ray beam through the interproximal regions.* Decreasing vertical angulation will not have an appreciable effect.
(d) *Direct the x-ray beam through the interproximal regions.* Making certain that no more than 1/8 inch of the film edge extends beyond the incisal-occlusal surfaces of the teeth will eliminate cut-off apices.
REF: p. 277

13. Short teeth with blunted roots appear on the film when:
   a. The vertical angulation is excessive.
   b. The vertical angulation is insufficient.
   c. The horizontal angulation is incorrect.
   d. There is a cone-cut.

Answer: a
Correct: Short teeth with blunted roots appear on the film when the vertical angulation is excessive.
Incorrect:
(b) Short teeth with blunted roots appear on the film when *the vertical angulation is excessive;* long, distorted teeth appear on the film when the vertical angulation is insufficient.
(c) Short teeth with blunted roots appear on the film when *the vertical angulation is excessive;* overlapped contacts appear on the film when the horizontal angulation is incorrect.
(d) Short teeth with blunted roots appear on the film when *the vertical angulation is excessive;* there is a cone-cut when a clear, rounded area appears on the film (if round collimator used).
REF: p. 277

14. Long, distorted teeth appear on the film when:
   a. The vertical angulation is excessive.
   b. The vertical angulation is insufficient.
   c. The horizontal angulation is incorrect.
   d. There is a cone-cut.

Answer: b
Correct: Long, distorted teeth appear on the film when the vertical angulation is insufficient.
Incorrect:
(a) Long, distorted teeth appear on the film when *the vertical angulation is insufficient.*
(c) Overlapped teeth appear on the film when *the horizontal angulation is incorrect.*

(d) A curved, unexposed area appears on the film when *there is a cone cut.*
REF: p. 277

15. A cone cut occurs when:
   a. The film is underexposed.
   b. The film is overexposed.
   c. The PID was not properly aligned with the periapical film holder.
   d. The exposure button was not depressed for a sufficient amount of time.

Answer: c
Correct: A cone-cut occurs when the PID (position-indicating device) was not properly aligned with the periapical film holder.
Incorrect:
(a) The film will appear light when it is underexposed.
(b) The film will appear dark when it is overexposed.
(d) The film will appear light when the exposure button is not depressed for a sufficient amount of time.
REF: p. 277

16. When the distal surfaces of the canines are not visible on a premolar bite-wing film, the solution is to:
   a. Change the horizontal angulation of the tubehead.
   b. Increase the vertical angulation of the tubehead.
   c. Decrease the vertical angulation of the tubehead.
   d. Position the anterior edge of the film at the midline of the mandibular canine.

Answer: d
Correct: When the distal surfaces of the canines are not visible on a premolar bite-wing film, the solution is to position the anterior edge of the film at the midline of the mandibular canine.
Incorrect:
(a) *Position the anterior edge of the film at the midline of the mandibular canine.* Changing the horizontal angulation of the tubehead will cause overlapping.
(b) *Position the anterior edge of the film at the midline of the mandibular canine.* Increasing the vertical angulation of the tubehead will cause distortion.
(c) *Position the anterior edge of the film at the midline of the mandibular canine.* Decreasing the vertical angulation of the tubehead will cause distortion.
REF: p. 279

17. When the third molar regions are not visible on a molar bite-wing film, the solution is to:
   a. Decrease the vertical angulation of the tubehead.
   b. Increase the vertical angulation of the tubehead.
   c. Position the anterior edge of the film at the midline of the mandibular first premolar.
   d. Position the anterior edge of the film at the midline of the mandibular second premolar.

140

Answer: d

Correct: When the third molar regions are not visible on a molar bite-wing film, the solution is to position the anterior edge of the film at the midline of the mandibular second premolar.

Incorrect:

(a) *Position the anterior edge of the film at the midline of the mandibular second premolar.* Decreasing the vertical angulation of the tubehead will cause distortion.

(b) *Position the anterior edge of the film at the midline of the mandibular second premolar.* Increasing the vertical angulation of the tubehead will cause distortion.

(c) *Position the anterior edge of the film at the midline of the mandibular second premolar.*

REF p. 279

18. With _____, images appear stretched and distorted.
    a. film creasing
    b. film bending
    c. double exposure
    d. patient movement

Answer: b

Correct: With film bending, images appear stretched and distorted.

Incorrect:

(a) *With film bending*, images appear stretched and distorted. Film creasing causes a distinct, dark line.

(c) *With film bending*, images appear stretched and distorted. Double exposure causes multiple images.

(d) *With film bending*, images appear stretched and distorted. Patient movement causes blurred images.

REF: p. 281

19. A thin radiolucent line appears on the film with:
    a. Film creasing
    b. Film bending
    c. Double exposure
    d. Patient movement

Answer: a

Correct: A thin radiolucent line appears on the film with film creasing.

Incorrect:

(b) A thin radiolucent line appears on the film with *film creasing*. Film bending causes stretched, distorted images.

(c) A thin radiolucent line appears on the film with *film creasing*. Double exposure causes multiple images.

(d) A thin radiolucent line appears on the film with *film creasing*. Patient movement causes blurred images.

REF: p. 281

20. The appearance of a patient's finger on the film is called a:
    a. Hemangioma
    b. Phalangioma
    c. Myxoma
    d. Pericytoma

Answer: b

Correct: The appearance of a patient's finger on the film is called a phalangioma.

Incorrect:

(a) The appearance of a patient's finger on the film is called a *phalangioma*.

(c) The appearance of a patient's finger on the film is called a *phalangioma*.

(d) The appearance of a patient's finger on the film is called a *phalangioma*.

REF: p. 282

21. What is the cause of a double exposure?
    a. Patient movement during film exposure
    b. Two radiographs were stuck together during film exposure
    c. A double packet of film was used
    d. The film was exposed in the patient's mouth twice

Answer: d

Correct: The cause of a double exposure is that *the film was exposed in the patient's mouth twice.*

Incorrect:

(a) *The film was exposed in the patient's mouth twice.* Patient movement causes blurring.

(b) *The film was exposed in the patient's mouth twice.* The emulsion is damaged when films are stuck together.

(c) *The film was exposed in the patient's mouth twice.* A double film packet produces two identical images.

REF: p. 282

22. To avoid a double exposure:
    a. Only expose and process one half of the patient's mouth at one time.
    b. Mark exposed films with indelible ink.
    c. Always separate exposed and unexposed films.
    d. Ask the patient to hold the unexposed films.

Answer: c

Correct: To avoid a double exposure, always separate exposed and unexposed films.

Incorrect:

(a) *Always separate exposed and unexposed films.* The recommended protocol is the entire mouth at one time.

(b) *Always separate exposed and unexposed films.* Exposed films are not marked.

(d) *Always separate exposed and unexposed films.* The patient is not asked to hold unexposed films.

REF: p. 282

23. Blurred images appear on the film when:
   a. There is patient movement.
   b. The film is reversed.
   c. There is a double exposure.
   d. The film is creased.

Answer: a
Correct: Blurred images appear on the film when *there is patient movement.*
Incorrect:
   (b) A herringbone appears on the film when thè *film is reversed.*
   (c) Multiple images appear on the film when *there is a double exposure.*
   (d) A thin radiolucent line appears on the film when *the film is creased.*
REF: p. 282

24. When the film is reversed, the image will be:
   a. Elongated
   b. Distorted
   c. Light with a herringbone pattern
   d. Blurred

Answer: c
Correct: When the film is reversed, the image will be light with a herringbone pattern.
Incorrect:
   (a) When the vertical angulation is insufficient, the image will be *elongated.*
   (b) When the film is curved, the image will be *distorted.*
   (c) When there is patient movement, the image will be *blurred.*
REF: p. 282

CHAPTER 21   OCCLUSAL AND LOCALIZATION TECHNIQUES

MULTIPLE CHOICE
1. The occlusal technique is used to examine:
   a. Interproximal areas
   b. Large areas of the upper or lower jaw
   c. Third molars
   d. For bone loss

Answer: b
Correct: The occlusal technique is used to examine *large areas of the upper or lower jaw.*
Incorrect:
   (a) The bite-wing technique is used to examine *interproximal areas.*
   (c) The periapical technique is used to examine *large areas of the upper or lower jaw.*
   (d) The bite-wing technique is used to examine *for bone loss.*
REF: p. 288

2. In adults, size _____ film is used in the occlusal examination.
   a. 0
   b. 1
   c. 2
   d. 4

Answer: d
Correct: In adults, size 4 film is used in the occlusal examination.
Incorrect:
   (a) Size 0 film is not typically used for adults for any projection.
   (b) In adults, size 1 film is used in anterior and posterior periapical and bite-wing films.
   (c) In adults, size 2 film is used in anterior and posterior periapical and bite-wing films.
REF: p. 288

3. In children, size _____ film is used in the occlusal examination.
   a. 0
   b. 1
   c. 2
   d. 4

Answer: c
Correct: In children, size 2 film is used in the occlusal examination.
Incorrect:
   (a) In children, size 0 film is used in anterior and posterior periapical and posterior bite-wing exams.
   (b) In children, size 1 film is used in anterior and posterior periapical and posterior bite-wing examinations.
   (d) In children, size 4 film is not used in the maxillary pediatric occlusal examination.
REF: p. 288

4. When the occlusal technique is used, a _____ to stabilize the film.
   a. Stabe bite-block is used
   b. hemostat is used
   c. patient gently bites on the surface of the film
   d. bite-wing tab is used

Answer: c
Correct: When the occlusal technique is used, a _____ to stabilize the film
Incorrect:
   (a) *A patient gently bites on the surface of the film* to stabilize the film. A Stabe Bite-Block is used with periapical films.
   (b) *A patient gently bites on the surface of the film* to stabilize the film. A haemostat is used with endodontic films.
   (d) *A patient gently bites on the surface of the film* to stabilize the film. A bite-wing tab is used with bite-wing films.
REF: p. 288

5. When using the occlusal technique, the film is positioned with the _____ side facing the arch that is being exposed, and the film is placed in the mouth _____.
   a. white; to the lingual of the teeth
   b. white; between the occlusal surfaces of the maxillary and mandibular teeth
   c. colored; to the lingual of the teeth
   d. colored; between the occlusal surfaces of the maxillary and mandibular teeth

Answer: b
Correct: When using the occlusal technique, the film is positioned with the white side facing the arch that is being exposed, and the film is placed in the mouth between the occlusal surfaces of the maxillary and mandibular teeth.
Incorrect:
   (a) When using the occlusal technique, the film is positioned with the white side facing the arch that is being exposed, and the film is placed in the mouth *between the occlusal surfaces of the maxillary and mandibular teeth.*
   (c) When using the occlusal technique, the film is positioned with the *white* side facing the arch that is being exposed, and the film is placed in the mouth *between the occlusal surfaces of the maxillary and mandibular teeth.*
   (d) When using the occlusal technique, the film is positioned with the *white* side facing the arch that is being exposed, and the film is placed in the mouth between the occlusal surfaces of the maxillary and mandibular teeth.
REF: p. 288

6. Which of the following is a maxillary occlusal projection, but *not* a mandibular occlusal projection?
   a. Topographic occlusal projection
   b. Lateral occlusal projection
   c. Cross-sectional occlusal projection
   d. Pediatric projection

Answer: b
Correct: The lateral occlusal projection is a maxillary occlusal projection, but *not* a mandibular occlusal projection.
Incorrect:
   (a) The *topographic occlusal projection* may be a maxillary or mandibular occlusal projection.
   (c) The *cross-sectional occlusal projection* is a mandibular occlusal projection.
   (d) The *pediatric projections* may be maxillary or mandibular occlusal projections.
REF: p. 289

7. Which occlusal projection is used to examine the palate and the anterior teeth of the maxilla?
   a. Topographic occlusal projection
   b. Lateral occlusal projection

   c. Cross-sectional occlusal projection
   d. Pediatric projection

Answer: a
Correct: The topographic occlusal projection is used to examine the palate and the anterior teeth of the maxilla.
Incorrect:
   (b) The *lateral occlusal projection* is used to examine the palatal roots of the molar teeth.
   (c) The *cross-sectional occlusal projection* is used to examine the buccal and lingual aspects of the mandible.
   (d) The *pedatric projection* is used to examine the anterior teeth of the maxilla or mandible in children younger than 5 years old.
REF: p. 289

8. Which occlusal projection is used to locate foreign bodies or salivary stones in the region of the floor of the mouth?
   a. Topographic occlusal projection
   b. Lateral occlusal projection
   c. Cross-sectional occlusal projection
   d. Pediatric projection

Answer: c
Correct: The cross-sectional occlusal projection is used to locate foreign bodies or salivary stones in the region of the floor of the mouth.
Incorrect:
   (a) The *mandibular topographic occlusal projection* is used to examine the anterior teeth of the mandible.
   (b) The *lateral occlusal projection,* a maxillary projection, is used to examine palatal roots of the molar teeth.
   (d) The *pediatric projection* is used to examine the anterior teeth of the maxilla or mandible in children.
REF: p. 289

9. The pediatric projection is recommended for use in children _____ years old or younger.
   a. 2
   b. 5
   c. 8
   d. 10

Answer: b
Correct: The pediatric projection is recommended for use in children 5 years old or younger.
Incorrect:
   (a) The pediatric projection is recommended for use in children *5 years old or younger.*
   (c) The pediatric projection is recommended for use in children *5 years old or younger.*
   (d) The pediatric projection is recommended for use in children *5 years old or younger.*
REF: p. 289

10. For the maxillary topographic occlusal projection, the central ray is directed at _____ degrees.
a. +30
b. +45
c. +65
d. −30

Answer: c
Correct: For the maxillary topographic occlusal projection, the central ray is directed at +65 degrees.
Incorrect:
(a) For the mandibular cross-sectional occlusal projection, the central ray is directed at 90 degrees.
(b) For the maxillary lateral occlusal projection, the central ray is directed at +60 degrees.
(d) For the mandibular pediatric occlusal projection, the central ray is directed at −55 degrees.
REF: p. 290

11. The dental radiograph is a _____-dimensional picture of a _____-dimensional object.
a. two; two
b. three; three
c. two; three
d. three; two

Answer: c
Correct: The dental radiograph is a two-dimensional picture of a three-dimensional object.
Incorrect:
(a) The dental radiograph is a two-dimensional picture of a *three*-dimensional object.
(b) The dental radiograph is a *two*-dimensional picture of a three-dimensional object.
(d) The dental radiograph is a *two*-dimensional picture of a *three*-dimensional object.
REF: p. 295

12. A radiograph depicts which of the following dimensions of an object?
(1) Length
(2) Width
(3) Depth
a. 1, 2, 3
b. 1, 2
c. 1, 3
d. 2, 3

Answer: b
Correct: A radiograph depicts length and width; the radiograph does not depict the buccal-lingual relationship (or depth).
Incorrect:
(a) A radiograph depicts *length* and *width;* it does not depict depth.

(c) A radiograph depicts *length* and *width;* it does not depict depth.
(d) A radiograph depicts *length* and *width,* it does not depict depth.
REF: p. 295

13. The buccal object rule depends on a _____ image shift when trying to locate vertically aligned images. With the buccal object rule, an object to the buccal of the reference object will move in the _____ direction as the shift.
a. vertical; same
b. vertical; opposite
c. horizontal; same
d. horizontal; opposite

Answer: d
Correct: The buccal object rule depends on a horizontal image shift when trying to locate vertically aligned images. With the buccal object rule, an object to the buccal of the reference object will move in the opposite direction as the shift.
Incorrect:
(a) The buccal object rule depends on a *horizontal* image shift when trying to locate vertically aligned images. With the buccal object rule, an object to the buccal of the reference object will move in the *opposite* direction as the shift.
(b) The buccal object rule depends on a *horizontal* image shift when trying to locate vertically aligned images. With the buccal object rule, an object to the buccal of the reference object will move in the opposite direction as the shift.
(c) The buccal object rule depends on a horizontal image shift when trying to locate vertically aligned images. With the buccal object rule, an object to the buccal of the reference object will move in the *opposite* direction as the shift.
REF: p. 296

14. The "S" in the mnemonic SLOB stands for:
a. Shift
b. Similar
c. Same
d. Some

Answer: c
Correct: The "S" in the mnemonic SLOB stands for same.
Incorrect:
(a) The "S" in the mnemonic SLOB stands for *same.*
(b) The "S" in the mnemonic SLOB stands for *same.*
(d) The "S" in the mnemonic SLOB stands for *same.*
REF: p. 296

15. According to the SLOB rule, when two radiographs are compared, the object that lies to the lingual appears to have moved in the same direction as the position-indicating device (PID), and the object that lies to the buccal appears to have moved in the opposite direction as the PID.
   a. Both statements are true.
   b. Both statements are false.
   c. The first statement is true; the second statement is false.
   d. The first statement is false; the second statement is true.

Answer: a
Correct: According to the SLOB rule, when two radiographs are compared, the object that lies to the lingual appears to have moved in the same direction as the PID, and the object that lies to the buccal appears to have moved in the opposite direction as the PID.
Incorrect:
   (b) According to the SLOB rule, when two radiographs are compared, the object that lies to the lingual appears to have moved in the *same* direction as the PID, and the object that lies to the buccal appears to have moved in the *opposite* direction as the PID.
   (c) According to the SLOB rule, when two radiographs are compared, the object that lies to the lingual appears to have moved in the *same* direction as the PID, and the object that lies to the buccal appears to have moved in the *opposite* direction as the PID.
   (d) According to the SLOB rule, when two radiographs are compared, the object that lies to the lingual appears to have moved in the *same* direction as the PID, and the object that lies to the buccal appears to have moved in the *opposite* direction as the PID.
REF: p. 296

16. When the right-angle technique is used, an occlusal film is exposed directing the central ray at _____ degrees to the film.
   a. 20
   b. 45
   c. 65
   d. 90

Answer: d
Correct: When the right-angle technique is used, an occlusal film is exposed directing the central ray at 90 degrees to the film.
Incorrect:
   (a) When the right-angle technique is used, an occlusal film is exposed directing the central ray at *90* degrees to the film.
   (b) When the right-angle technique is used, an occlusal film is exposed directing the central ray at *90* degrees to the film.

   (c) When the right-angle technique is used, an occlusal film is exposed directing the central ray at *90* degrees to the film.
REF: pp. 296-297

17. For the maxillary pediatric occlusal projection, position the PID so that the central ray is directed at _____ degrees toward the center of the film.
   a. +20
   b. +45
   c. +60
   d. +90

Answer: c
Correct: For the maxillary pediatric occlusal projection, position the PID so that the central ray is directed at +60 degrees toward the center of the film.
Incorrect:
   (a) For the maxillary pediatric occlusal projection, position the PID so that the central ray is directed at *+60* degrees toward the center of the film.
   (b) For the maxillary pediatric occlusal projection, position the PID so that the central ray is directed at *+60* degrees toward the center of the film.
   (d) For the maxillary pediatric occlusal projection, position the PID so that the central ray is directed at *+60* degrees toward the center of the film.
REF: p. 292

18. For the mandibular topographic occlusal projection, position the PID so that the central ray is directed at _____ degrees toward the center of the film.
   a. +55
   b. −55
   c. +90
   d. −90

Answer: b
Correct: For the mandibular topographic occlusal projection, position the PID so that the central ray is directed at −55 degrees toward the center of the film.
Incorrect:
   (a) For the mandibular topographic occlusal projection, position the PID so that the central ray is directed at *−55* degrees toward the center of the film.
   (c) For the mandibular topographic occlusal projection, position the PID so that the central ray is directed at *−55* degrees toward the center of the film.
   (d) For the mandibular topographic occlusal projection, position the PID so that the central ray is directed at *−55* degrees toward the center of the film.
REF: p. 293

145

MULTIPLE CHOICE

1. Advantages of panoramic films over intraoral peri-apical films include visualization of:
(1) Impacted third molar teeth
(2) Jaw fractures
(3) Large lesions in the posterior mandible
    a. 1, 2, 3
    b. 1, 2
    c. 1, 3
    d. 2, 3

Answer: a
Correct: Advantages of panoramic films over intraoral periapical films include visualization of impacted third molar teeth, jaw fractures, and large lesions in the posterior mandible.
Incorrect:
    (b) Advantages of panoramic films over intraoral periapical films include visualization of impacted third molar teeth, jaw fractures, *and large lesions in the posterior mandible.*
    (c) Advantages of panoramic films over intraoral periapical films include visualization of impacted third molar teeth, *jaw fractures,* and large lesions in the posterior mandible.
    (d) Advantages of panoramic films over intraoral periapical films include visualization of *impacted third molar teeth,* jaw fractures, and large lesions in the posterior mandible.
REF: p. 305

2. A panoramic film is _____ film(s) taken using an _____ technique.
    a. a series of; intraoral
    b. a series of; extraoral
    c. a single; intraoral
    d. a single; extraoral

Answer: d
Correct: A panoramic film is single film taken using an extraoral technique.
Incorrect:
    (a) A panoramic film is *single* film taken using an *extraoral* technique.
    (b) A panoramic film is *single* film taken using an extraoral technique.
    (c) A panoramic film is single film taken using an *extraoral* technique.
REF: p. 305

3. In panoramic radiography, the _____ rotates around the patient.
    a. film
    b. tubehead
    c. tubehead and film
    d. dental chair

Answer: c
Correct: In panoramic radiography, the tubehead and film rotates around the patient.
Incorrect:
    (a) In panoramic radiography the *tubehead,* as well as the film, rotates around the patient.
    (b) In panoramic radiography the *film,* as well as the tubehead, rotates around the patient.
    (d) In panoramic radiography the *dental chair* does not rotate.
REF: p. 306

4. The panoramic film is typically used to evaluate and diagnose:
    a. Caries
    b. Periodontal disease
    c. Impacted teeth
    d. Periapical lesions

Answer: c
Correct: The panoramic film is typically used to evaluate and diagnose impacted teeth.
Incorrect:
    (a) The panoramic film is typically used to *evaluate and diagnose impacted teeth;* it is not recommended that the panoramic film be used to evaluate and diagnose caries.
    (b) The panoramic film is typically used to *evaluate and diagnose impacted teeth;* it is not recommended that the panoramic film be used to evaluate and diagnose periodontal disease.
    (d) The panoramic film is typically used to *evaluate and diagnose impacted teeth;* it is not recommended that the panoramic film be used to evaluate and diagnose periapical lesions.
REF: p. 306

5. In panoramic radiography, the x-ray tube rotates around the patient's head in one direction while the film rotates _____ direction.
    a. horizontally in the same
    b. horizontally in the opposite
    c. vertically in the same
    d. vertically in the opposite

Answer: b
Correct: In panoramic radiography, the x-ray tube rotates around the patient's head in one direction while the film rotates horizontally in the opposite direction.
Incorrect:
    (a) In panoramic radiography, the x-ray tube rotates around the patient's head in one direction while the film rotates *in the opposite* and not same direction.
    (c) In panoramic radiography, the x-ray tube rotates around the patient's head in one direction while the film rotates *horizontally* rather than vertically in the opposite and not same direction.

(d) In panoramic radiography, the x-ray tube rotates around the patient's head in one direction while the film rotates *horizontally* rather than vertically.

REF: p. 306

6. In panoramic radiography, the movement of the film and the tubehead produces an image through the process known as:
   a. Scanography
   b. Digitizing
   c. Scintillation
   d. Tomography

Answer: d

Correct: In panoramic radiography, the movement of the film and the tubehead produces an image through the process known as tomography.

Incorrect:
   (a) In panoramic radiography, the movement of the film and the tubehead produces an image through the process known as *tomography.*
   (b) In panoramic radiography, the movement of the film and the tubehead produces an image through the process known as *tomography.*
   (c) In panoramic radiography, the movement of the film and the tubehead produces an image through the process known as *tomography.*

REF: p. 306

7. In panoramic radiography, the pivotal point, or axis, around which the cassette carrier and x-ray tubehead rotate is termed a:
   a. Terminal hinge axis
   b. Rotation center
   c. Tipping point
   d. Germinal center

Answer: b

Correct: In panoramic radiography, the pivotal point, or axis, around which the cassette carrier and x-ray tubehead rotate is termed a rotation center.

Incorrect:
   (a) In panoramic radiography, the pivotal point, or axis, around which the cassette carrier and x-ray tubehead rotate is termed a *rotation center.*
   (c) In panoramic radiography, the pivotal point, or axis, around which the cassette carrier and x-ray tubehead rotate is termed a *rotation center.*
   (d) In panoramic radiography, the pivotal point, or axis, around which the cassette carrier and x-ray tubehead rotate is termed a *rotation center.*

REF: p. 306

8. The rotational change in a panoramic machine allows the image layer to conform to the _____ shape of the dental arches.
   a. square
   b. tapering
   c. ovoid
   d. elliptical

Answer: d

Correct: The rotational change in a panoramic machine allows the image layer to conform to the elliptical shape of the dental arches.

Incorrect:
   (a) The rotational change in a panoramic machine allows the image layer to conform to the *elliptical* shape of the dental arches
   (b) The rotational change in a panoramic machine allows the image layer to conform to the *elliptical* shape of the dental arches.
   (c) The rotational change in a panoramic machine allows the image layer to conform to the *elliptical* shape of the dental arches.

REF: p. 306

9. In panoramic radiography, the _____ is a theoretical concept used to determine where the dental arches must be positioned to achieve the clearest image.
   a. waypoint
   b. focal trough
   c. neutral zone
   d. home zone

Answer: b

Correct: In panoramic radiography, the _____ is a theoretical concept used to determine where the dental arches must be positioned to achieve the clearest image.

Incorrect:
   (a) In panoramic radiography, the *focal trough* is a theoretical concept used to determine where the dental arches must be positioned to achieve the clearest image.
   (c) In panoramic radiography, the *focal trough* is a theoretical concept used to determine where the dental arches must be positioned to achieve the clearest image.
   (d) In panoramic radiography, the *focal trough* is a theoretical concept used to determine where the dental arches must be positioned to achieve the clearest image.

REF: p. 306

10. Structures are clearly demonstrated on a panoramic radiograph in a _____ zone.
    a. two-dimensional straight
    b. two-dimensional curved
    c. three-dimensional straight
    d. three-dimensional curved

Answer: d

Correct: Structures are clearly demonstrated on a panoramic radiograph in a three-dimensional curved zone.

Incorrect:
    (a) Structures are clearly demonstrated on a panoramic radiograph in a *three-dimensional curved* zone.
    (b) Structures are clearly demonstrated on a panoramic radiograph in a *three-dimensional curved* zone.

147

(c) Structures are clearly demonstrated on a pano-ramic radiograph in a *three-dimensional curved zone.*

REF: p. 306

11. The closer the rotation center is to the teeth, the wider the focal trough. In most panoramic machines, the focal trough is wide in the anterior region and narrow in the posterior region.
   a. Both statements are true.
   b. Both statements are false.
   c. The first statement is true; the second statement is false.
   d. The first statement is false; the second statement is true.

Answer: b
Correct: The closer the rotation center is to the teeth, the *narrower* the focal trough. In most panoramic machines, the focal trough is *narrow* in the anterior region and *wide* in the posterior region.
Incorrect:
   (a) The closer the rotation center is to the teeth, the *narrower* the focal trough. In most panoramic machines, the focal trough is *narrow* in the anterior region and *wide* in the posterior region.
   (c) The closer the rotation center is to the teeth, the *narrower* the focal trough. In most panoramic machines, the focal trough is *narrow* in the anterior region and *wide* in the posterior region.
   (d) The closer the rotation center is to the teeth, the *narrower* the focal trough. In most panoramic machines, the focal trough is *narrow* in the anterior region and *wide* in the posterior region.

REF: p. 306

12. Panoramic units may differ in the:
   (1) Number of the rotation centers
   (2) The size and shape of the focal trough
   (3) The type of film transport mechanism used
      a. 1, 2, 3
      b. 1, 2
      c. 1, 3
      d. 2, 3

Answer: a
Correct: Panoramic units may differ in the number of the rotation centers, the size and shape of the focal trough, and the type of film transport mechanism used.
Incorrect:
   (b) Panoramic units may differ in the number of the rotation centers, the size and shape of the focal trough, *and the type of film transport mechanism used.*
   (c) Panoramic units may differ in the number of the rotation centers, *the size and shape of the focal trough,* and the type of film transport mechanism used.

(d) Panoramic units may differ in the *number of the rotation centers,* the size and shape of the focal trough, and the type of film transport mechanism used.

REF: p. 307

13. Which component in the panoramic x-ray machine tubehead is most different from that found in an intraoral x-ray machine tubehead?
   a. Filament
   b. Target
   c. Heat sink
   d. Collimator

Answer: d
Correct: The collimator in the panoramic x-ray machine tubehead is most different from that found in an intraoral x-ray machine tubehead.
Incorrect:
   (a) The *collimator* in the panoramic x-ray machine tubehead is most different from that found in an intraoral x-ray machine tubehead.
   (b) The *collimator* in the panoramic x-ray machine tubehead is most different from that found in an intraoral x-ray machine tubehead.
   (c) The *collimator* in the panoramic x-ray machine tubehead is most different from that found in an intraoral x-ray machine tubehead.

REF: p. 309

14. The collimator used in the panoramic x-ray machine is a _____ plate.
   a. aluminum
   b. silver
   c. lead
   d. copper

Answer: c
Correct: The collimator used in the panoramic x-ray ma-chine is a lead plate.
Incorrect:
   (a) The collimator used in the panoramic x-ray machine is a *lead* plate.
   (b) The collimator used in the panoramic x-ray machine is a *lead* plate.
   (d) The collimator used in the panoramic x-ray machine is a *lead* plate.

REF: p. 309

15. The collimator used in panoramic radiography has an opening in the shape of a _____ slit.
   a. narrow horizontal
   b. narrow vertical
   c. wide horizontal
   d. wide vertical

Answer: b
Correct: The collimator used in panoramic radiography has an opening in the shape of a narrow vertical slit.

Incorrect:

(a) The collimator used in panoramic radiography has an opening in the shape of a *narrow vertical* slit.

(c) The collimator used in panoramic radiography has an opening in the shape of a *narrow vertical* slit.

(d) The collimator used in panoramic radiography has an opening in the shape of a *narrow vertical* slit.

REF: p. 309

16. The vertical angulation in the tubehead of the panoramic unit:
    a. Is fixed in position so that the x-ray beam is directed slightly upward
    b. Is fixed in position so that the x-ray beam is directed slightly downward
    c. Can be adjusted according to the size of the patient
    d. Can be adjusted for maxillary or mandibular films

Answer: a

Correct: The vertical angulation in the tubehead of the panoramic unit is fixed in position so that the x-ray beam is directed slightly upward.

Incorrect:

(b) The vertical angulation in the tubehead of the panoramic unit *is directed slightly upward* rather than downward.

(c) The vertical angulation in the tubehead of the panoramic unit *is directed slightly upward*; it cannot be adjusted according to the size of the patient.

(d) The vertical angulation in the tubehead of the panoramic unit *is directed slightly upward*; it cannot be adjusted for maxillary or mandibular films.

REF: p. 309

17. The tubehead of the panoramic unit always rotates _____ the patient's head as the film rotates _____ of the patient.
    a. behind; behind
    b. in front; in front
    c. behind; in front
    d. in front; behind

Answer: c

Correct: The tubehead of the panoramic unit always rotates behind the patient's head as the film rotates in front of the patient.

Incorrect:

(a) The tubehead of the panoramic unit always rotates behind the patient's head as the film rotates *in front* of the patient.

(b) The tubehead of the panoramic unit always rotates *behind* the patient's head as the film rotates in front of the patient.

(d) The tubehead of the panoramic unit always rotates *behind* the patient's head as the film rotates *in front* of the patient.

REF: p. 309

18. In panoramic radiography, which of the following exposure factors *cannot* be changed?
    a. Milliamperage
    b. Kilovoltage
    c. Exposure time
    d. Both a and c

Answer: c

Correct: In panoramic radiography, the exposure time cannot be changed.

Incorrect:

(a) In panoramic radiography the *exposure time* cannot be changed, but milliamperage can.

(b) In panoramic radiography the *exposure time* cannot be changed, but kilovoltage can.

(d) Choice a is true, but choice c is false; in panoramic radiography the *exposure time* cannot be changed.

REF: p. 309

19. Panoramic screen film is exposed by:
    a. Photons
    b. Electrons
    c. Intensifying screens in a cassette holder
    d. A shutter in the cassette with visible light

Answer: c

Correct: Panoramic screen film is exposed by intensifying screens in a cassette holder.

Incorrect:

(a) Panoramic screen film is exposed by *intensifying screens in a cassette holder*.

(b) Panoramic screen film is exposed by *intensifying screens in a cassette holder*.

(d) Panoramic screen film is exposed by *intensifying screens in a cassette holder*.

REF: p. 310

20. Green-sensitive film must be paired with intensifying screens that produce _____ light.
    a. yellow
    b. blue
    c. red
    d. green

Answer: d

Correct: Green-sensitive film must be paired with intensifying screens that produce green light.

Incorrect:

(a) Green-sensitive film must be paired with intensifying screens that produce *green* light.

(b) Green-sensitive film must be paired with intensifying screens that produce *green* light.

(c) Green-sensitive film must be paired with intensifying screens that produce *green* light.

REF: p. 310

21. Rare earth screens emit _____ light and are considered faster than calcium tungstate screens, which emit _____ light.
   a. blue; green
   b. blue; blue
   c. green; green
   d. green; blue

Answer: d

Correct: Rare earth screens emit green light and are considered faster than calcium tungstate screens, which emit blue light.

Incorrect:
   (a) Rare earth screens emit *green* light and are considered faster than calcium tungstate screens, which emit *blue* light.
   (b) Rare earth screens emit *green* light and are considered faster than calcium tungstate screens, which emit *blue* light.
   (c) Rare earth screens emit *green* light and are considered faster than calcium tungstate screens, which emit *blue* light.

REF: p. 310

22. A cassette has _____ intensifying screen(s).
   a. one
   b. two
   c. three
   d. four

Answer: b

Correct: A cassette has two intensifying screens; one screen is placed on either side of the film.

Incorrect:
   (a) A cassette has *two* intensifying screens.
   (c) A cassette has *two* intensifying screens.
   (d) A cassette has *two* intensifying screens.

REF: p. 310

23. A ghost image occurs when:
   a. The patient moves while the film is being exposed.
   b. The film is reversed after being removed from the film carrier.
   c. All metallic or radiodense objects are not removed before the exposure of a panoramic film.
   d. The patient raises his or her hand while an exposure is being made.

Answer: c

Correct: A ghost image occurs when all metallic or radiodense objects are not removed before the exposure of a panoramic film.

Incorrect:
   (a) Blurring occurs when the patient moves while the film is being exposed.
   (b) Reversing a film after it is removed from the film carrier does not cause a ghost image.

   (d) Patient hand movement does not cause a ghost image.

REF: p. 313

24. A ghost image appears _____ than its actual counterpart.
   a. smaller
   b. lower
   c. more indistinct
   d. more distinct

Answer: c

Correct: A ghost image appears more indistinct than its actual counterpart.

Incorrect:
   (a) A ghost image appears *more indistinct* than its actual counterpart.
   (b) A ghost image appears *more indistinct* than its actual counterpart.
   (d) A ghost image appears *more indistinct* than its actual counterpart.

REF: p. 313

25. A lead apron _____ a thyroid collar should be used when exposing a panoramic film, and the patient should be told to raise the tongue up to the _____.
   a. without; palate
   b. without; occlusal plane
   c. with; palate
   d. with; occlusal plane

Answer: a

Correct: A lead apron without a thyroid collar should be used when exposing a panoramic film, and the patient should be told to raise the tongue up to the palate.

Incorrect:
   (b) A lead apron *without* a thyroid collar should be used when exposing a panoramic film, and the patient should be told to raise the tongue up to the *palate,* not the occlusal plane.
   (c) A lead apron *without* a thyroid collar should be used when exposing a panoramic film, and the patient should be told to raise the tongue up to the *palate*.
   (d) A lead apron *without* a thyroid collar should be used when exposing a panoramic film, and the patient should be told to raise the tongue up to the *palate*, not the occlusal plane.

REF: p. 313

26. If the patient's lips are not closed on the bite-block during the exposure of a panoramic film, a _____ shadow results that obscures the anterior teeth.
   a. light radiopaque
   b. dark radiopaque
   c. light radiolucent
   d. dark radiolucent

Answer: d

Correct: If the patient's lips are not closed on the bite-block during the exposure of a panoramic film, a dark radiolucent shadow results that obscures the anterior teeth.

Incorrect:

(a) If the patient's lips are not closed on the bite-block during the exposure of a panoramic film, a *dark radiolucent* shadow results that obscures the anterior teeth.

(b) If the patient's lips are not closed on the bite-block during the exposure of a panoramic film, a *dark radiolucent* shadow results that obscures the anterior teeth.

(c) If the patient's lips are not closed on the bite-block during the exposure of a panoramic film, a *dark radiolucent* shadow results that obscures the anterior teeth.

REF: p. 313

27. A "reverse smile line" is seen on the radiograph if the patient's:
    a. Chin is tipped down
    b. Chin is tipped up
    c. Teeth are positioned too far back on the bite-block
    d. Teeth are positioned too far forward on the bite-block

Answer: b

Correct: A "reverse smile line" is seen if the patient's chin is tipped up.

Incorrect:

(a) A "reverse smile line" is seen if the patient's *chin is tipped up,* not down.

(c) The anterior teeth will appear "fat" if the teeth are positioned too far back on the bite-block.

(d) The anterior teeth will appear "skinny" if the teeth are positioned too far forward on the bite-block.

REF: p. 314

28. An "exaggerated smile line" is seen on the radiograph if the patient's:
    a. Chin is tipped down
    b. Chin is tipped up
    c. Teeth are positioned too far back on the bite-block
    d. Teeth are positioned too far forward on the bite-block

Answer: a

Correct: An "exaggerated smile line" is seen on the radiograph if the patient's chin is tipped down.

Incorrect:

(b) An "exaggerated smile line" is seen on the radiograph if the patient's *chin is tipped down,* not up.

(c) The anterior teeth will appear "fat" if the teeth are positioned too far forward on the bite-block.

(d) The anterior teeth will appear "skinny" if the teeth are positioned too far forward on the bite-block.

REF: p. 315

29. The anterior teeth will appear "skinny" if the:
    a. Chin is tipped down
    b. Chin is tipped up
    c. Teeth are positioned too far back on the bite-block
    d. Teeth are positioned too far forward on the bite-block

Answer: d

Correct: The anterior teeth will appear "skinny" if the teeth are positioned too far forward on the bite-block.

Incorrect:

(a) An "exaggerated smile line" is seen on the radiograph if the patient's chin is tipped down.

(b) A "reverse smile line" is seen if the patient's chin is tipped up.

(c) The anterior teeth will appear "fat" if the *teeth are positioned too far forward on the bite-block.*

REF: p. 315

30. The anterior teeth will appear "fat" if the:
    a. Chin is tipped down
    b. Chin is tipped up
    c. Teeth are positioned too far back on the bite-block
    d. Teeth are positioned too far forward on the bite-block

Answer: c

Correct: The anterior teeth will appear "fat" if the teeth are positioned too far back on the bite-block.

Incorrect:

(a) An "exaggerated smile line" is seen on the radiograph if the patient's chin is tipped down.

(b) A "reverse smile line" is seen if the patient's chin is tipped up.

(d) The anterior teeth will appear "skinny" if the teeth are positioned too far forward on the bite-block.

REF: p. 315

31. A disadvantage of panoramic dental radiography when contrasted with intraoral dental radiography is:
    a. Panoramic radiography results in higher exposure to the patient than intraoral radiography.
    b. Fewer anatomic structures can be viewed on a panoramic film than on a complete intraoral radiographic series.
    c. The images seen on a panoramic radiograph are not as sharp as those on intraoral radiographs because of the intensifying screens.
    d. The exposure of a panoramic radiograph is readily accepted by the patient because there is no discomfort involved.

Answer: c
Correct: A disadvantage of panoramic dental radiography when contrasted with intraoral dental radiography is the images seen on a panoramic radiograph are not as sharp as those on intraoral radiographs because of the intensifying screens.
Incorrect:
  (a) Panoramic radiography results in lower exposure to the patient than intraoral radiography.
  (b) More anatomic structures can be viewed on a panoramic film than on a complete intraoral radiographic series.
  (d) This is an advantage rather than disadvantage of panoramic radiography.
REF: p. 319

CHAPTER 23   EXTRAORAL RADIOGRAPHY

MULTIPLE CHOICE

1. An extraoral radiograph is placed _____ the mouth during x-ray exposure. Extraoral radiography is used to image _____ areas of the skull or jaws.
   a. outside; small
   b. outside; large
   c. inside; small
   d. inside; large

Answer: b
Correct: An extraoral radiograph is placed outside the mouth during x-ray exposure. Extraoral radiography is used to image large areas of the skull or jaws.
Incorrect:
  (a) An extraoral radiograph is placed outside the mouth during x-ray exposure. Extraoral radiography is used to image *large* areas of the skull or jaws.
  (c) An extraoral radiograph is placed *outside* the mouth during x-ray exposure. Extraoral radiography is used to image *large* areas of the skull or jaws.
  (d) An extraoral radiograph is placed *outside* the mouth during x-ray exposure. Extraoral radiography is used to image large areas of the skull or jaws.
REF: p. 324

2. Extraoral films are primarily used in which of the following specialty areas?
   a. Endodontics
   b. Periodontics
   c. Oral surgery
   d. Pediatric dentistry

Answer: c
Correct: Extraoral films are primarily used in oral surgery.
Incorrect:
  (a) Intraoral films are primarily used in endodontics.
  (b) Intraoral films are primarily used in periodontics.

  (d) Intraoral films are primarily used in pediatric dentistry.
REF: p. 324

3. The most common extraoral film is the _____ projection.
   a. lateral cephalometric
   b. posteroanterior
   c. Waters
   d. panoramic radiograph

Answer: d
Correct: The most common extraoral film is the panoramic radiograph projection.
Incorrect:
  (a) The most common extraoral film is the *panoramic radiograph* projection.
  (b) The most common extraoral film is the *panoramic radiograph* projection.
  (c) The most common extraoral film is the *panoramic radiograph* projection.
REF: p. 324

4. The extraoral film is typically used to evaluate:
   a. gutta percha root canal fillings
   b. the integrity of the crest of alveolar bone
   c. the temporomandibular joint area
   d. interproximal decay

Answer: c
Correct: The extraoral film is typically used to evaluate the temporomandibular joint area.
Incorrect:
  (a) The extraoral film is typically used to evaluate *the temporomandibular joint area.*
  (b) The extraoral film is typically used to evaluate *the temporomandibular joint area.*
  (d) The extraoral film is typically used to evaluate *the temporomandibular joint area.*
REF: p. 324

5. Extraoral radiographs may be used in conjunction with intraoral films. The images seen on extraoral film are not as defined or sharp as the images seen on an intraoral radiograph.
   a. Both statements are true.
   b. Both statements are false.
   c. The first statement is true; the second statement is false.
   d. The first statement is false; the second statement is true.

Answer: a
Correct: Extraoral radiographs may be used in conjunction with intraoral films. The images seen on extraoral film are not as defined or sharp as the images seen on an intraoral radiograph.

Incorrect:

 (b) Extraoral radiographs may be used in conjunction with intraoral films. The images seen on extraoral film are not as defined or sharp as the images seen on an intraoral radiograph.

 (c) Extraoral radiographs may be used in conjunction with intraoral films. *The images seen on extraoral film are not as defined or sharp as the images seen on an intraoral radiograph.*

 (d) *Extraoral radiographs may be used in conjunction with intraoral films.* The images seen on extraoral film are not as defined or sharp as the images seen on an intraoral radiograph.

REF: p. 324

6. Which of the following is the most commonly used extraoral film size?
 a. 3×5
 b. 4×6
 c. 5×7
 d. 10×12

Answer: c

Correct: The 5×7 is the most commonly used extraoral film size.

Incorrect:

 (a) The 5×7 is the most commonly used extraoral film size.

 (b) The 5×7 is the most commonly used extraoral film size.

 (d) The 5×7 is the most commonly used extraoral film size.

REF: p. 325

7. An occlusal film (size _____) may be used for some extraoral radiographs.
 a. 0
 b. 1
 c. 2
 d. 4

Answer: d

Correct: An occlusal film (size 4) may be used for some extraoral radiographs.

Incorrect:

 (a) An occlusal film (size *4*) may be used for some extraoral radiographs; size 0 is too small.

 (b) An occlusal film (size *4*) may be used for some extraoral radiographs; size 1 is too small.

 (c) An occlusal film (size *4*) may be used for some extraoral radiographs; size 2 is too small.

REF: p. 326

8. An occlusal film _____ be used for some extraoral radiographs. When used extraorally, it covers a _____ area than a screen film
 a. may; smaller
 b. may not; smaller

 c. may; larger
 d. may not; larger

Answer: a

Correct: An occlusal film may be used for some extraoral radiographs. When used extraorally, it covers a smaller area than a screen film.

Incorrect:

 (b) An occlusal film *may* be used for some extraoral radiographs. When used extraorally, it covers a smaller area than a screen film.

 (c) An occlusal film may be used for some extraoral radiographs. When used extraorally, it covers a *smaller* area than a screen film.

 (d) An occlusal film *may* be used for some extraoral radiographs. When used extraorally, it covers a *smaller* area than a screen film.

REF: p. 326

9. The front side of the cassette is typically constructed of _____ and permits the passage of the x-ray beam, whereas the back side is made of _____ to reduce scatter radiation.
 a. metal; metal
 b. plastic; plastic
 c. plastic; metal
 d. metal; plastic

Answer: c

Correct: The front side of the cassette is typically constructed of plastic and permits the passage of the x-ray beam, whereas the back side is made of metal to reduce scatter radiation.

Incorrect:

 (a) The front side of the cassette is typically constructed of *plastic* and permits the passage of the x-ray beam, whereas the back side is made of metal to reduce scatter radiation.

 (b) The front side of the cassette is typically constructed of plastic and permits the passage of the x-ray beam, whereas the back side is made of *metal* to reduce scatter radiation.

 (d) The front side of the cassette is typically constructed of *plastic* and permits the passage of the x-ray beam, whereas the back side is made of *metal* to reduce scatter radiation.

REF: p. 326

10. Which of the following is the fastest recommended screen and screen film combination?
 a. Calcium tungstate screen with blue light
 b. Calcium tungstate screen with green light
 c. Rare earth screen with blue light
 d. Rare earth screen with green light

Answer: d

Correct: The *rare earth screen with green light* is the fastest recommended screen and screen film combination.

Incorrect:

(a) The *rare earth screen with green light* is the fastest recommended screen and screen film combination.

(b) The *rare earth screen with green light* is the fastest recommended screen and screen film combination.

(c) The *rare earth screen with green light* is the fastest recommended screen and screen film combination.

REF: p. 326

11. A(n) _____ is a device used to reduce the amount of scatter radiation that reaches an extraoral film during exposure.
    a. collimator
    b. grid
    c. cassette
    d. intensifying screen

Answer: b

Correct: A grid is a device used to reduce the amount of scatter radiation that reaches an extraoral film during exposure.

Incorrect:

(a) A collimator is a device used to restrict the size and shape of the x-ray beam.

(c) A cassette is a device used to hold the extraoral film and intensifying screens.

(d) An intensifying screen is a device that converts x-ray energy into visible light.

REF: p. 326

12. Scatter radiation:
    a. Increases film fog
    b. Increases film contrast
    c. Reduces film contrast
    d. Both a and c

Answer: d

Correct: Scatter radiation increases film fog and reduces film contrast.

Incorrect:

(a) Scatter radiation *increases film fog* and *reduces film contrast*.

(b) Scatter radiation *increases film fog* and *reduces film contrast*.

(c) Scatter radiation *increases film fog* and *reduces film contrast*.

REF: p. 326

13. A grid can be used to _____ film fog and _____ the contrast of the radiographic image.
    a. decrease; decrease
    b. increase; increase
    c. decrease; increase
    d. increase; decrease

Answer: c

Correct: A grid can be used to decrease film fog and increase the contrast of the radiographic image.

Incorrect:

(a) A grid can be used to *decrease* film fog and *increase* the contrast of the radiographic image.

(b) A grid can be used to *decrease* film fog and increase the contrast of the radiographic image.

(d) A grid can be used to *decrease* film fog and *increase* the contrast of the radiographic image.

REF: p. 326

14. A grid is composed of a series of:
    a. Wire mesh that is similar to the screen in a window or door
    b. Copper wires around an armature
    c. Thin lead strips
    d. Thick lead strips

Answer: c

Correct: A grid is composed of a series of thin lead strips.

Incorrect:

(a) A grid is composed of a series of *thin lead strips*.

(b) A grid is composed of a series of *thin lead strips*.

(d) A grid is composed of a series of *thin lead strips*.

REF: p. 326

15. The grid is placed between the _____ and the _____.
    a. aluminum filter; PID
    b. PID; patient's head
    c. patient's head; film
    d. film; cassette

Answer: c

Correct: The grid is placed between the patient's head and the film.

Incorrect:

(a) The grid is placed between the *patient's head* and the *film*.

(b) The grid is placed between the *patient's head* and the *film*.

(d) The grid is placed between the *patient's head* and the *film*.

REF: p. 326

16. To compensate for the strips found in the grid, _____ must be used to expose a film.
    a. increased kilovoltage
    b. increased milliamperage
    c. increased exposure time
    d. decreased exposure time

Answer: c

Correct: To compensate for the strips found in the grid, increased exposure time must be used to expose a film.

Incorrect:

(a) To compensate for the strips found in the grid, *increased exposure time* must be used to expose a film.

(b) To compensate for the strips found in the grid, *increased exposure time* must be used to expose a film.

(d) To compensate for the strips found in the grid, *increased exposure time* must be used to expose a film.

REF: p. 326

17. Lateral jaw radiography:
    a. Requires the use of a special x-ray unit
    b. Provides for more diagnostic information than a panoramic radiograph
    c. Is used to examine the anterior portion of the mandible
    d. Is valuable for patients with limited jaw opening because of a fracture or swelling

Answer: d

Correct: Lateral jaw radiography is valuable for patients with limited jaw opening because of a fracture or swelling.

Incorrect:
(a) Lateral jaw radiography *does not* require the use of a special x-ray unit.
(b) Lateral jaw radiography provides for *less* diagnostic information than a panoramic radiograph.
(c) Lateral jaw radiography is used to examine the *posterior* portion of the mandible.

REF: p. 327

18. Which of the following choices is a lateral jaw projection?
    a. Lateral cephalometric projection
    b. Reverse Towne projection
    c. Waters projection
    d. Body of mandible projection

Answer: d

Correct: The body of mandible projection is a lateral jaw projection.

Incorrect:
(a) The *body of mandible projection* is a lateral jaw projection; the lateral cephalometric projection is considered to be skull radiography.
(b) The *body of mandible projection* is a lateral jaw projection; the reverse Towne projection is considered to be skull radiography.
(c) The *body of mandible projection* is a lateral jaw projection; the Waters projection is considered to be skull radiography.

REF: p. 327

19. Which of the following projections would be best for evaluating impacted third molars?
    a. Body of the mandible projection
    b. Ramus of the mandible projection
    c. Reverse Towne projection
    d. Waters projection

Answer: b

Correct: The ramus of the mandible projection would be best for evaluating impacted third molars.

Incorrect:
(a) The *body of the mandible projection* is best for evaluating teeth in the body of the mandible.
(c) The *reverse Towne projection* is best for evaluating fractures of the condylar neck and ramus area.
(d) The *Waters projection* is best for evaluating the maxillary sinuses.

REF: p. 327

20. For the _____ projection, the patient's head is tipped toward the side being imaged.
    a. body of the mandible
    b. lateral cephalometric
    c. reverse Towne
    d. Waters

Answer: a

Correct: For the body of the mandible projection, the patient's head is tipped toward the side being imaged.

Incorrect:
(b) For the *lateral cephalometric* projection, the left side of the patient's head is positioned adjacent to the cassette.
(c) For the *reverse Towne* projection, the patient's head is tipped down and the mouth opened as wide as possible.
(d) For the *Waters* projection, the patient's head faces the cassette and the patient elevates his or her chin.

REF: p. 327

21. The beam should be directed _____ degrees for the ramus of the mandible projection.
    a. downward at 15 to 20
    b. upward at 15 to 20
    c. downward at 45
    d. upward at 45

Answer: b

Correct: The beam should be directed *upward at 15 to 20* degrees for the ramus of the mandible projection.

Incorrect:
(a) The beam should be directed *upward at 15 to 20* degrees for the ramus of the mandible projection.
(c) The beam should be directed *upward at 15 to 20* degrees for the ramus of the mandible projection.
(d) The beam should be directed *upward at 15 to 20* degrees for the ramus of the mandible projection.

REF: p. 328

155

22. The left side of the patient's head is positioned adjacent to the cassette for the _____ projection.
   a. lateral cephalometric
   b. posteroanterior
   c. Waters
   d. submentovertex

Answer: a
Correct: The left side of the patient's head is positioned adjacent to the cassette for the lateral cephalometric projection.
Incorrect:
   (b) The patient faces the cassette for the *posteroanterior* projection.
   (c) The patient faces the cassette and elevates the chin for the *Waters* projection.
   (d) The patient's head and neck are tipped back far as possible for the *submentovertex* projection.
REF: p. 331

23. The patient's head and neck are tipped back as far as possible for the _____ projection.
   a. lateral cephalometric
   b. posteroanterior
   c. Waters
   d. submentovertex

Answer: d
Correct: The patient's head and neck are tipped back as far as possible for the submentovertex projection.
Incorrect:
   (a) The left side of the patient's head is positioned adjacent to the cassette for the *lateral cephalometric* projection.
   (b) The patient faces the cassette for the *posteroanterior* projection.
   (c) The patient faces the cassette and elevates the chin for the *Waters* projection.
REF: p. 331

24. Which of the following projections is used to evaluate fractures of the zygomatic arch?
   a. lateral cephalometric
   b. posteroanterior
   c. Waters
   d. submentovertex

Answer: d
Correct: The submentovertex projection is used to evaluate fractures of the zygomatic arch.
Incorrect:
   (a) The *lateral cephalometric* projection is used to evaluate facial growth and development, trauma, disease, and developmental abnormalities.
   (b) The *posteroanterior* projection is used to evaluate facial growth and development, trauma, disease, and developmental abnormalities.
   (c) The *Waters* projection is used to evaluate the maxillary sinus area.
REF: p. 331

25. The purpose of the _____ projection is to identify fractures of the condylar neck and ramus area.
   a. reverse Towne projection
   b. posteroanterior
   c. Waters
   d. submentovertex

Answer: a
Correct: The purpose of the reverse Towne projection projection is to identify fractures of the condylar neck and ramus area.
Incorrect:
   (b) The purpose of the *posteroanterior* projection is to evaluate facial growth and development, trauma, disease, and developmental abnormalities.
   (c) The purpose of the *Waters* projection is to evaluate the maxillary sinus area.
   (d) The purpose of the *submentovertex* projection is to evaluate fractures of the zygomatic arch.
REF: p. 334

26. For the _____ projection, the patient faces the cassette with the head tipped down and the mouth open as wide as possible.
   a. Waters
   b. posteroanterior
   c. reverse Towne projection
   d. submentovertex

Answer: c
Correct: For the reverse Towne projection, the patient faces the cassette with the head tipped down and the mouth open as wide as possible.
Incorrect:
   (a) For the *Waters* projection, the patient faces the cassette and elevates the chin.
   (b) For the *posteroanterior* projection, the patient faces the cassette but the head is not tipped.
   (d) For the *submentovertex* projection, the patient faces the cassette with the head tipped down and the mouth open as wide as possible.
REF: p. 337

27. The purpose of the transcranial projection is to evaluate the articular eminence and _____ surface of the condyle.
   a. anterior
   b. posterior
   c. superior
   d. inferior

Answer: c
Correct: The purpose of the transcranial projection is to evaluate the articular eminence and superior surface of the condyle.
Incorrect:
   (a) The purpose of the transcranial projection is to evaluate the articular eminence and *superior* surface of the condyle.

(b) The purpose of the transcranial projection is to evaluate the articular eminence and *superior* surface of the condyle.

(d) the purpose of the transcranial projection is to evaluate the articular eminence and *superior* surface of the condyle.

REF: p. 337

28. For the transcranial projection, the central ray is directed toward a point _____ inches above and 0.5 inches behind the opening of the ear canal.
   a. 0.5
   b. 1.0
   c. 2.0
   d. 4.0

Answer: c
Correct: For the transcranial projection, the central ray is directed toward a point 2.0 inches above and 0.5 inches behind the opening of the ear canal.
Incorrect:
   (a) For the transcranial projection, the central ray is directed toward a point *2.0* inches above and 0.5 inches behind the opening of the ear canal.
   (b) For the transcranial projection, the central ray is directed toward a point *2.0* inches above and 0.5 inches behind the opening of the ear canal.
   (d) For the transcranial projection, the central ray is directed toward a point *2.0* inches above and 0.5 inches behind the opening of the ear canal.
REF: p. 337

29. Cone-beam technology uses a _____-degree rotational field around the patient's head.
   a. 45
   b. 90
   c. 180
   d. 360

Answer: d
Correct: Cone-beam technology uses a 360-degree rotational field around the patient's head.
Incorrect:
   (a) Cone-beam technology uses a *360*-degree rotational field around the patient's head.
   (b) Cone-beam technology uses a *360*-degree rotational field around the patient's head.
   (c) Cone-beam technology uses a *360*-degree rotational field around the patient's head.
REF: p. 338

30. Cone-beam technology:
   a. Is a two-dimensional imaging device
   b. Uses more radiation than medical CT

c. Provides digital information for reconstruction of the image via the computer
d. Is steadily decreasing in popularity

Answer: c
Correct: Cone-beam technology *provides digital information for reconstruction of the image via the computer.*
Incorrect:
   (a) Cone-beam technology *provides digital information for reconstruction of the image via the computer.*
   (b) Cone-beam technology *provides digital information for reconstruction of the image via the computer.*
   (d) Cone-beam technology *provides digital information for reconstruction of the image via the computer.*
REF: p. 338

CHAPTER 24   DIGITAL RADIOGRAPHY

MULTIPLE CHOICE
1. Digital radiography uses _____ to produce an image.
   a. an x-ray processor
   b. radiographic film
   c. processing chemistry
   d. an electronic sensor and computerized imaging system

Answer: d
Correct: Digital radiography uses an electronic sensor and computerized imaging system to produce an image.
Incorrect:
   (a) An x-ray processor is not used in digital radiography.
   (b) Radiographic film is not used in digital radiography.
   (c) Processing chemistry is not used in digital radiography.
REF: p. 344

2. With digital radiography, the term _____ is used to describe the pictures that are produced.
   a. radiograph
   b. x-ray film
   c. image
   d. phosphor

Answer: c
Correct: With digital radiography, the term *image* is used to describe the pictures that are produced.
Incorrect:
   (a) The term *radiograph* is not used to describe pictures in digital radiography.

(b) The term *x-ray film* is not used to describe pictures in digital radiography.
(d) The term *phosphor* is not used to describe pictures in digital radiography.

REF: p. 345

3. Exposure times are _____ than that required for conventional radiography.
   a. 10% to 20% less
   b. 10% to 20% more
   c. 50% to 80% less
   d. 50% to 80% more

Answer: c
Correct: Exposure times are 50% to 80% less than that required for conventional radiography.
Incorrect:
   (a) Exposure times are *50% to 80% less* than that required for conventional radiography.
   (b) Exposure times are *50% to 80% less* than that required for conventional radiography.
   (d) Exposure times are *50% to 80% less* than that required for conventional radiography.

REF: p. 346

4. Most digital radiography systems use a _____ as the x-radiation source.
   a. flat-bed scanner
   b. conventional dental x-ray unit
   c. commercial analog intraoral camera
   d. commercial digital intraoral camera

Answer: b
Correct: Most digital radiography systems use a conventional dental x-ray unit as the x-radiation source.
Incorrect:
   (a) Most digital radiography systems use a *conventional dental x-ray unit* as the x-radiation source.
   (c) Most digital radiography systems use a *conventional dental x-ray unit* as the x-radiation source.
   (d) Most digital radiography systems use a *conventional dental x-ray unit* as the x-radiation source.

REF: p. 347

5. In order to be used for digital radiography, the x-ray unit timer must be adapted to allow exposures in a time frame of _____ a second.
   a. 1/5
   b. 1/10
   c. 1/15
   d. 1/100

Answer: d
Correct: In order to be used for digital radiography, the x-ray unit timer must be adapted to allow exposures in a time frame of 1/100 a second
Incorrect:
   (a) In order to be used for digital radiography, the x-ray unit timer must be adapted to allow exposures in a time frame of *1/100* a second.

(b) In order to be used for digital radiography, the x-ray unit timer must be adapted to allow exposures in a time frame of *1/100* a second.
(c) In order to be used for digital radiography, the x-ray unit timer must be adapted to allow exposures in a time frame of *1/100* a second.

REF: p. 347

6. Which of the following direct types of sensors do *not* require a computer to process the images?
   a. Charged-coupled device
   b. Complementary metal oxide semiconductor/active pixel sensor
   c. Charge injection device
   d. Both a and c

Answer: c
Correct: The charge injection device type of sensor does not require a computer to process the images.
Incorrect:
   (a) The *charge injection device* type of sensor does not require a computer to process the images.
   (b) The *charge injection device* type of sensor does not require a computer to process the images.
   (d) The *charge injection device* type of sensor does not require a computer to process the images.

REF: p. 348

7. The electrons that make up the silicon charge-coupled device (CCD) can be visualized as being divided into an arrangement of blocks or picture elements known as:
   a. A field arrangement
   b. Pixels
   c. Phosphors
   d. A grid

Answer: b
Correct: The electrons that make up the silicon CCD can be visualized as being divided into an arrangement of blocks or picture elements known as pixels.
Incorrect:
   (a) The electrons that make up the silicon CCD can be visualized as being divided into an arrangement of blocks or picture elements known as *pixels*.
   (c) The electrons that make up the silicon CCD can be visualized as being divided into an arrangement of blocks or picture elements known as *pixels*.
   (d) The electrons that make up the silicon CCD can be visualized as being divided into an arrangement of blocks or picture elements known as *pixels*.

REF: p. 347

8. The human eye can appreciate _____ shades of gray.
   a. 16
   b. 32
   c. 64
   d. 256

Answer: b
Correct: The human eye can appreciate 32 shades of gray.
Incorrect:
    (a) The human eye can appreciate *32* shades of gray.
    (c) The human eye can appreciate *32* shades of gray.
    (d) The human eye can appreciate *32* shades of gray.
REF: p. 348

9. A six bit-depth image has a gray-scale combination that equals _____ shades of gray.
    a. 16
    b. 64
    c. 128
    d. 256

Answer: b
Correct: A six bit-depth image has a gray-scale combination that equals 64 shades of gray.
Incorrect:
    (a) A six bit-depth image has a gray-scale combination that equals *64* shades of gray.
    (c) A six bit-depth image has a gray-scale combination that equals *64* shades of gray.
    (d) A six bit-depth image has a gray-scale combination that equals *64* shades of gray.
REF: p. 348

10. _____ digital imaging involves digitizing an existing x-ray film using a CCD camera. Indirect digital imaging is _____ to direct digital imaging.
    a. Indirect; inferior
    b. Indirect; superior
    c. Direct; inferior
    d. Direct; superior

Answer: a
Correct: Indirect digital imaging involves digitizing an existing x-ray film using a CCD camera. Indirect digital imaging is inferior to direct digital imaging.
Incorrect:
    (b) Indirect digital imaging involves digitizing an existing x-ray film using a CCD camera. Indirect digital imaging is *inferior* to direct digital imaging.
    (c) *Indirect* digital imaging involves digitizing an existing x-ray film using a CCD camera. Indirect digital imaging is inferior to direct digital imaging.
    (d) *Indirect* digital imaging involves digitizing an existing x-ray film using a CCD camera. Indirect digital imaging is *inferior* to direct digital imaging.
REF: p. 350

11. Storage phosphor imaging:
    a. Is a form of direct digital imaging
    b. Is a wired digital radiography system
    c. Uses a sensor with a fiber-optic cable
    d. Uses a reusable imaging plate

Answer: d
Correct: Storage phosphor imaging uses a reusable imaging plate.
Incorrect:
    (a) Storage phosphor imaging is a form of indirect digital imaging.
    (b) Storage phosphor imaging is a wireless digital radiography system.
    (c) Storage phosphor imaging *utilizes a reusable imaging plate* instead of a sensor with a fiber optic cable.
REF: p. 350

12. Radiographic images are cleared from the storage phosphor imaging plates by:
    a. Being processed in an x-ray processing machine
    b. Being autoclaved
    c. Exposure to viewbox light for several minutes
    d. Being placed in a microwave oven for 1 minute

Answer: c
Correct: Radiographic images are cleared from the storage phosphor imaging plates by exposure to viewbox light for several minutes.
Incorrect:
    (a) Radiographic images are cleared from the storage phosphor imaging plates by *exposure to viewbox light for several minutes*.
    (b) Radiographic images are cleared from the storage phosphor imaging plates by *exposure to viewbox light for several minutes*.
    (d) Radiographic images are cleared from the storage phosphor imaging plates by *exposure to viewbox light for several minutes*.
REF: p. 350

13. Advantages of digital radiography include:
    a. All sensors can be autoclaved
    b. Increased speed of image viewing
    c. Color radiography rather than black and white
    d. Low initial setup costs

Answer: b
Correct: Advantages of digital radiography include increased speed of image viewing.
Incorrect:
    (a) Advantages of digital radiography include *increased speed of image viewing;* not all sensors can be autoclaved.
    (c) Advantages of digital radiography include *increased speed of image viewing;* the radiographs still are black and white, not color.
    (d) Advantages of digital radiography include *increased speed of image viewing;* high initial setup costs are a barrier to implementation.
REF: p. 352

159

14. A primary advantage to digital radiography is the superior gray-scale resolution that results. Digital radiography uses up to 32 shades of gray.
   a. Both statements are true.
   b. Both statements are false.
   c. The first statement is true; the second statement is false.
   d. The first statement is false; the second statement is true.

Answer: c
Correct: A primary advantage to digital radiography is the superior gray-scale resolution that results. Digital radiography uses up to *256* shades of gray.
Incorrect:
   (a) A primary advantage to digital radiography is the superior gray-scale resolution that results. Digital radiography uses up to *256* shades of gray.
   (b) A primary advantage to digital radiography is the *superior* gray-scale resolution that results. Digital radiography uses up to *256* shades of gray.
   (d) A primary advantage to digital radiography is the *superior* gray-scale resolution that results. Digital radiography uses up to *256* shades of gray.
REF: p. 351

15. Conventional dental x-ray film has a resolution of _____ lp/mm.
   a. 6 to 8
   b. 8 to 12
   c. 12 to 20
   d. 20 to 50

Answer: c
Correct: Conventional dental x-ray film has a resolution of 12 to 20 lp/mm.
Incorrect:
   (a) Conventional dental x-ray film has a resolution of *12 to 20* lp/mm.
   (b) Conventional dental x-ray film has a resolution of *12 to 20* lp/mm.
   (d) Conventional dental x-ray film has a resolution of *12 to 20* lp/mm.
REF: p. 353

16. Sensors that cannot be sterilized:
   a. Should be disposed of between patients
   b. Are wiped off with a surface disinfectant (iodophor) between patients
   c. Require complete coverage with disposable plastic sleeves for each patient
   d. Are placed in an immersion disinfectant for an appropriate amount of time between each patient

Answer: c
Correct: Sensors that cannot be sterilized require complete coverage with disposable plastic sleeves for each patient.

Incorrect:
   (a) Sensors that cannot be sterilized *require complete coverage with disposable plastic sleeves for each patient.*
   (b) Sensors that cannot be sterilized *require complete coverage with disposable plastic sleeves for each patient.*
   (d) Sensors that cannot be sterilized *require complete coverage with disposable plastic sleeves for each patient.*
REF: p. 353

17. It is questionable whether digital images can be used as evidence in lawsuits, because:
   a. The images are inferior to conventional film.
   b. Digitized images cannot be transported across state lines.
   c. The original digital image can be enhanced.
   d. A "hard copy" of the image does not exist.

Answer: c
Correct: It is questionable whether digital images can be used as evidence in lawsuits, because the original digital image can be enhanced.
Incorrect:
   (a) It is questionable whether digital images can be used as evidence in lawsuits, because *the original digital image can be enhanced.*
   (b) It is questionable whether digital images can be used as evidence in lawsuits, because *the original digital image can be enhanced.*
   (d) It is questionable whether digital images can be used as evidence in lawsuits, because *the original digital image can be enhanced.*
REF: p. 353

CHAPTER 25 RADIOGRAPHY OF PATIENTS WITH SPECIAL NEEDS

MULTIPLE CHOICE
   1. The gag reflex is elicited by stimulation of the sensitive tissues of the:
   a. Larynx
   b. Pharynx
   c. Soft palate
   d. Hard palate

Answer: c
Correct: The gag reflex is elicited by stimulation of the sensitive tissues of the soft palate.
Incorrect:
   (a) The gag reflex is elicited by stimulation of the sensitive tissues of the *soft palate.*
   (b) The gag reflex is elicited by stimulation of the sensitive tissues of the *soft palate.*
   (d) The gag reflex is elicited by stimulation of the sensitive tissues of the *soft palate.*
REF: p. 358

2. The gag reflex is a(n) _____ effort, preceded by _____ of respiration.
   a. voluntary; an increased rate
   b. involuntary; cessation
   c. voluntary; cessation
   d. involuntary; an increased rate

Answer: b
Correct: The gag reflex is an involuntary effort, preceded by cessation of respiration.
Incorrect:
   (a) The gag reflex is an *involuntary* effort, preceded by *cessation* of respiration.
   (c) The gag reflex is an *involuntary* effort, preceded by cessation of respiration.
   (d) The gag reflex is an involuntary effort, preceded by *cessation* of respiration.
REF: p. 358

3. Which film placement is most likely to elicit the gag reflex?
   a. Maxillary premolar
   b. Maxillary molar
   c. Mandibular premolar
   d. Mandibular molar

Answer: b
Correct: The maxillary molar film placement is most likely to elicit the gag reflex.
Incorrect:
   (a) The *maxillary molar* film placement is most likely to elicit the gag reflex.
   (c) The *maxillary molar* film placement is most likely to elicit the gag reflex.
   (d) The *maxillary molar* film placement is most likely to elicit the gag reflex.
REF: p. 358

4. Which of the following choices would represent the suggested film placement sequence for a patient who is likely to gag?
   (1) Anterior
   (2) Premolar
   (3) Molar
      a. 1, 2, 3
      b. 2, 1, 3
      c. 2, 3, 1
      d. 3, 1, 2

Answer: a
Correct: Anterior, premolar, and then molar film placement would represent the suggested sequence for a patient who is likely to gag.
Incorrect:
   (b) *Anterior, premolar, and then molar* film placement would represent the suggested sequence for a patient who is likely to gag.
   (c) *Anterior, premolar, and then molar* film placement would represent the suggested sequence for a patient who is likely to gag.

   (d) *Anterior, premolar, and then molar* film placement would represent the suggested sequence for a patient who is likely to gag.
REF: p. 358

5. Suggestions to avoid stimulating the gag reflex include:
   a. Sliding the film along the palate
   b. Placing the film slowly to avoid stimulating the patient
   c. Demonstrating film placement
   d. Waiting for 30 seconds before exposing each film

Answer: c
Correct: Suggestions to avoid stimulating the gag reflex include demonstrating film placement.
Incorrect:
   (a) It is suggested that film should be firmly brought into contact with palatal tissues to avoid the gag reflex.
   (b) It is suggested that film be placed quickly to avoid the gag reflex.
   (d) It is suggested that exposing the film as quickly as possible can help to avoid the gag reflex.
REF: p. 358

6. When intraoral films are impossible to obtain, the radiographer should:
   a. Skip radiographs.
   b. Use an injection of local anesthetic on the patient's throat and try again.
   c. Use extraoral films to obtain diagnostic information.
   d. Use an intraoral digital film sensor rather than conventional film.

Answer: c
Correct: When intraoral films are impossible to obtain, the radiographer should use extraoral films to obtain diagnostic information
Incorrect:
   (a) When intraoral films are impossible to obtain, the radiographer should *use extraoral films to obtain diagnostic information*.
   (b) When intraoral films are impossible to obtain, the radiographer should *use extraoral films to obtain diagnostic information*.
   (d) When intraoral films are impossible to obtain, the radiographer should *use extraoral films to obtain diagnostic information*.
REF: p. 359

7. If the patient gags, the dental radiographer must:
   a. Bring up the subject of gagging.
   b. Remove the film as quickly as possible.
   c. Wait 30 seconds before removing the film so the patient can acclimate to its presence.
   d. Wait until the patient removes the film.

Answer: b

Correct: If the patient gags, the dental radiographer must remove the film as quickly as possible.

Incorrect:
- (a) If the patient gags, the dental radiographer must *remove the film as quickly as possible.*
- (c) If the patient gags, the dental radiographer must *remove the film as quickly as possible.*
- (d) If the patient gags, the dental radiographer must *remove the film as quickly as possible.*

REF: p. 359

8. To help reduce the gag reflex:
   a. Tell the patient to hold his or her breath.
   b. Do not try to distract the patient.
   c. Use the term "gagging" when talking with the patient.
   d. Try to reduce tactile stimuli.

Answer: d

Correct: To help reduce the gag reflex, try to reduce tactile stimuli.

Incorrect:
- (a) To help reduce the gag reflex, try to reduce tactile stimuli; do not tell the patient to hold his or her breath.
- (b) To help reduce the gag reflex, try to reduce tactile stimuli; distracting the patient is a good idea.
- (c) To help reduce the gag reflex, try to reduce tactile stimuli; avoid using the term "gagging."

REF: p. 359

9. Which of the following suggestions are intended to help reduce the gag reflex?
   a. Instructing the patient to breathe rapidly through the nose.
   b. Asking the patient to suspend an arm or leg in the air.
   c. Placing a small amount of baking soda on the tongue.
   d. Asking the patient to perform jumping jacks for 5 minutes in the treatment room.

Answer: b

Correct: Asking the patient to suspend an arm or leg in the air is a suggestion intended to help reduce the gag reflex.

Incorrect:
- (a) *Asking the patient to suspend an arm or leg in the air* is a suggestion intended to help reduce the gag reflex; instructing the patient to breathe *slowly* through the nose is another.
- (c) *Asking the patient to suspend an arm or leg in the air* is a suggestion intended to help reduce the gag reflex; placing a small amount of *table salt* on the tip of the tongue is another.
- (d) *Asking the patient to suspend an arm or leg in the air* is a suggestion intended to help reduce the gag reflex; asking the patient to perform jumping

jacks for 5 minutes in the treatment room is *not* a suggestion.

REF: p. 359

10. A person with a physical disability may have problems with:
    (1) Vision
    (2) Hearing
    (3) Mobility
       a. 1, 2, 3
       b. 1, 2
       c. 1, 3
       d. 2, 3

Answer: a

Correct: A person with a physical disability may have problems with vision, hearing, and mobility.

Incorrect:
- (b) A person with a physical disability may have problems with vision, hearing, *and mobility.*
- (c) A person with a physical disability may have problems with vision, *hearing,* and mobility.
- (d) A person with a physical disability may have problems with *vision,* hearing, and mobility.

REF: p. 360

11. If a person is blind or visually impaired, the dental radiographer must:
    a. Communicate using clear visual explanations
    b. Communicate using clear verbal explanations
    c. Not explain each procedure before performing it
    d. Gesture to another person in the presence of a person who is blind

Answer: b

Correct: If a person is blind or visually impaired, the dental radiographer must communicate using clear verbal explanations.

Incorrect:
- (a) If a person is blind or visually impaired, the dental radiographer must *communicate using clear verbal explanations;* visual explanations will not work.
- (c) If a person is blind or visually impaired, the dental radiographer must *communicate using clear verbal explanations;* the radiographer also must explain each procedure before performing it.
- (d) If a person is blind or visually impaired, the dental radiographer must *communicate using clear verbal explanations;* the radiographer must *never* gesture to another person in the presence of a person who is blind.

REF: p. 360

12. A developmental disability is a substantial impairment of mental or physical functioning that occurs before age _____ years and is of indefinite duration.
    a. 12
    b. 18
    c. 19
    d. 22

Answer: d

Correct: A developmental disability is a substantial impairment of mental or physical functioning that occurs before age 22 years and is of indefinite duration.

Incorrect:

(a) A developmental disability is a substantial impairment of mental or physical functioning that occurs before age *22* years and is of indefinite duration.

(b) A developmental disability is a substantial impairment of mental or physical functioning that occurs before age *22* years and is of indefinite duration.

(c) A developmental disability is a substantial impairment of mental or physical functioning that occurs before age *22* years and is of indefinite duration.

REF: p. 360

13. In treating children with a primary or transitional dentition, the bisecting technique is preferred, because the small size of the mouth precludes the placement of a film beyond the apical regions of the teeth.
   a. Both statements are true.
   b. Both statements are false.
   c. The first statement is true; the second statement is false.
   d. The first statement is false; the second statement is true.

Answer: a

Correct: In treating children with a primary or transitional dentition, the bisecting technique is preferred, because the small size of the mouth precludes the placement of a film beyond the apical regions of the teeth.

Incorrect:

(b) In treating children with a primary or transitional dentition, the bisecting technique is preferred, because the small size of the mouth precludes the placement of a film beyond the apical regions of the teeth.

(c) In treating children with a primary or transitional dentition, the bisecting technique is preferred, *because the small size of the mouth precludes the placement of a film beyond the apical regions of the teeth.*

(d) In treating children with a primary or transitional dentition, *the bisecting technique is preferred,* because the small size of the mouth precludes the placement of a film beyond the apical regions of the teeth.

REF: p. 361

14. _____ periapical films can be used to examine the edentulous arches.
   a. Eight
   b. Twelve
   c. Fourteen
   d. Eighteen

Answer: c

Correct: Fourteen periapical films can be used to examine the edentulous arches.

Incorrect:

(a) *Fourteen* periapical films can be used to examine the edentulous arches.

(b) *Fourteen* periapical films can be used to examine the edentulous arches.

(d) *Fourteen* periapical films can be used to examine the edentulous arches.

REF: p. 363

15. Size _____ film is typically used for the edentulous examination.
   a. 0
   b. 1
   c. 2
   d. 4

Answer: c

Correct: Size 2 film is typically used for the edentulous examination.

Incorrect:

(a) Size *2* film is typically used for the edentulous examination.

(b) Size *2* film is typically used for the edentulous examination.

(d) Size *2* film is typically used for the edentulous examination.

REF: p. 363

16. For a periapical examination in an edentulous patient, the film should be positioned so that approximately _____ of it extends beyond the edentulous ridge.
   a. one eighth
   b. one quarter
   c. one third
   d. half

Answer: c

Correct: For a periapical examination in an edentulous patient, the film should be positioned so that approximately one third of it extends beyond the edentulous ridge.

Incorrect:

(a) For a periapical examination in an edentulous patient, the film should be positioned so that approximately *one third* of it extends beyond the edentulous ridge.

(b) For a periapical examination in an edentulous patient, the film should be positioned so that approximately *one third* of it extends beyond the edentulous ridge.

(d) For a periapical examination in an edentulous patient, the film should be positioned so that approximately *one third* of it extends beyond the edentulous ridge.

REF: p. 363

163

17. If the alveolar ridges of the patient are severely resorbed, the _____ technique is recommended for a periapical examination.
   a. bisecting
   b. paralleling
   c. occlusal
   d. interproximal

Answer: a
Correct: If the alveolar ridges of the patient are severely resorbed, the bisecting technique is recommended for a periapical examination.
Incorrect:
   (b) If the alveolar ridges of the patient are severely resorbed, the *bisecting* technique is recommended for a periapical examination.
   (c) If the alveolar ridges of the patient are severely resorbed, the *bisecting* technique is recommended for a periapical examination.
   (d) If the alveolar ridges of the patient are severely resorbed, the *bisecting* technique is recommended for a periapical examination.
REF: p. 363

18. The mixed occlusal and periapical examination consists of _____ size 4 films and _____ size 2 films.
   a. two; four
   b. two; two
   c. four; four
   d. four; two

Answer: a
Correct: The mixed occlusal and periapical examination consists of two size 4 films and four size 2 films.
Incorrect:
   (b) The mixed occlusal and periapical examination consists of *two* size 4 films and *four* size 2 films.
   (c) The mixed occlusal and periapical examination consists of *two* size 4 films and *four* size 2 films.
   (d) The mixed occlusal and periapical examination consists of *two* size 4 films and *four* size 2 films.
REF: pp. 363-364

CHAPTER 26   NORMAL ANATOMY: INTRAORAL FILMS

MULTIPLE CHOICE
1. Cortical bone is also referred to as:
   a. Trabecular
   b. Spongy
   c. Cancellous
   d. Compact bone

Answer: d
Correct: Cortical bone is also referred to as compact bone.
Incorrect:
   (a) Cortical bone is also referred to as *compact bone;* trabecular bone is cancellous, spongy bone.
   (b) Cortical bone is also referred to as *compact bone;* trabecular bone is cancellous, spongy bone.
   (c) Cortical bone is also referred to as *compact bone;* trabecular bone is cancellous, spongy bone.
REF: p. 369

2. _____ bone appears predominantly radiopaque, and _____ bone appears predominantly radiolucent.
   a. Cortical; cancellous
   b. Cancellous; cortical
   c. Trabecular; compact
   d. Spongy; cortical

Answer: a
Correct: Cortical bone appears predominantly radiopaque, and cancellous bone appears predominantly radiolucent.
Incorrect:
   (b) *Cancellous* bone appears predominately radiolucent. *Cortical* bone appears predominately radiopaque.
   (c) *Trabecular* bone appears predominately radiolucent. *Compact* bone appears predominately radiopaque.
   (d) *Spongy* bone appears predominately radiolucent. *Cortical* bone appears predominately radiopaque.
REF: p. 369

3. The _____ the trabeculations, the _____ radiolucent the area of cancellous bone appears.
   a. smaller; more
   b. larger; more
   c. larger; less
   d. Both a and b

Answer: b
Correct: The larger the trabeculations, the more radiolucent the area of cancellous bone appears.
Incorrect:
   (a) The *larger* the trabeculations, the *more* radiolucent the area of cancellous bone appears.
   (c) The *larger* the trabeculations, the *more* radiolucent the area of cancellous bone appears.
   (d) The *larger* the trabeculations, the *more* radiolucent the area of cancellous bone appears.
REF: p. 369

4. Cancellous bone is the soft, _____ bone located between two layers of _____ cortical bone.
   a. spongy; spongy
   b. dense; dense
   c. spongy; dense
   d. dense; spongy

Answer: c
Correct: Cancellous bone is the soft, spongy bone located between two layers of dense cortical bone.
Incorrect:
   (a) Cancellous bone is the soft, *spongy* bone located between two layers of *dense* cortical bone.

(b) Cancellous bone is the soft, *spongy* bone located between two layers of *dense* cortical bone.

(d) Cancellous bone is the soft, *spongy* bone located between two layers of *dense* cortical bone.

REF: p. 369

5. Which type of bone is composed of bony trabeculae?
   a. Cortical
   b. Dense
   c. Compact
   d. Cancellous

Answer: d

Correct: Cancellous bone is composed of bony trabeculae.

Incorrect:
   (a) *Cancellous* bone is composed of bony trabeculae.
   (b) *Cancellous* bone is composed of bony trabeculae.
   (c) *Cancellous* bone is composed of bony trabeculae.

REF: p. 369

6. A ridge is defined as a _____ of bone.
   a. linear prominence or projection
   b. sharp, thornlike projection
   c. small bump or nodule
   d. rounded prominence

Answer: a

Correct: A ridge is defined as a linear prominence or projection of bone.

Incorrect:
   (b) A ridge is defined as a *linear prominence or projection* of bone.
   (c) A ridge is defined as a *linear prominence or projection* of bone.
   (d) A ridge is defined as a *linear prominence or projection* of bone.

REF: p. 370

7. A _____ is defined as a marked prominence or projection of bone.
   a. process
   b. ridge
   c. spine
   d. tubercle

Answer: a

Correct: A process is defined as a marked prominence or projection of bone.

Incorrect:
   (b) A *ridge* is defined as a linear prominence or projection of bone.
   (c) A *spine* is defined as a sharp, thornlike projection of bone.
   (d) A *tubercle* is defined as a small bump or nodule of bone.

REF: p. 370

8. A _____ is a tubelike passageway through bone that contains nerves and blood vessels.
   a. canal
   b. foramen
   c. fossa
   d. sinus

Answer: a

Correct: A canal is a tubelike passageway through bone that contains nerves and blood vessels.

Incorrect:
   (b) A *foramen* is an opening or hole in bone that permits the passage of nerves and blood vessels.
   (c) A *fossa* is a broad, shallow, scooped-out or depressed area of bone.
   (d) A *sinus* is a hollow space, cavity, or recess in bone.

REF: p. 371

9. A foramen is a(n):
   a. Opening or hole in bone that permits the passage of nerves and blood vessels
   b. Broad, shallow, scooped-out or depressed area of bone
   c. Hollow space, cavity, or recess in bone
   d. Sharp, thornlike projection of bone

Answer: a

Correct: A foramen is an opening or hole in bone that permits the passage of nerves and blood vessels.

Incorrect:
   (b) A *fossa* is a broad, shallow, scooped-out or depressed area of bone.
   (c) A *sinus* is a hollow space, cavity, or recess in bone.
   (d) A *spine* is defined as a sharp, thornlike projection of bone.

REF: p. 371

10. A suture is a(n):
    a. Movable joint between any two bones in the body
    b. Immovable joint between any two bones in the body
    c. Movable joint between two bones in the skull
    d. Immovable joint between two bones in the skull

Answer: d

Correct: A suture is an immovable joint between two bones in the skull.

Incorrect:
    (a) A suture is *an immovable joint between two bones in the skull.*
    (b) A suture is *an immovable joint between two bones in the skull.*
    (c) A suture is *an immovable joint between two bones in the skull.*

REF: p. 372

11. A _____ is a bony wall or partition that divides two spaces or cavities.
 a. process
 b. ridge
 c. septum
 d. spine

Answer: c
Correct: A septum is a bony wall or partition that divides two spaces or cavities.
Incorrect:
 (a) A *septum* is a bony wall or partition that divides two spaces or cavities.
 (b) A *septum* is a bony wall or partition that divides two spaces or cavities.
 (d) A *septum* is a bony wall or partition that divides two spaces or cavities.
REF: p. 372

12. Which of the following radiographic landmarks would appear radiolucent?
 a. Septum
 b. Suture
 c. Tubercle
 d. Tuberosity

Answer: b
Correct: A suture would appear radiolucent.
Incorrect:
 (a) A *septum* appears radiopaque.
 (c) A *tubercle* appears radiopaque.
 (d) A *tuberosity* appears radiopaque.
REF: p. 373

13. The _____ is an opening or hole in bone that is located in the midline of the anterior portion of the hard palate directly posterior to the maxillary central incisors.
 a. mental foramen
 b. foramen ovale
 c. greater palatine foramen
 d. incisive foramen

Answer: d
Correct: The incisive foramen is an opening or hole in bone that is located in the midline of the anterior portion of the hard palate directly posterior to the maxillary central incisors.
Incorrect:
 (a) The *mental foramen* is an opening or hole in bone on the external surface of the mandible in the region of the mandibular premolars.
 (b) The *foramen ovale* is an opening or hole in bone located on the base of the skull.
 (c) The *greater palatine foramen* is an opening or hole in bone that is located in the posterior corner of the hard palate anterior to hamulus.
 373

14. The _____ nerve exits the maxilla through the incisive foramen.
 a. anterior superior alveolar
 b. middle superior alveolar
 c. posterior superior alveolar
 d. nasopalatine

Answer: d
Correct: The nasopalatine nerve exits the maxilla through the incisive foramen.
Incorrect:
 (a) The *nasopalatine* nerve exits the maxilla through the incisive foramen.
 (b) The *nasopalatine* nerve exits the maxilla through the incisive foramen.
 (c) The *nasopalatine* nerve exits the maxilla through the incisive foramen.
REF: p. 373

15. On a _____ periapical radiograph the incisive foramen appears as a small, ovoid or round, _____ area located between the roots of the central incisors.
 a. maxillary; radiopaque
 b. maxillary; radiolucent
 c. mandibular; radiopaque
 d. mandibular; radiolucent

Answer: b
Correct: On a maxillary periapical radiograph the incisive foramen appears as a small, ovoid or round, radiolucent area located between the roots of the central incisors.
Incorrect:
 (a) On a *maxillary* periapical radiograph the incisive foramen appears as a small, ovoid or round, *radiolucent* area located between the roots of the central incisors.
 (c) On a *maxillary* periapical radiograph the incisive foramen appears as a small, ovoid or round, *radiolucent* area located between the roots of the central incisors.
 (d) On a *maxillary* periapical radiograph the incisive foramen appears as a small, ovoid or round, *radiolucent* area located between the roots of the central incisors.
REF: p. 373

16. The superior foramina of the incisive canal are _____ tiny openings or holes in bone.
 a. two
 b. four
 c. six
 d. eight

Answer: a
Correct: The superior foramina of the incisive canal are two tiny openings or holes in bone.
Incorrect:
(b) The superior foramina of the incisive canal are *two* tiny openings or holes in bone.
(c) The superior foramina of the incisive canal are *two* tiny openings or holes in bone.
(d) The superior foramina of the incisive canal are *two* tiny openings or holes in bone.
REF: p. 374

17. The superior foramina of the incisive canal are located on the _____ of the nasal cavity.
   a. lateral wall
   b. medial wall
   c. floor
   d. roof

Answer: c
Correct: The superior foramina of the incisive canal are located on the floor of the nasal cavity.
Incorrect:
(a) The superior foramina of the incisive canal are located on the *floor* of the nasal cavity.
(b) The superior foramina of the incisive canal are located on the *floor* of the nasal cavity.
(d) The superior foramina of the incisive canal are located on the *floor* of the nasal cavity.
REF: p. 374

18. On a periapical radiograph the superior foramina appear as radiolucencies located superior to apices of the:
   a. Maxillary canines
   b. Maxillary central incisors
   c. Mandibular canines
   d. Mandibular central incisors

Answer: b
Correct: On a periapical radiograph the superior foramina appear as radiolucencies located superior to apices of the maxillary central incisors.
Incorrect:
(a) On a periapical radiograph the superior foramina appear as radiolucencies located superior to apices of the maxillary *central incisors*.
(c) On a periapical radiograph the superior foramina appear as radiolucencies located superior to apices of the *maxillary central incisors*.
(d) On a periapical radiograph the superior foramina appear as radiolucencies located superior to apices of the *maxillary* central incisors.
REF: p. 375

19. The median palatal suture is located between the two _____ of the maxilla.
   a. inferior nasal conchae
   b. nasal cavities

   c. palatine processes
   d. maxillary sinuses

Answer: c
Correct: The median palatal suture is located between the two palatine processes of the maxilla.
Incorrect:
(a) The median palatal suture is located between the two *palatine processes* of the maxilla.
(b) The median palatal suture is located between the two *palatine processes* of the maxilla.
(d) The median palatal suture is located between the two *palatine processes* of the maxilla.
REF: p. 375

20. On a periapical radiograph the median palatal suture appears as a thin _____ line between the _____.
   a. radiopaque; maxillary lateral incisor and cuspid
   b. radiolucent; maxillary lateral incisor and cuspid
   c. radiopaque; maxillary central incisors
   d. radiolucent; maxillary central incisors

Answer: d
Correct: On a periapical radiograph the median palatal suture appears as a thin radiolucent line between the maxillary central incisors.
Incorrect:
(a) On a periapical radiograph the median palatal suture appears as a thin *radiolucent* line between the maxillary *central incisors*.
(b) On a periapical radiograph the median palatal suture appears as a thin radiolucent line between the maxillary *central incisors*.
(c) On a periapical radiograph the median palatal suture appears as a thin *radiolucent* line between the maxillary central incisors.
REF: p. 375

21. The lateral fossa is located between the:
   a. Maxillary canine and lateral incisor
   b. Mandibular canine and lateral incisor
   c. Maxillary canine and first premolar
   d. Mandibular canine and first premolar

Answer: a
Correct: The lateral fossa is located between the maxillary canine and lateral incisor.
Incorrect:
(b) The lateral fossa is located between the *maxillary* canine and lateral incisor.
(c) The lateral fossa is located between the maxillary canine and *lateral incisor*.
(d) The lateral fossa is located between the *maxillary* canine and *lateral incisor*.
REF: p. 375

167

Test Bank

22. On a radiograph the lateral fossa appears as a _____ area of _____ appearance depending on the anatomy of the individual.
a. radiopaque; consistent
b. radiolucent; consistent
c. radiopaque; variable
d. radiolucent; variable

Answer: d
Correct: On a radiograph the lateral fossa appears as a radiolucent area of variable appearance depending on the anatomy of the individual.
Incorrect:
(a) On a radiograph the lateral fossa appears as a *radiolucent* area of *variable* appearance depending on the anatomy of the individual.
(b) On a radiograph the lateral fossa appears as a radiolucent area of *variable* appearance depending on the anatomy of the individual.
(c) On a radiograph the lateral fossa appears as a *radiolucent* area of variable appearance depending on the anatomy of the individual.
REF: pp. 375-376

23. The lateral walls of the nasal cavity are formed by the _____ bone and the maxillae.
a. temporal
b. sphenoid
c. ethmoid
d. zygomatic

Answer: c
Correct: The lateral walls of the nasal cavity are formed by the ethmoid bone and the maxillae.
Incorrect:
(a) The lateral walls of the nasal cavity are formed by the *ethmoid* bone and the maxillae.
(b) The lateral walls of the nasal cavity are formed by the *ethmoid* bone and the maxillae.
(d) The lateral walls of the nasal cavity are formed by the *ethmoid* bone and the maxillae.
REF: p. 376

24. On a maxillary periapical radiograph the nasal septum may be superimposed over the:
a. Canine
b. Median palatal suture
c. Greater palatine foramen
d. Genial tubercles

Answer: b
Correct: On a maxillary periapical radiograph the nasal septum may be superimposed over the median palatal suture.
Incorrect:
(a) On a maxillary periapical radiograph the nasal septum may be superimposed over the *median palatal suture*.

(c) On a maxillary periapical radiograph the nasal septum may be superimposed over the *median palatal suture*.
(d) On a maxillary periapical radiograph the nasal septum may be superimposed over the *median palatal suture*.
REF: p. 376

25. On a maxillary periapical radiograph the floor of the nasal cavity appears as a _____ band of bone _____ the maxillary incisors.
a. radiolucent; above
b. radiolucent; below
c. radiopaque; above
d. radiopaque; below

Answer: a
Correct: On a maxillary periapical radiograph the floor of the nasal cavity appears as a radiolucent band of bone above the maxillary incisors.
Incorrect:
(b) On a maxillary periapical radiograph the floor of the nasal cavity appears *above*, not below, the maxillary incisors.
(c) On a maxillary periapical radiograph the floor of the nasal cavity appears as a *radiolucent*, not radiopaque, band of bone.
(d) On a maxillary periapical radiograph the floor of the nasal cavity appears as a *radiolucent*, not radiopaque, band of bone *above*, not below, the maxillary incisors.
REF: p. 377

26. The anterior nasal spine is located at the _____ portion of the nasal cavity.
a. anterior and superior
b. anterior and inferior
c. posterior and superior
d. posterior and inferior

Answer: b
Correct: The anterior nasal spine is located at the anterior and inferior portion of the nasal cavity.
Incorrect:
(a) The anterior nasal spine is located at the anterior and *inferior* portion of the nasal cavity.
(c) The anterior nasal spine is located at the *anterior and inferior* portion of the nasal cavity.
(d) The anterior nasal spine is located at the *anterior* and inferior portion of the nasal cavity.
REF: p. 377

27. On a maxillary periapical radiograph the anterior nasal spine appears as a _____-shaped radiopaque area located at the intersection of the floor of the nasal cavity and the nasal septum.
a. T
b. U
c. V
d. I

Answer: c

Correct: On a maxillary periapical radiograph the anterior nasal spine appears as a V-shaped radiopaque area located at the intersection of the floor of the nasal cavity and the nasal septum.

Incorrect:
- (a) On a maxillary periapical radiograph the anterior nasal spine appears as a *V*-shaped radiopaque area located at the intersection of the floor of the nasal cavity and the nasal septum.
- (b) On a maxillary periapical radiograph the anterior nasal spine appears as a *V*-shaped radiopaque area located at the intersection of the floor of the nasal cavity and the nasal septum.
- (d) On a maxillary periapical radiograph the anterior nasal spine appears as a *V*-shaped radiopaque area located at the intersection of the floor of the nasal cavity and the nasal septum.

REF: p. 377

---

28. The inferior nasal conchae extend from the:
   a. Medial walls of the maxillary sinus
   b. Lateral walls of the maxillary sinus
   c. Medial walls of the nasal cavity
   d. Lateral walls of the nasal cavity

Answer: d

Correct: The inferior nasal conchae extend from the lateral walls of the nasal cavity.

Incorrect:
- (a) The inferior nasal conchae extend from the *lateral walls of the nasal cavity*.
- (b) The inferior nasal conchae extend from the lateral walls of the *nasal cavity*.
- (c) The inferior nasal conchae extend from the *lateral walls* of the nasal cavity.

REF: p. 377

---

29. On a maxillary periapical radiograph the inferior nasal conchae appear as a _____ mass within the nasal cavity.
   a. well-demarcated radiolucent
   b. well-demarcated radiopaque
   c. diffuse radiolucent
   d. diffuse radiopaque

Answer: d

Correct: On a maxillary periapical radiograph the inferior nasal conchae appear as a diffuse radiopaque mass within the nasal cavity.

Incorrect:
- (a) On a maxillary periapical radiograph the inferior nasal conchae appear as a *diffuse radiopaque* mass within the nasal cavity.
- (b) On a maxillary periapical radiograph the inferior nasal conchae appear as a *diffuse* radiopaque mass within the nasal cavity.
- (c) On a maxillary periapical radiograph the inferior nasal conchae appear as a diffuse *radiopaque* mass within the nasal cavity.

REF: p. 378

---

30. The maxillary sinuses are located above the _____ teeth.
   a. incisor
   b. premolar
   c. molar
   d. premolar and molar

Answer: d

Correct:

Incorrect: The maxillary sinuses are located above the premolar and molar teeth.
- (a) The maxillary sinuses are located above the *premolar and molar* teeth.
- (b) The maxillary sinuses are located above the premolar *and molar* teeth.
- (c) The maxillary sinuses are located above the *premolar and* molar teeth.

REF: p. 379

---

31. Bony septa and nutrient canals may be seen within the walls of the:
   a. Median palatal suture
   b. Maxillary sinus
   c. Incisive foramen
   d. Anterior nasal spine

Answer: b

Correct: Bony septa and nutrient canals may be seen within the walls of the maxillary sinus.

Incorrect:
- (a) Bony septa and nutrient canals may be seen within the walls of the *maxillary sinus*.
- (c) Bony septa and nutrient canals may be seen within the walls of the *maxillary sinus*.
- (d) Bony septa and nutrient canals may be seen within the walls of the *maxillary sinus*.

REF: p. 380

---

32. The inverted Y refers to the intersection of the maxillary sinus and the:
   a. Median palatal suture
   b. Anterior nasal spine
   c. Incisive foramen
   d. Nasal cavity

Answer: d

Correct: The inverted Y refers to the intersection of the maxillary sinus and the nasal cavity.

Incorrect:
- (a) The inverted Y refers to the intersection of the maxillary sinus and the *nasal cavity*.
- (b) The inverted Y refers to the intersection of the maxillary sinus and the *nasal cavity*.
- (c) The inverted Y refers to the intersection of the maxillary sinus and the *nasal cavity*.

REF: p. 380

---

33. The inverted Y is a _____ line above the maxillary _____.
   a. radiopaque; canine
   b. radiopaque; first molar

c. radiolucent; canine
d. radiolucent; first molar

Answer: a
Correct: The inverted Y is a radiopaque line above the maxillary canine.
Incorrect:
(b) The inverted Y is a radiopaque line above the maxillary *canine.*
(c) The inverted Y is a *radiopaque* line above the maxillary canine.
(d) The inverted Y is a *radiopaque* line above the maxillary *canine.*
REF: p. 380

34. The maxillary tuberosity appears as a _____ bulge distal to the _____ molar region.
    a. radiolucent; first
    b. radiolucent; third
    c. radiopaque; first
    d. radiopaque; third

Answer: d
Correct: The maxillary tuberosity appears as a radiopaque bulge distal to the third molar region.
Incorrect:
(a) The maxillary tuberosity appears as a *radiopaque* bulge distal to the *third* molar region.
(b) The maxillary tuberosity appears as a *radiopaque* bulge distal to the third molar region.
(c) The maxillary tuberosity appears as a radiopaque bulge distal to the *third* molar region.
REF: p. 380

35. The hamulus extends from the:
    a. Medial pterygoid plate of the sphenoid bone
    b. Lateral pterygoid plate of the sphenoid bone
    c. Styloid process
    d. Maxillary tuberosity

Answer: a
Correct: The hamulus extends from the *medial pterygoid plate of the sphenoid bone.*
Incorrect:
(b) The hamulus extends from the *medial pterygoid plate of the sphenoid bone.*
(c) The hamulus extends from the *medial pterygoid plate of the sphenoid bone.*
(d) The hamulus extends from the *medial pterygoid plate of the sphenoid bone.*
REF: p. 381

36. On a maxillary periapical radiograph the zygomatic process appears as a _____ to the maxillary first molar region.
    a. radiolucency located inferior
    b. radiopacity located superior
    c. radiolucency located superior
    d. radiopacity located inferior

Answer: b
Correct: On a maxillary periapical radiograph the zygomatic process appears as a radiopacity located superior to the maxillary first molar region.
Incorrect:
(a) On a maxillary periapical radiograph the zygomatic process appears as a *radiopacity located superior* to the maxillary first molar region.
(c) On a maxillary periapical radiograph the zygomatic process appears as a *radiopacity* located superior to the maxillary first molar region.
(d) On a maxillary periapical radiograph the zygomatic process appears as a radiopacity *located superior* to the maxillary first molar region.
REF: p. 381

37. The _____ is the portion of the mandible that encases and supports the teeth.
    a. ramus
    b. coronoid process
    c. body
    d. alveolar process

Answer: d
Correct: The alveolar process is the portion of the mandible that encases and supports the teeth.
Incorrect:
(a) The *ramus* is the vertical portion of the mandible that is found posterior to the third molar.
(b) The *coronoid process* is the prominence of bone at the anterior ramus of the mandible.
(c) The *body* of the mandible is the horizontal, U-shaped portion that extends from ramus to ramus.
REF: p. 383

38. The genial tubercles serve as attachments for the _____ muscles.
    a. digastric and genioglossus
    b. genioglossus and geniohyoid
    c. geniohyoid and digastric
    d. mylohyoid and geniohyoid

Answer: b
Correct: The genial tubercles serve as attachments for the genioglossus and geniohyoid muscles.
Incorrect:
(a) The genial tubercles serve as attachments for the *genioglossus and geniohyoid* muscles.
(c) The genial tubercles serve as attachments for the *genioglossus and geniohyoid* muscles.
(d) The genial tubercles serve as attachments for the *genioglossus* and geniohyoid muscles.
REF: p. 383

39. On a periapical radiograph the genial tubercles appear as a ring-shaped _____ the apices of the mandibular incisors.
    a. radiolucency below
    b. radiolucency above
    c. radiopacity below
    d. radiopacity above

Answer: c

Correct: On a periapical radiograph the genial tubercles appear as a ring-shaped radiopacity below the apices of the mandibular incisors.

Incorrect:
- (a) On a periapical radiograph the genial tubercles appear as a ring-shaped *radiopacity* below the apices of the mandibular incisors.
- (b) On a periapical radiograph the genial tubercles appear as a ring-shaped *radiopacity below* the apices of the mandibular incisors.
- (d) On a periapical radiograph the genial tubercles appear as a ring-shaped radiopacity *below* the apices of the mandibular incisors.

REF: p. 383

40. The lingual foramen is surrounded by the:
    - a. Mental foramen
    - b. Genial tubercles
    - c. Anterior nasal spine
    - d. Internal oblique ridge

Answer: b

Correct: The lingual foramen is surrounded by the genial tubercles.

Incorrect:
- (a) The lingual foramen is surrounded by the *genial tubercles.*
- (c) The lingual foramen is surrounded by the *genial tubercles.*
- (d) The lingual foramen is surrounded by the *genial tubercles.*

REF: p. 383

41. Interdental nutrient canals are most often seen in the:
    - a. Anterior maxilla
    - b. Anterior mandible
    - c. Posterior maxilla
    - d. Posterior mandible

Answer: b

Correct: Interdental nutrient canals are most often seen in the anterior mandible.

Incorrect:
- (a) Interdental nutrient canals are most often seen in the anterior *mandible.*
- (c) Interdental nutrient canals are most often seen in the *anterior mandible.*
- (d) Interdental nutrient canals are most often seen in the *anterior* mandible.

REF: p. 384

42. Nutrient canals appear as _____ lines on a periapical radiograph.
    - a. vertical radiolucent
    - b. horizontal radiolucent
    - c. vertical radiopaque
    - d. horizontal radiopaque

Answer: a

Correct: Nutrient canals appear as vertical radiolucent lines on a periapical radiograph.

Incorrect:
- (b) Nutrient canals appear as *vertical* radiolucent lines on a periapical radiograph.
- (c) Nutrient canals appear as vertical *radiolucent* lines on a periapical radiograph.
- (d) Nutrient canals appear as *vertical radiolucent* lines on a periapical radiograph.

REF: p. 384

43. The mental ridge is located on the _____ portion of the mandible.
    - a. external surface of the anterior
    - b. internal surface of the anterior
    - c. external surface of the posterior
    - d. internal surface of the posterior

Answer: a

Correct: The mental ridge is located on the external surface of the anterior portion of the mandible.

Incorrect:
- (b) The mental ridge is located on the *external surface* of the anterior portion of the mandible.
- (c) The mental ridge is located on the external surface of the *anterior* portion of the mandible.
- (d) The mental ridge is located on the *external surface of the anterior* portion of the mandible.

REF: p. 384

44. Radiographically, the mental ridge often appears superimposed over the _____ teeth.
    - a. maxillary anterior
    - b. maxillary posterior
    - c. mandibular anterior
    - d. mandibular posterior

Answer: c

Correct: Radiographically, the mental ridge often appears superimposed over the mandibular anterior teeth.

Incorrect:
- (a) Radiographically, the mental ridge often appears superimposed over the *mandibular* anterior teeth.
- (b) Radiographically, the mental ridge often appears superimposed over the *mandibular anterior* teeth.
- (d) Radiographically, the mental ridge often appears superimposed over the mandibular *anterior* teeth.

REF: p. 384

45. The mental fossa is located _____ the mental ridge in the mandibular _____ region.
    - a. above; incisor
    - b. below; incisor
    - c. above; premolar
    - d. below; premolar

Answer: a

Correct: The mental fossa is located above the mental ridge in the mandibular incisor region.

Incorrect:

(b) The mental fossa is located *above* the mental ridge in the mandibular incisor region.

(c) The mental fossa is located above the mental ridge in the mandibular *incisor* region.

(d) The mental fossa is located *above* the mental ridge in the mandibular *incisor* region.

REF: p. 384

---

46. The _____ is an opening or hole in bone located on the external surface of the mandible in the region of the mandibular premolars.
   a. nutrient canal
   b. mental fossa
   c. lingual foramen
   d. mental foramen

Answer: d

Correct: The mental foramen is an opening or hole in bone located on the external surface of the mandible in the region of the mandibular premolars.

Incorrect:

(a) The *nutrient canal* is one of a group of tiny canals most often seen in the anterior mandible.

(b) The *mental fossa* is located on the external surface of the anterior mandible.

(c) The *lingual foramen* is located on the internal surface of the mandible.

REF: p. 385

---

47. The mental foramen is frequently misdiagnosed as a _____ because of its apical location.
   a. dentigerous cyst
   b. radicular cyst
   c. periapical granuloma
   d. odontoma

Answer: c

Correct: The mental foramen is frequently misdiagnosed as a periapical granuloma because of its apical location.

Incorrect:

(a) The mental foramen is frequently misdiagnosed as a *periapical granuloma* because of its apical location.

(b) The mental foramen is frequently misdiagnosed as a *periapical granuloma* because of its apical location.

(d) The mental foramen is frequently misdiagnosed as a *periapical granuloma* because of its apical location.

REF: p. 385

---

48. The _____ is a linear prominence of bone extending from the molar region downward on the internal surface of the mandible.
   a. external oblique ridge
   b. mylohyoid ridge
   c. internal oblique ridge
   d. symphysis

Answer: b

Correct: The mylohyoid ridge is a linear prominence of bone extending from the molar region downward on the internal surface of the mandible.

Incorrect:

(a) The *external oblique ridge* is a linear prominence of bone located on the external surface of body of the mandible.

(c) The *internal oblique ridge* is a linear prominence of bone located on the internal surface of the mandible that extends downward and forward from the ramus.

(d) The *symphysis* is located at the midline of the mandible.

REF: pp. 385-386

---

49. On radiographs the mylohyoid ridge is a _____ band that may appear to be continuous with the _____.
   a. radiolucent; internal oblique ridge
   b. radiolucent; external oblique ridge
   c. radiopaque; internal oblique ridge
   d. radiopaque; external oblique ridge

Answer: c

Correct: On radiographs the mylohyoid ridge is a radiopaque band that may appear to be continuous with the internal oblique ridge.

Incorrect:

(a) On radiographs the mylohyoid ridge is a *radiopaque* band that may appear to be continuous with the internal oblique ridge.

(b) On radiographs the mylohyoid ridge is a *radiopaque* band that may appear to be continuous with the *internal oblique ridge.*

(d) On radiographs the mylohyoid ridge is a radiopaque band that may appear to be continuous with the *internal oblique ridge.*

REF: p. 386

---

50. On a mandibular periapical radiograph the mandibular canal appears as a _____ band. It appears below or superimposed over the apices of the mandibular _____ teeth.
   a. radiolucent; incisor
   b. radiolucent; molar
   c. radiopaque; incisor
   d. radiopaque; molar

Answer: b
Correct: On a mandibular periapical radiograph the-mandibular canal appears as a radiolucent band. It appears below or superimposed over the apices of the mandibular molar teeth.
Incorrect:
(a) On a mandibular periapical radiograph the mandibular canal appears as a radiolucent band. It appears below or superimposed over the apices of the mandibular *molar* teeth.
(c) On a mandibular periapical radiograph the mandibular canal appears as a *radiolucent* band. It appears below or superimposed over the apices of the mandibular *molar* teeth.
(d) On a mandibular periapical radiograph the mandibular canal appears as a *radiolucent* band. It appears below or superimposed over the apices of the mandibular molar teeth.
REF: p. 386

51. The internal oblique ridge may end in the region of the mandibular _____ molar, or it may continue on as the _____ ridge.
    a. first; mylohyoid
    b. third; mylohyoid
    c. first; external oblique
    d. third; external oblique

Answer: b
Correct: The internal oblique ridge may end in the region of the mandibular third molar, or it may continue on as the mylohyoid ridge.
Incorrect:
(a) The internal oblique ridge may end in the region of the mandibular *third* molar, or it may continue on as the mylohyoid ridge.
(c) The internal oblique ridge may end in the region of the mandibular *third* molar, or it may continue on as the *mylohyoid* ridge.
(d) The internal oblique ridge may end in the region of the mandibular third molar, or it may continue on as the *mylohyoid* ridge.
REF: p. 387

52. When the internal and external oblique ridges appear separate, the _____ band is the external oblique ridge.
    a. superior radiopaque
    b. superior radiolucent
    c. inferior radiopaque
    d. inferior radiolucent

Answer: a
Correct: When the internal and external oblique ridges appear separate, the superior radiopaque band is the external oblique ridge.
Incorrect:
(b) When the internal and external oblique ridges appear separate, the *superior radiopaque* band is the external oblique ridge.

(c) When the internal and external oblique ridges appear separate, the *superior radiopaque* band is the external oblique ridge.
(d) When the internal and external oblique ridges appear separate, the *superior radiopaque* band is the external oblique ridge.
REF: pp. 387-388

53. The external oblique ridge typically ends in the _____ molar region.
    a. maxillary first
    b. mandibular first
    c. maxillary third
    d. mandibular third

Answer: d
Correct: The external oblique ridge typically ends in the mandibular third molar region.
Incorrect:
(a) The external oblique ridge typically ends in the *mandibular third* molar region.
(b) The external oblique ridge typically ends in the mandibular *third* molar region.
(c) The external oblique ridge typically ends in the *mandibular* third molar region.
REF: p. 388

54. The _____ is found in the submandibular fossa.
    a. inferior alveolar nerve
    b. submandibular salivary gland
    c. mylohyoid muscle
    d. lingual nerve

Answer: b
Correct: The submandibular salivary gland is found in the submandibular fossa.
Incorrect:
(a) The *submandibular salivary gland* is found in the submandibular fossa.
(c) The *submandibular salivary gland* is found in the submandibular fossa.
(d) The *submandibular salivary gland* is found in the submandibular fossa.
REF: p. 388

55. On a periapical radiograph the submandibular fossa appears as a _____ area in the molar region _____ the mylohyoid ridge.
    a. radiopaque; above
    b. radiopaque; below
    c. radiolucent; above
    d. radiolucent; below

Answer: d
Correct: On a periapical radiograph the submandibular fossa appears as a radiolucent area in the molar region below the mylohyoid ridge.

Incorrect:
  (a) On a periapical radiograph the submandibular fossa appears as a *radiolucent* area in the molar region *below* the mylohyoid ridge.
  (b) On a periapical radiograph the submandibular fossa appears as a *radiolucent* area in the molar region below the mylohyoid ridge.
  (c) On a periapical radiograph the submandibular fossa appears as a radiolucent area in the molar region *below* the mylohyoid ridge.
REF: p. 388

56. The coronoid process may be seen on a _____ periapical film.
  a. maxillary incisor
  b. maxillary molar
  c. mandibular incisor
  d. mandibular molar

Answer: b
Correct: The coronoid process may be seen on a maxillary molar periapical film.
Incorrect:
  (a) The coronoid process may be seen on a maxillary *molar* periapical film.
  (c) The coronoid process may be seen on a *maxillary molar* periapical film.
  (d) The coronoid process may be seen on a *maxillary* molar periapical film.
REF: p. 388

57. Which of the following tooth structures is most radiopaque?
  a. Enamel
  b. Dentin
  c. Cementum
  d. Pulp

Answer: a
Correct: Enamel is the most radiopaque tooth structure.
Incorrect:
  (b) *Enamel* is more radiopaque than dentin.
  (c) *Enamel* is more radiopaque than cementum.
  (d) *Enamel* is more radiopaque than pulp.
REF: p. 389

58. Which of the following tooth structures is most radiolucent?
  a. Enamel
  b. Dentin
  c. Cementum
  d. Pulp

Answer: d
Correct: Pulp is the most radiolucent tooth structure.
Incorrect:
  (a) *Pulp* is more radiolucent than enamel.
  (b) *Pulp* is more radiolucent than dentin.
  (c) *Pulp* is more radiolucent than cementum.
REF: p. 389

59. The _____ is the wall of the tooth socket that surrounds the root of a tooth.
  a. alveolar crest
  b. residual ridge
  c. periodontal ligament space
  d. lamina dura

Answer: d
Correct: The lamina dura is the wall of the tooth socket that surrounds the root of a tooth.
Incorrect:
  (a) The *lamina dura* is the wall of the tooth socket that surrounds the root of a tooth.
  (b) The *lamina dura* is the wall of the tooth socket that surrounds the root of a tooth.
  (c) The *lamina dura* is the wall of the tooth socket that surrounds the root of a tooth.
REF: p. 390

60. On a dental radiograph the alveolar crest is typically located _____ mm below the junction of the crown and the root surfaces.
  a. 0.5 to 1.0
  b. 1.5 to 2.0
  c. 2.0 to 3.0
  d. 1.5 to 3.0

Answer: b
Correct:
Incorrect: On a dental radiograph the alveolar crest is typically located 1.5 to 2.0 mm below the junction of the crown and the root surfaces.
  (a) On a dental radiograph the alveolar crest is typically located *1.5 to 2.0* mm below the junction of the crown and the root surfaces.
  (c) On a dental radiograph the alveolar crest is typically located *1.5 to 2.0* mm below the junction of the crown and the root surfaces.
  (d) On a dental radiograph the alveolar crest is typically located 1.5 to *2.0* mm below the junction of the crown and the root surfaces.
REF: p. 390

61. On a dental radiograph the periodontal ligament space (PDL) space appears as a _____ line around the root of a tooth.
  a. thin radiopaque
  b. thin radiolucent
  c. wide radiopaque
  d. wide radiolucent

Answer: b
Correct: On a dental radiograph the PDL space appears as a thin radiolucent line around the root of a tooth.
Incorrect:
  (a) On a dental radiograph the PDL space appears as a thin *radiolucent* line around the root of a tooth.
  (c) On a dental radiograph the PDL space appears as a *thin radiolucent* line around the root of a tooth.

(d) On a dental radiograph the PDL space appears as a *thin* radiolucent line around the root of a tooth.
REF: p. 391

62. The alveolar crest in the posterior region tends to appear _____ dense and _____ radiopaque than the alveolar crest seen in the anterior region.
   a. less; less
   b. more; more
   c. less; more
   d. more; less

Answer: a
Correct: The alveolar crest in the posterior region tends to appear less dense and less radiopaque than the alveolar crest seen in the anterior region.
Incorrect:
   (b) The alveolar crest in the posterior region tends to appear *less* dense and *less* radiopaque than the alveolar crest seen in the anterior region.
   (c) The alveolar crest in the posterior region tends to appear less dense and *less* radiopaque than the alveolar crest seen in the anterior region.
   (d) The alveolar crest in the posterior region tends to appear *less* dense and less radiopaque than the alveolar crest seen in the anterior region.
REF: p. 391

CHAPTER 27   FILM MOUNTING AND VIEWING

MULTIPLE CHOICE
1. Radiographs are intended to be placed in a film holder in:
   a. The order in which they were exposed
   b. The order in which they were processed
   c. Anatomic order
   d. The order prescribed by the ADA nomenclature

Answer: c
Correct: Radiographs are intended to be placed in a film holder in anatomic order.
Incorrect:
   (a) Radiographs are intended to be placed in a film holder in *anatomic order*. They are not placed in the film holder in the order in which they were exposed.
   (b) Radiographs are intended to be placed in a film holder in *anatomic order*. They are not placed in the film holder in the order in which they were processed.
   (d) Radiographs are intended to be placed in a film holder in *anatomic order*. They are not placed in the film holder in the order prescribed by the ADA nomenclature.
REF: p. 394

2. In dental radiography, film mounting is the placement of radiographs:
   a. On a viewbox
   b. In a supporting structure or holder
   c. In the patient's mouth
   d. In the processor

Answer: b
Correct: In dental radiography, film mounting is the placement of radiographs in a supporting structure or holder.
Incorrect:
   (a) In dental radiography, film mounting is the placement of radiographs *in a supporting structure or holder*. They are examined on a viewbox.
   (c) In dental radiography, film mounting is the placement of radiographs *in a supporting structure or holder*. They are placed in the patient's mouth for exposure.
   (d) In dental radiography, film mounting is the placement of radiographs *in a supporting structure or holder*. They are placed in the processor for processing.
REF: p. 394

3. A film mount may be made of:
   (1) Cardboard
   (2) Lead foil
   (3) Plastic
   (4) Vinyl
      a. 1, 2, 3, 4
      b. 1, 2, 4
      c. 1, 3, 4
      d. 3, 4

Answer: c
   Correct: A film mount may be made of cardboard, plastic, or vinyl.
   Incorrect:
   (a) A film mount may be made of *cardboard, plastic, or vinyl*. They are not made of lead foil, which is a component of the film package.
   (b) A film mount may be made of *cardboard, plastic, or vinyl*. They are not made of lead foil, which is a component of the film package.
   (d) A film mount may be made of *cardboard*, plastic, or vinyl.
REF: p. 394

4. An opaque film mount is preferred because it:
   a. Increases the contrast of the radiograph
   b. Increases the density of the radiograph
   c. Decreases the density of the radiograph
   d. Masks the light around each radiograph

Answer: d
Correct: An opaque film mount is preferred because it masks the light around each radiograph.

Incorrect:

(a) An opaque film mount is preferred because it *masks the light around each radiograph*. The contrast is a property of the radiograph itself.

(b) An opaque film mount is preferred because it *masks the light around each radiograph*. The density is a property of the radiograph itself.

(c) An opaque film mount is preferred because it *masks the light around each radiograph*. The density is a property of the radiograph itself.

REF: p. 394

5. When radiographs are viewed, subtle changes in density and contrast are easier to detect if:
   a. The treatment room lights are left on.
   b. Extraneous light is eliminated.
   c. The viewbox light is turned off.
   d. Films are held up by the operator and viewed through ceiling lights.

Answer: b

Correct: When radiographs are viewed, subtle changes in density and contrast are easier to detect if extraneous light is eliminated.

Incorrect:

(a) When radiographs are viewed, subtle changes in density and contrast are easier to detect if *extraneous light is eliminated*. Treatment room lights are a source of extraneous light.

(c) When radiographs are viewed, subtle changes in density and contrast are easier to detect if *extraneous light is eliminated*. Backlighting, as from the viewbox, is preferred.

(d) When radiographs are viewed, subtle changes in density and contrast are easier to detect if *extraneous light is eliminated*. Viewing films through ceiling lights is discouraged.

REF: p. 394

6. When all the windows of the film mount are not filled with radiographs, the text recommends placing _____ in the unused frames.
   a. masking tape
   b. nothing
   c. black opaque paper
   d. an unexposed film

Answer: c

Correct: When all the windows of the film mount are not filled with radiographs, the text recommends placing black opaque paper in the unused frames.

Incorrect:

(a) When all the windows of the film mount are not filled with radiographs, the text recommends placing *black opaque paper* in the unused frames. Masking tape would be difficult to place and remove and is not suggested.

(b) When all the windows of the film mount are not filled with radiographs, the text recommends

placing *black opaque paper* in the unused frames. Not placing anything fails to eliminate extraneous light.

(d) When all the windows of the film mount are not filled with radiographs, the text recommends placing *black opaque paper* in the unused frames. Using an unexposed film would eliminate extraneous light but would be wasteful.

REF: p. 394

7. According to the text, the size of the film mount should correspond to the size of the:
   a. Patient chart
   b. Mailing envelopes
   c. Viewbox
   d. Processor

Answer: c

Correct: According to the text, the size of the film mount should correspond to the size of the viewbox.

Incorrect:

(a) According to the text, the size of the film mount should correspond to the size of the *viewbox*. The patient chart can accommodate a wide variety of film mounts.

(b) According to the text, the size of the film mount should correspond to the size of the *viewbox*. It is important to purchase mailing envelopes that can hold the largest size of mount used in the dental office.

(d) According to the text, the size of the film mount should correspond to the size of the *viewbox*. It does not bear any correlation to the size or capacity of the processor.

REF: p. 394

8. Who among the following categories of dental professionals is qualified to mount dental radiographs?
   (1) Dentist
   (2) Dental hygienist
   (3) Dental assistant
      a. 1, 2, 3
      b. 1, 2
      c. 2, 3
      d. 1 only

Answer: a

Correct: The dentist, dental hygienist, and dental assistant are all qualified to mount dental radiographs.

Incorrect:

(b) The dentist, dental hygienist, and *dental assistant* are all qualified to mount dental radiographs. A dental assistant with knowledge of normal anatomic landmarks is qualified.

(c) The *dentist,* dental hygienist, and dental assistant are all qualified to mount dental radiographs. In many offices the dental hygienist and dental assistant mount most of the dental radiographs, but the dentist may do so on occasion.

(d) The dentist, *dental hygienist, and dental assistant* are all qualified to mount dental radiographs.

REF: p. 394

9. The dental radiographer should always mount films _____ after processing.
   a. immediately
   b. 24 hours
   c. 3 days
   d. 1 week

Answer: a

Correct: The dental radiographer should always mount films immediately after processing.

Incorrect:
   (b) The dental radiographer should always mount films *immediately* after processing. The longer the period between processing and mounting, the greater is the risk of loss or damage to the films.
   (c) The dental radiographer should always mount films *immediately* after processing. The longer the period between processing and mounting, the greater is the risk of loss or damage to the films.
   (d) The dental radiographer should always mount films *immediately* after processing. The longer the period between processing and mounting, the greater is the risk of loss or damage to the films.

REF: p. 394

10. Mounted radiographs increase:
   a. Chances of error in determining the patient's right and left sides
   b. Handling of individual films
   c. Chances of damage to the emulsion
   d. Accessibility for interpretation

Answer: d

Correct: Mounted radiographs increase accessibility for interpretation.

Incorrect:
   (a) Mounted radiographs increase *accessibility for interpretation*. They decrease the chances of error in determining the patient's right and left sides.
   (b) Mounted radiographs increase *accessibility for interpretation*. They decrease the handling of individual films.
   (c) Mounted radiographs increase *accessibility for interpretation*. They decrease chances of damage to the emulsion.

REF: p. 395

11. The film mount should be labeled _____ the films are mounted. A(n) _____ can be used to label film mounts.
   a. before; special marking pencil
   b. after; special marking pencil
   c. before; ink pen
   d. after; standard graphite pencil

Answer: a

Correct: The film mount should be labeled before the films are mounted. A special marking pencil can be used to label film mounts.

Incorrect:
   (b) The film mount should be labeled *before* the films are mounted. A *special marking pencil* can be used to label film mounts.
   (c) The film mount should be labeled before the films are mounted. A *special marking pencil* can be used to label film mounts. Mounts can be reused, and it is difficult to erase mounts marked with an ink pen.
   (d) The film mount should be labeled *before* the films are mounted. A *special marking pencil* can be used to label film mounts.

REF: p. 395

12. It is desirable that radiographs be identified with each of the following pieces of information, but it is critical that they be labeled with the:
   a. Patient's name and date of exposure
   b. Number of films
   c. Dentist's name
   d. Radiographer's name

Answer: a

Correct: It is desirable that radiographs be identified with each of the following pieces of information, but it is critical that they be labeled with the patient's name and date of exposure. Any person who has worked in a dental office knows the frustration of trying to identify a loose film that has popped out of the film mount and is found on the counter or floor.

Incorrect:
   (b) It is desirable that radiographs be identified with each of the following pieces of information, but it is critical that they be labeled with the *patient's name and date of exposure*. Although the number of films can be counted, and the dentist's and radiographer's names can usually be determined from memory or work schedules, the films are useless if the patient's name and the date of exposure cannot be determined.
   (c) It is desirable that radiographs be identified with each of the following pieces of information, but it is critical that they be labeled with the *patient's name and date of exposure*. Although the number of films can be counted, and the dentist's and radiographer's names can usually be determined from memory or work schedules, the films are useless if the patient's name and the date of exposure cannot be determined.
   (d) It is desirable that radiographs be identified with each of the following pieces of information, but it is critical that they are labeled with the *patient's name and date of exposure*. Although the number of films can be counted, and the dentist's and

radiographer's names can usually be determined from memory or work schedules, the films are useless if the patient's name and the date of exposure cannot be determined.

REF: p. 395

13. In the labial mounting method, radiographs are placed in the film mount with the _____ side of the identification dot facing the viewer. They are then viewed from the _____ aspect.
   a. depressed; labial
   b. depressed; lingual
   c. raised; labial
   d. raised; lingual

Answer: c

Correct: In the labial mounting method, radiographs are placed in the film mount with the raised side of the identification dot facing the viewer. They are then viewed from the labial aspect.

Incorrect:
   (a) In the labial mounting method, radiographs are placed in the film mount with the *raised* side of the identification dot facing the viewer. They are then viewed from the labial aspect.
   (b) In the labial mounting method, radiographs are placed in the film mount with the *raised* side of the identification dot facing the viewer. They are then viewed from the *labial* aspect.
   (c) In the labial mounting method, radiographs are placed in the film mount with the *raised* side of the identification dot facing the viewer. They are then viewed from the *labial* aspect.
   (d) In the labial mounting method, radiographs are placed in the film mount with the raised side of the identification dot facing the viewer. They are then viewed from the *labial* aspect.

REF: p. 397

14. With the lingual mounting method, films are viewed from the _____ aspect. The lingual method _____ recommended.
   a. labial; is
   b. labial; is not
   c. lingual; is
   d. lingual; is not

Answer: d

Correct: With the lingual mounting method, films are viewed from the lingual aspect. The lingual method is not recommended.

Incorrect:
   (a) With the lingual mounting method, films are viewed from the *lingual* aspect. The lingual method *is not* recommended.
   (b) With the lingual mounting method, films are viewed from the *lingual* aspect. The lingual method is not recommended.

(c) With the lingual mounting method, films are viewed from the lingual aspect. The lingual method *is not* recommended.

REF: p. 397

15. Suggestions for mounting radiographs include mounting bite-wing radiographs with the curve of Spee directed _____ toward the distal and remembering that most maxillary molars have _____ roots.
   a. upward; two
   b. upward; three
   c. downward; two
   d. downward; three

Answer: b

Correct: Suggestions for mounting radiographs include mounting bite-wing radiographs with the curve of Spee directed upward toward the distal and remembering that most maxillary molars have three roots.

Incorrect:
   (a) Suggestions for mounting radiographs include mounting bite-wing radiographs with the curve of Spee directed upward toward the distal and remembering that most maxillary molars have *three* roots.
   (c) Suggestions for mounting radiographs include mounting bite-wing radiographs with the curve of Spee directed *upward* toward the distal and remembering that most maxillary molars have *three* roots.
   (d) Suggestions for mounting radiographs include mounting bite-wing radiographs with the curve of Spee directed *upward* toward the distal and remembering that most maxillary molars have three roots.

REF: p. 401

16. Although all members of the dental team may interpret dental radiographs, it is the responsibility of the _____ to establish a final or definitive interpretation and diagnosis.
   a. dentist or dental hygienist
   b. dentist or dental assistant
   c. dental hygienist or dental assistant
   d. dentist

Answer: d

Correct: Although all members of the dental team may interpret dental radiographs, it is the responsibility of the dentist to establish a final or definitive interpretation and diagnosis.

Incorrect:
   (a) Although all members of the dental team may interpret dental radiographs, it is the responsibility of the *dentist* to establish a final or definitive interpretation and diagnosis.
   (b) Although all members of the dental team may interpret dental radiographs, it is the responsibility

of the *dentist* to establish a final or definitive interpretation and diagnosis.

(c) Although all members of the dental team may interpret dental radiographs, it is the responsibility of the *dentist* to establish a final or definitive interpretation and diagnosis.

REF: p. 401

17. The text recommends viewing radiographs _____ in a room with _____ lighting.
a. as many times as necessary; bright
b. as many times as necessary; dimmed
c. a single time; bright
d. a single time; dimmed

Answer: b
Correct: The text recommends viewing radiographs as many times as necessary in a room with dimmed lighting.
Incorrect:
(a) The text recommends viewing radiographs as many times as necessary in a room with *dimmed* lighting.
(c) The text recommends viewing radiographs *as many times as necessary* in a room with *dimmed* lighting.
(d) The text recommends viewing radiographs *as many times as necessary* in a room with dimmed lighting.

REF: p. 401

CHAPTER 28 NORMAL ANATOMY: PANORAMIC FILMS

MULTIPLE CHOICE

1. Which of the following radiographs allows the dental professional to view the largest area of the mandible and maxilla on a single film?
a. Four bite-wing films
b. 18-film periapical series
c. 21-film periapical series
d. Panoramic

Answer: d
Correct: The panoramic radiograph allows the dental professional to view the largest area of the mandible and maxilla on a single film.
Incorrect:
(a) The *panoramic* radiograph allows the dental professional to view the largest area of the mandible and maxilla on a single film. Bite-wing films do not permit visualization of the apical area.
(b) The *panoramic* radiograph allows the dental professional to view the largest area of the mandible and maxilla on a single film. An 18-film periapical series does not permit visualization of the entire maxilla and mandible.
(c) The *panoramic* radiograph allows the dental professional to view the largest area of the mandible and maxilla on a single film. A 21-film periapical series does not permit visualization of the entire maxilla and mandible.

REF: p. 407

2. The _____ forms the floor of the orbit of the eyes, the sides and floor of the nasal cavity, and the hard palate.
a. maxillary sinus
b. maxilla
c. incisive foramen
d. infraorbital foramen

Answer: b
Correct: The maxilla forms the floor of the orbit of the eyes, the sides and floor of the nasal cavity, and the hard palate.
Incorrect:
(a) The *maxilla* forms the floor of the orbit of the eyes, the sides and floor of the nasal cavity, and the hard palate. The maxillary sinuses are paired cavities or compartments of bone located within the maxilla.
(c) The *maxilla* forms the floor of the orbit of the eyes, the sides and floor of the nasal cavity, and the hard palate. The incisive foramen is an opening or hole in bone located at the midline of the anterior portion of the hard palate.
(d) The *maxilla* forms the floor of the orbit of the eyes, the sides and floor of the nasal cavity, and the hard palate. The infraorbital foramen is a hole or opening in bone found inferior to the border of the orbit.

REF: p. 407

3. The mastoid process is a marked prominence of bone located _____ to the temporomandibular joint (TMJ).
a. anterior and superior
b. anterior and inferior
c. posterior and superior
d. posterior and inferior

Answer: d
Correct: The mastoid process is a marked prominence of bone located posterior and inferior to the TMJ.
Incorrect:
(a) The mastoid process is a marked prominence of bone located *posterior and inferior* to the TMJ.
(b) The mastoid process is a marked prominence of bone located *posterior and inferior* to the TMJ.
(c) The mastoid process is a marked prominence of bone located *posterior and inferior* to the TMJ.

REF: p. 407

4. The mastoid process is a rounded _____ that _____ seen on periapical radiographs.
a. radiolucency; is
b. radiolucency; is not
c. radiopacity; is
d. radiopacity; is not

Answer: d

Correct: The mastoid process is a rounded radiopacity that is not seen on periapical radiographs.

Incorrect:
(a) The mastoid process is a rounded *radiopacity* that *is not* seen on periapical radiographs.
(b) The mastoid process is a rounded *radiopacity* that is not seen on periapical radiographs.
(c) The mastoid process is a rounded radiopacity that *is not* seen on periapical radiographs.

REF: p. 407

5. Which of the following structures is part of the sphenoid bone?
   a. Glenoid fossa
   b. Articular eminence
   c. Lateral pterygoid plate
   d. Styloid process

Answer: c

Correct: The lateral pterygoid plate is part of the sphenoid bone.

Incorrect:
(a) The *lateral pterygoid plate* is part of the sphenoid bone. The glenoid fossa is part of the temporal bone.
(b) The *lateral pterygoid plate* is part of the sphenoid bone. The articular eminence is part of the temporal bone.
(d) The *lateral pterygoid plate* is part of the sphenoid bone. The styloid process is part of the temporal bone.

REF: p. 408

6. Which of the following structures may be seen on periapical radiographs?
   a. Mastoid process
   b. Styloid process
   c. External auditory meatus
   d. Maxillary tuberosity

Answer: d

Correct: The maxillary tuberosity may be seen on periapical radiographs.

Incorrect:
(a) The *maxillary tuberosity* may be seen on periapical radiographs. The mastoid process is not seen on periapical radiographs, but may be seen on panoramic radiographs.
(b) The *maxillary tuberosity* may be seen on periapical radiographs. The styloid process is not seen on periapical radiographs, but may be seen on panoramic radiographs.
(c) The *maxillary tuberosity* may be seen on periapical radiographs. The external auditory meatus is not seen on periapical radiographs, but may be seen on panoramic radiographs.

REF: pp. 407-408

7. The _____ is a hole or opening in the temporal bone located superior and anterior to the mastoid process.

a. glenoid fossa
b. articular eminence
c. external auditory meatus
d. infraorbital foramen

Answer: c

Correct: The external auditory meatus is a hole or opening in the temporal bone located superior and anterior to the mastoid process.

Incorrect:
(a) The *external auditory meatus* is a hole or opening in the temporal bone located superior and anterior to the mastoid process. The glenoid fossa is a concave, depressed area of the temporal bone located anterior to the mastoid process and the external auditory meatus.
(b) The *external auditory meatus* is a hole or opening in the temporal bone located superior and anterior to the mastoid process. The articular eminence is a rounded projection of the temporal bone located anterior to the glenoid fossa.
(d) The *external auditory meatus* is a hole or opening in the temporal bone located superior and anterior to the mastoid process. The infraorbital foramen is a hole or opening in bone found inferior to the border of the orbit.

REF: p. 407

8. The glenoid fossa is a _____ area.
   a. convex, raised
   b. convex, depressed
   c. concave, raised
   d. concave, depressed

Answer: d

Correct: The glenoid fossa is a concave, depressed area.

Incorrect:
(a) The glenoid fossa is a *concave, depressed* area.
(b) The glenoid fossa is a *concave,* depressed area.
(c) The glenoid fossa is a concave, *depressed* area.

REF: p. 407

9. The _____ rests in the glenoid fossa.
   a. styloid process
   b. mastoid process
   c. mandibular condyle
   d. coronoid process

Answer: c

Correct: The mandibular condyle rests in the glenoid fossa.

Incorrect:
(a) The *mandibular condyle* rests in the glenoid fossa. The styloid process extends down from the inferior surface of the temporal bone.
(b) The *mandibular condyle* rests in the glenoid fossa. The mastoid process is part of the temporal bone.
(d) The *mandibular condyle* rests in the glenoid fossa. The coronoid process extends from the anterior portion of the mandible.

REF: p. 407

10. On a panoramic radiograph the articular eminence appears as a rounded radiopaque projection of the bone located _____ to the glenoid fossa.
   a. anterior
   b. posterior
   c. superior
   d. inferior

Answer: a

Correct: On a panoramic radiograph the articular eminence appears as a rounded radiopaque projection of the bone located anterior to the glenoid fossa.

Incorrect:
   (b) On a panoramic radiograph the articular eminence appears as a rounded radiopaque projection of the bone located *anterior* to the glenoid fossa.
   (c) On a panoramic radiograph the articular eminence appears as a rounded radiopaque projection of the bone located *anterior* to the glenoid fossa.
   (d) On a panoramic radiograph the articular eminence appears as a rounded radiopaque projection of the bone located *anterior* to the glenoid fossa.

REF: p. 408

11. The lateral pterygoid plate is a wing-shaped bony projection of the _____ bone.
   a. temporal
   b. frontal
   c. occipital
   d. sphenoid

Answer: d

Correct: The lateral pterygoid plate is a wing-shaped bony projection of the sphenoid bone.

Incorrect:
   (a) The lateral pterygoid plate is a wing-shaped bony projection of the *sphenoid* bone.
   (b) The lateral pterygoid plate is a wing-shaped bony projection of the *sphenoid* bone.
   (c) The lateral pterygoid plate is a wing-shaped bony projection of the *sphenoid* bone.

REF: p. 408

12. The pterygomaxillary fissure is a narrow space or cleft that separates the _____ and the maxilla.
   a. medial pterygoid plate
   b. lateral pterygoid plate
   c. hamulus
   d. coronoid notch

Answer: b

Correct: The pterygomaxillary fissure is a narrow space or cleft that separates the lateral pterygoid plate and the maxilla.

Incorrect:
   (a) The pterygomaxillary fissure is a narrow space or cleft that separates the *lateral* pterygoid plate and the maxilla.

   (c) The pterygomaxillary fissure is a narrow space or cleft that separates the *lateral pterygoid plate* and the maxilla.
   (d) The pterygomaxillary fissure is a narrow space or cleft that separates the *lateral pterygoid plate* and the maxilla.

REF: p. 408

13. Which of the following structures appears as a radiolucency on panoramic radiographs?
   a. Lateral pterygoid plate
   b. Medial pterygoid plate
   c. Pterygomaxillary fissure
   d. Coronoid process

Answer: c

Correct: The pterygomaxillary fissure appears as a radiolucency on panoramic radiographs. A fissure is a narrow space or cleft, so a greater number of photons would pass through this area of decreased density and interact with the halide in the film.

Incorrect:
   (a) The *pterygomaxillary fissure* appears as a radiolucency on panoramic radiographs. The lateral pterygoid plate is a wing-shaped bony projection of the sphenoid bone located distal to the maxillary tuberosity region. On a panoramic radiograph the lateral pterygoid plate appears as a radiopaque projection of bone distal to the maxillary tuberosity region.
   (b) The *pterygomaxillary fissure* appears as a radiolucency on panoramic radiographs. The medial pterygoid plate is a bony projection that lies medial to and is obscured by the lateral pterygoid plate on panoramic radiographs.
   (d) The *pterygomaxillary fissure* appears as a radiolucency on panoramic radiographs. The coronoid process is a marked prominence of bone found on the anterior superior ramus of the mandible. On a panoramic radiograph the coronoid process appears as a triangular radiopacity posterior to the maxillary tuberosity region.

REF: p. 408

14. Which of the following structures appears as a radiopaque bulge distal to the third molar region?
   a. Hamulus
   b. Maxillary tuberosity
   c. Coronoid process
   d. External auditory meatus

Answer: b

Correct: The maxillary tuberosity appears as a radiopaque bulge distal to the third molar region.

Incorrect:
   (a) The *maxillary tuberosity* appears as a radiopaque bulge distal to the third molar region. The hamulus is a small, hooklike projection of bone that extends from the medial pterygoid plate of the

sphenoid bone. The hamulus is located posterior to the maxillary tuberosity. On a panoramic radiograph the hamulus appears as a radiopaque hooklike projection posterior to the maxillary tuberosity area.

(c) The *maxillary tuberosity* appears as a radiopaque bulge distal to the third molar region. The coronoid process is a marked prominence of bone found on the anterior superior ramus of the mandible. On a panoramic radiograph the coronoid process appears as a triangular radiopacity posterior to the maxillary tuberosity region.

(d) The *maxillary tuberosity* appears as a radiopaque bulge distal to the third molar region. The external auditory meatus is a hole or opening in the temporal bone located superior and anterior to the mastoid process. On a panoramic radiograph the external auditory meatus appears as a round-to-ovoid radiolucency anterior and superior to the mastoid process.

REF: p. 408

15. The infraorbital foramen may be superimposed over the _____ on a panoramic radiograph.
   a. mental foramen
   b. maxillary sinus
   c. frontal sinus
   d. external auditory meatus

Answer: b

Correct: The infraorbital foramen may be superimposed over the maxillary sinus on a panoramic radiograph.

Incorrect:

(a) The infraorbital foramen may be superimposed over the *maxillary sinus* on a panoramic radiograph. The infraorbital foramen is a hole of opening in bone found inferior to the border of the orbit. The mental foramen is an opening or hole in bone located on the external surface of the mandible in the region of the mandibular premolars; thus the infraorbital foramen would not be superimposed over the mental foramen on a panoramic radiograph.

(c) The infraorbital foramen may be superimposed over the *maxillary sinus* on a panoramic radiograph. The infraorbital foramen is a hole of opening in bone found inferior to the border of the orbit. The frontal sinus is superior to the orbit; thus the infraorbital foramen would not be superimposed over the frontal sinus on a panoramic radiograph.

(d) The infraorbital foramen may be superimposed over the *maxillary sinus* on a panoramic radiograph. The infraorbital foramen is a hole of opening in bone found inferior to the border of the orbit. The external auditory meatus is a hole or opening in the temporal bone located superior and anterior to the mastoid process; thus the infraorbital foramen would not be superimposed

over the external auditory meatus on a panoramic radiograph.

REF: p. 409

16. Only the _____ border of the orbit is visible on most panoramic radiographs.
   a. inferior
   b. lateral
   c. medial
   d. superior

Answer: a

Correct: Only the inferior border of the orbit is visible on most panoramic radiographs.

Incorrect:

(b) Only the *inferior* border of the orbit is visible on most panoramic radiographs.

(c) Only the *inferior* border of the orbit is visible on most panoramic radiographs.

(d) Only the *inferior* border of the orbit is visible on most panoramic radiographs.

REF: p. 409

17. On a panoramic radiograph the incisive foramen appears as a small, ovoid or round area located:
   a. Near the apex of the mandibular first premolar
   b. Between the roots of the maxillary central incisors
   c. Inferior to the orbit
   d. Superior to the maxillary sinuses

Answer: b

Correct: On a panoramic radiograph the incisive foramen appears as a small, ovoid or round area located between the roots of the maxillary central incisors.

Incorrect:

(a) On a panoramic radiograph the incisive foramen appears as a small, ovoid or round area located *between the roots of the maxillary central incisors*. The mental foramen is located near the apex of the mandibular first premolar.

(c) On a panoramic radiograph the incisive foramen appears as a small, ovoid or round area located *between the roots of the maxillary central incisors*. The infraorbital foramen is located inferior to the orbit.

(d) On a panoramic radiograph the incisive foramen appears as a small, ovoid or round area located *between the roots of the maxillary central incisors*. The orbit is located superior to the maxillary sinuses.

REF: p. 409

18. The anterior nasal spine is a sharp bony projection of the maxilla located at the _____ portion of the nasal cavity.
   a. anterior and superior
   b. anterior and inferior
   c. posterior and superior
   d. posterior and inferior

Answer: b
Correct: The anterior nasal spine is a sharp bony projection of the maxilla located at the anterior and inferior portion of the nasal cavity.
Incorrect:
  (a) The anterior nasal spine is a sharp bony projection of the maxilla located at the anterior and *inferior* portion of the nasal cavity.
  (c) The anterior nasal spine is a sharp bony projection of the maxilla located at the *anterior and inferior* portion of the nasal cavity.
  (d) The anterior nasal spine is a sharp bony projection of the maxilla located at the *anterior* and inferior portion of the nasal cavity.
REF: p. 409

19. The nasal cavity is also known as the:
  a. Nasal spine
  b. Nasal septum
  c. Zygoma
  d. Nasal fossa

Answer: d
Correct: The nasal cavity is also known as the nasal fossa.
Incorrect:
  (a) The nasal cavity is also known as the *nasal fossa*.
  (b) The nasal cavity is also known as the *nasal fossa*.
  (c) The nasal cavity is also known as the *nasal fossa*.
REF: p. 409

20. The nasal _____ is a vertical bony wall or partition that divides the nasal cavity into the right and left nasal fossae.
  a. spine
  b. cavity
  c. hard palate
  d. septum

Answer: d
Correct: The nasal septum is a vertical bony wall or partition that divides the nasal cavity into the right and left nasal fossae.
Incorrect:
  (a) The nasal *septum* is a vertical bony wall or partition that divides the nasal cavity into the right and left nasal fossae.
  (b) The nasal *septum* is a vertical bony wall or partition that divides the nasal cavity into the right and left nasal fossae.
  (c) The nasal *septum* is a vertical bony wall or partition that divides the nasal cavity into the right and left nasal fossae.
REF: p. 409

21. On a panoramic radiograph the zygomatic process of the maxilla appears as a _____ -shaped radiopacity.
  a. J
  b. Y
  c. U
  d. Both a and c

Answer: d
Correct: On a panoramic radiograph, the zygomatic process of the maxilla appears as a J- or U-shaped radiopacity.
Incorrect:
  (a) Choice a is correct, but choice c is also true. On a panoramic radiograph the zygomatic process of the maxilla appears as a *J-or U*-shaped radiopacity.
  (b) On a panoramic radiograph the zygomatic process of the maxilla appears as a *J- or U*-shaped radiopacity.
  (c) Choice c is correct, but choice a is also true. On a panoramic radiograph the zygomatic process of the maxilla appears as a *J-or U*-shaped radiopacity.
REF: p. 409

22. The hamulus extends from the:
  a. Medial pterygoid plate of the sphenoid bone
  b. Lateral pterygoid plate of the sphenoid bone
  c. Coronoid process
  d. Styloid process

Answer: a
Correct: The hamulus extends from the medial pterygoid plate of the sphenoid bone.
Incorrect:
  (b) The hamulus extends from the *medial pterygoid plate of the sphenoid bone.*
  (c) The hamulus extends from the *medial pterygoid plate of the sphenoid bone.*
  (d) The hamulus extends from the *medial pterygoid plate of the sphenoid bone.*
REF: pp. 409-410

23. Which of the following structures may be seen on both periapical and panoramic radiographs?
  a. Mandibular condyle
  b. Coronoid notch
  c. Mandibular foramen
  d. Mental foramen

Answer: d
Correct: The mental foramen may be seen on both periapical and panoramic radiographs.
Incorrect:
  (a) The *mental foramen* may be seen on both periapical and panoramic radiographs. The mandibular condyle is not seen on periapical films, but can be viewed on panoramic radiographs.
  (b) The *mental foramen* may be seen on both periapical and panoramic radiographs. The coronoid notch is not seen on periapical films, but can be viewed on panoramic radiographs.
  (c) The *mental foramen* may be seen on both periapical and panoramic radiographs. The mandibular foramen is not seen on periapical films, but can be viewed on panoramic radiographs.
REF: pp. 410-412

24. On a panoramic radiograph the coronoid notch appears as a _____ to the coronoid process.
a. concavity located mesial
b. concavity located distal
c. convexity located mesial
d. convexity located distal

Answer: b
Correct: On a panoramic radiograph the coronoid notch appears as a concavity located distal to the coronoid process.
Incorrect:
(a) On a panoramic radiograph the coronoid notch appears as a concavity *located distal* to the coronoid process.
(c) On a panoramic radiograph the coronoid notch appears as a *concavity located distal* to the coronoid process.
(d) On a panoramic radiograph the coronoid notch appears as a *concavity* located distal to the coronoid process.
REF: p. 411

25. The _____ is a marked prominence of bone found on the anterior superior ramus of the mandible.
a. mandibular condyle
b. coronoid notch
c. coronoid process
d. lingula

Answer: c
Correct: The coronoid process is a marked prominence of bone found on the anterior superior ramus of the mandible.
Incorrect:
(a) The *coronoid process* is a marked prominence of bone found on the anterior superior ramus of the mandible. The mandibular condyle is a rounded projection of bone extending from the posterior superior border of the ramus of the mandible.
(b) The *coronoid process* is a marked prominence of bone found on the anterior superior ramus of the mandible. The coronoid notch is a scooped-out concavity of bone located distal to the coronoid process of the mandible.
(d) The *coronoid process* is a marked prominence of bone found on the anterior superior ramus of the mandible. The lingula is a small, tongue-shaped projection of bone seen adjacent to the mandibular foramen.
REF: p. 412

26. The _____ is an opening or hole in bone located on the external surface of the mandible in the region of the mandibular premolars.
a. mandibular foramen
b. lingula
c. mandibular canal
d. mental foramen

Answer: d
Correct: The mental foramen is an opening or hole in bone located on the external surface of the mandible in the region of the mandibular premolars.
Incorrect:
(a) The *mental foramen* is an opening or hole in bone located on the external surface of the mandible in the region of the mandibular premolars. The mandibular foramen is a round or ovoid hole in bone on the lingual aspect of the ramus of the mandible.
(b) The *mental foramen* is an opening or hole in bone located on the external surface of the mandible in the region of the mandibular premolars. The lingula is a small, tongue-shaped projection of bone seen adjacent to the mandibular foramen on the lingual surface of the mandible.
(c) The *mental foramen* is an opening or hole in bone located on the external surface of the mandible in the region of the mandibular premolars. The mandibular canal is a tubelike passageway through bone that travels the length of the mandible.
REF: p. 412

27. The _____ foramen is a tiny opening or hole in bone located on the internal surface of the mandible near the midline.
a. lingual
b. mental
c. incisive
d. mandibular

Answer: a
Correct: The lingual foramen is a tiny opening or hole in bone located on the internal surface of the mandible near the midline.
Incorrect:
(b) The *lingual* foramen is a tiny opening or hole in bone located on the internal surface of the mandible near the midline. The mental foramen is an opening or hole in bone located on the external surface of the mandible in the region of the mandibular premolars.
(c) The *lingual* foramen is a tiny opening or hole in bone located on the internal surface of the mandible near the midline. The incisive foramen (nasopalatine foramen) is an opening or hole in bone located at the midline of the anterior portion of the hard palate directly posterior to the maxillary central incisors.
(d) The *lingual* foramen is a tiny opening or hole in bone located on the internal surface of the mandible near the midline. The mandibular foramen is a round or ovoid hole in bone on the lingual aspect of the ramus of the mandible.
REF: p. 412

28. On a panoramic radiograph the _____ air space appears as a diagonal radiolucency located superior to the radiopaque shadow of the soft palate and uvula.
a. palatoglossal
b. nasopharyngeal
c. glossopharyngeal
d. Both a and b

Answer: b
Correct: On a panoramic radiograph the nasopharyngeal air space appears as a diagonal radiolucency located superior to the radiopaque shadow of the soft palate and uvula.
Incorrect:
(a) On a panoramic radiograph the *nasopharyngeal* air space appears as a diagonal radiolucency located superior to the radiopaque shadow of the soft palate and uvula. The palatoglossal air space is found between the palate and the tongue and appears as a horizontal radiolucent band located above the apices of the maxillary teeth.
(c) On a panoramic radiograph the *nasopharyngeal* air space appears as a diagonal radiolucency located superior to the radiopaque shadow of the soft palate and uvula. The glossopharyngeal air space is the portion of the pharynx located posterior to the tongue and oral cavity and appears as a vertical radiolucent band superimposed over the ramus of the mandible.
(d) On a panoramic radiograph the *nasopharyngeal* air space appears as a diagonal radiolucency located superior to the radiopaque shadow of the soft palate and uvula. The palatoglossal air space is found between the palate and the tongue and appears as a horizontal radiolucent band located above the apices of the maxillary teeth.
REF: p. 413

29. On a panoramic radiograph the ear is viewed superimposed over the:
a. Anterior teeth
b. Styloid process
c. Incisive foramen
d. Mandibular canal

Answer: b
Correct: On a panoramic radiograph the ear is viewed superimposed over the styloid process.
Incorrect:
(a) On a panoramic radiograph the ear is viewed superimposed over the *styloid process.*
(c) On a panoramic radiograph the ear is viewed superimposed over the *styloid process.*
(d) On a panoramic radiograph the ear is viewed superimposed over the *styloid process.*
REF: p. 416

CHAPTER 29   INTRODUCTION TO RADIOGRAPHIC INTERPRETATION

MULTIPLE CHOICE
1. The definition of *interpret* is to:
a. Establish a diagnosis
b. Offer an explanation
c. Process radiographs
d. Mount radiographs

Answer: b
Correct: The definition of *interpret* is to offer an explanation.
Incorrect:
(a) The definition of *interpret* is *to offer an explanation.* It is not synonymous with establishing a diagnosis.
(c) The definition of *interpret* is *to offer an explanation.* It is not synonymous with establishing a diagnosis. Processing radiographs is not the same as interpreting them.
(d) The definition of *interpret* is *to offer an explanation.* It is not synonymous with establishing a diagnosis. Mounting radiographs is not the same as interpreting them.
REF: p. 421

2. Radiographic interpretation enables the dental professional to play a vital role in the detection of _____ of the teeth and jaws that cannot be identified clinically.
(1) lesions
(2) diseases
(3) conditions
a. 1, 2, 3
b. 1, 2
c. 1, 3
d. 1 only

Answer: a
Correct: Radiographic interpretation enables the dental professional to play a vital role in the detection of lesions, diseases, and conditions of the teeth and jaws that cannot be identified clinically.
Incorrect:
(b) All three choices are correct. Radiographic interpretation enables the dental professional to play a vital role in the detection of lesions, diseases, and *conditions* of the teeth and jaws that cannot be identified clinically.
(c) All three choices are correct. Radiographic interpretation enables the dental professional to play a vital role in the detection of lesions, *diseases,* and conditions of the teeth and jaws that cannot be identified clinically.
(d) All three choices are correct. Radiographic interpretation enables the dental professional to play a vital role in the detection of lesions, *diseases, and conditions* of the teeth and jaws that cannot be identified clinically.
REF: p. 421

3. To interpret films, the dental radiographer must be confident in the identification and recognition of the following:
   (1) Normal anatomy
   (2) Dental caries
   (3) Periodontal disease
   (4) Traumatic injuries and periapical lesions
      a. 1, 2, 3, 4
      b. 1, 2, 3
      c. 2, 3, 4
      d. 1, 2, 4

Answer: a
Correct: To interpret films, the dental radiographer must be confident in the identification and recognition of the following: normal anatomy, dental caries, periodontal disease, and traumatic injuries and periapical lesions.
Incorrect:
   (b) All the choices are correct. To interpret films, the dental radiographer must be confident in the identification and recognition of the following: normal anatomy, dental caries, periodontal disease, and *traumatic injuries and periapical lesions.*
   (c) All the choices are correct. To interpret films, the dental radiographer must be confident in the identification and recognition of the following: *normal anatomy,* dental caries, periodontal disease, and traumatic injuries and periapical lesions.
   (d) All the choices are correct. To interpret films, the dental radiographer must be confident in the identification and recognition of the following: normal anatomy, dental caries, *periodontal disease,* and traumatic injuries and periapical lesions.
REF:

4. In the dental setting, *interpretation* refers to an explanation of what is viewed on a radiograph, whereas the term *diagnosis* refers to the identification of disease by examination or analysis.
   a. Both statements are true.
   b. Both statements are false.
   c. The first statement is true; the second statement is false.
   d. The first statement is false; the second statement is true.

Answer: a
Correct: In the dental setting, *interpretation* refers to an explanation of what is viewed on a radiograph, whereas the term *diagnosis* refers to the identification of disease by examination or analysis.
Incorrect:
   (b) In the dental setting, *interpretation* refers to an explanation of what is viewed on a radiograph, whereas the term *diagnosis* refers to the identification of disease by examination or analysis.
   (c) In the dental setting, *interpretation* refers to an explanation of what is viewed on a radiograph,

whereas the term *diagnosis* refers to the identification of disease by examination or analysis.
   (d) In the dental setting, *interpretation* refers to an explanation of what is viewed on a radiograph, whereas the term *diagnosis* refers to the identification of disease by examination or analysis.
REF: p. 421

5. According to the text, ideally, dental radiographs should be reviewed and interpreted immediately after mounting:
   a. Alone in a quiet room in the evening
   b. In the presence of the patient
   c. Even if processing and mounting take place a week after the films were exposed
   d. Only when it is convenient

Answer: b
Correct: According to the text, ideally, dental radiographs should be reviewed and interpreted immediately after mounting in the presence of the patient.
Incorrect:
   (a) According to the text, ideally, dental radiographs should be reviewed and interpreted immediately after mounting *in the presence of the patient.*
   (c) According to the text, ideally, dental radiographs should be reviewed and interpreted immediately after mounting *in the presence of the patient.*
   (d) According to the text, ideally, dental radiographs should be reviewed and interpreted immediately after mounting *in the presence of the patient.*
REF: p. 422

6. In the dental setting, most films are examined in the:
   a. Business office
   b. Darkroom
   c. Operatory at chairside
   d. Reception room

Answer: c
Correct: In the dental setting, most films are examined in the operatory at chairside.
Incorrect:
   (a) In the dental setting, most films are examined in the *operatory.* The business office is not the best area for examination of dental radiographs; the lighting is not appropriate, and there are privacy concerns. Dental radiographs are best interpreted by the dental professional on a viewbox in a room with dimmed lighting; however, examination in the operatory allows for immediate review and interpretation after mounting in the presence of the patient.
   (b) In the dental setting, most films are examined in the *operatory.* The darkroom itself is not the best area for examination of dental radiographs because the light from the viewbox will fog and ruin unfixed films. Dental radiographs are best interpreted by the dental professional on a viewbox in a room with dimmed lighting; however,

examination in the operatory allows for review and interpretation immediately after mounting in the presence of the patient.

(d) In the dental setting, most films are examined in the *operatory*. The reception room is not an acceptable area for examination of dental radiographs; the lighting is not appropriate, and there are privacy concerns. Dental radiographs are best interpreted by the dental professional on a view-box in a room with dimmed lighting; however, examination in the operatory allows for immediate review and interpretation after mounting in the presence of the patient.

REF: p. 422

CHAPTER 30   DESCRIPTIVE TERMINOLOGY

MULTIPLE CHOICE

1. A(n) _____ is an image that is produced on photosensitive film.
   a. x-ray
   b. radiograph
   c. photon
   d. electron

Answer: b
Correct: A radiograph is an image that is produced on photosensitive film.
Incorrect:
   (a) A *radiograph* is an image that is produced on photosensitive film. An x-ray refers to the beam of energy, or radiation.
   (c) A *radiograph* is an image that is produced on photosensitive film. A photon interacts with the halide to produce a radiographic image.
   (d) A *radiograph* is an image that is produced on photosensitive film. An electron interacts with the target to produce the photons that interact with the film to create a radiographic image.
REF: p. 425

2. A radiograph should *not* be referred to as a(n):
   a. Radiogram
   b. Roentgenogram
   c. X-ray
   d. X-ray film

Answer: c
Correct: A radiograph should *not* be referred to as an x-ray.
Incorrect:
   (a) A radiograph should *not* be referred to as an x-ray. An x-ray refers to the beam of energy, or radiation, and not to the image produced on photosensitive film by exposing the film to x-rays and then processing the film so that a negative is produced. "Radiogram" is an acceptable but antiquated synonym for radiograph.
   (b) A radiograph should *not* be referred to as an x-ray. An x-ray refers to the beam of energy, or radiation, and not to the image produced on photosensitive film by exposing the film to x-rays and then processing the film so that a negative is produced. "Roentgenogram" is an acceptable but antiquated synonym for radiograph.
   (d) A radiograph should *not* be referred to as an *x-ray*. An x-ray refers to the beam of energy, or radiation, and not to the image produced on photosensitive film by exposing the film to x-rays and then processing the film so that a negative is produced. X-ray film is an acceptable synonym for radiograph.
REF: p. 425

3. An x-ray is:
   a. An image that is produced on photosensitive film
   b. A beam of energy that has the power to penetrate substances
   c. A radiograph
   d. The actual film exposed

Answer: b
Correct: An x-ray is a beam of energy that has the power to penetrate substances.
Incorrect:
   (a) An x-ray is *a beam of energy that has the power to penetrate substances*. An x-ray beam does not have mass and is described in terms of photons or waves. A radiograph is an image that is produced on photosensitive film by exposing the film to x-rays and then processing the film so that a negative is produced. A radiograph has mass.
   (c) An x-ray is *a beam of energy that has the power to penetrate substances*. A radiograph is an image that is produced on photosensitive film by exposing the film to x-rays and then processing the film so that a negative is produced. A radiograph has mass.
   (d) An x-ray is *a beam of energy that has the power to penetrate substances*. A radiograph is an image that is produced on photosensitive film by exposing the film to x-rays and then processing the film so that a negative is produced. A radiograph has mass.
REF: p. 425

4. A radiograph appears _____ where the tissues are soft or thin.
   a. radiopaque
   b. white
   c. light
   d. black or dark

Answer: d
Correct: A radiograph appears black or dark where the tissues are soft or thin.
Incorrect:
   (a) A radiograph appears *black or dark* (radiolucent) where the tissues are soft or thin. More photons pass through tissue that is soft or thin rather than

hard or thick to expose the halide of the film. In contrast, the film would appear white or light (radiopaque) where tissues are thick or hard. Fewer photons pass through thick or hard tissue to expose the halide of the film. The unexposed halide is washed off during processing, leaving light areas on the radiograph.

(b) A radiograph appears *black or dark* (radiolucent) where the tissues are soft or thin. More photons pass through tissue that is soft or thin rather than hard or thick to expose the halide of the film. In contrast, the film would appear white or light (radiopaque) where tissues are thick or hard. Fewer photons pass through thick or hard tissue to expose the halide of the film. The unexposed halide is washed off during processing, leaving light areas on the radiograph.

(c) A radiograph appears *black or dark* (radiolucent) where the tissues are soft or thin. More photons pass through tissue that is soft or thin rather than hard or thick to expose the halide of the film. In contrast, the film would appear white or light (radiopaque) where tissues are thick or hard. Fewer photons pass through thick or hard tissue to expose the halide of the film. The unexposed halide is washed off during processing, leaving light areas on the radiograph.

REF: p. 425

5. Most structures radiographed _____ exhibit uniform thickness and therefore appear _____.
   a. do; white
   b. do not; gray
   c. do; black
   d. do not; white

Answer: b
Correct: Most structures radiographed do not exhibit uniform thickness and therefore appear gray.
Incorrect:
   (a) Most structures radiographed *do not* exhibit uniform thickness and therefore appear *gray*.
   (c) Most structures radiographed *do not* exhibit uniform thickness and therefore appear *gray*.
   (d) Most structures radiographed do not exhibit uniform thickness and therefore appear *gray*.

REF: p. 425

6. Dental caries appears _____ because the area of the tooth with caries is _____ dense than surrounding structures.
   a. radiopaque; more
   b. radiopaque; less
   c. radiolucent; more
   d. radiolucent; less

Answer: d
Correct: Dental caries appears radiolucent because the area of the tooth with caries is less dense than surrounding structures.

Incorrect:
   (a) Dental caries appears *radiolucent* because the area of the tooth with caries is *less* dense than surrounding structures.
   (b) Dental caries appears *radiolucent* because the area of the tooth with caries is less dense than surrounding structures.
   (c) Dental caries appears radiolucent because the area of the tooth with caries is *less* dense than surrounding structures.

REF: pp. 425-426

7. Which of the following structures would appear the most radiopaque?
   a. Dental pulp
   b. Metallic restoration
   c. Periodontal ligament space
   d. Air space

Answer: b
Correct: A metallic restoration would appear the most radiopaque.
Incorrect:
   (a) A *metallic restoration* would appear the most radiopaque. Dental pulp appears radiolucent.
   (c) A *metallic restoration* would appear the most radiopaque. The periodontal ligament space appears radiolucent.
   (d) A *metallic restoration* would appear the most radiopaque. An air space appears radiolucent.

REF: p. 426

8. Which of the following is an example of a radiopaque structure?
   a. Dental pulp
   b. Dentin
   c. Periodontal ligament space
   d. Soft tissue

Answer: b
Correct: Dentin is an example of a radiopaque structure.
Incorrect:
   (a) *Dentin* is an example of a radiopaque structure. Dental pulp is radiolucent.
   (c) *Dentin* is an example of a radiopaque structure. The periodontal ligament space is radiolucent.
   (d) *Dentin* is an example of a radiopaque structure. Soft tissue is radiolucent.

REF: p. 426

9. Which of the following terms is used to classify a radiolucent lesion?
   a. Target lesion
   b. Multifocal confluent
   c. Ground glass
   d. Moth-eaten pattern

Answer: d
Correct: Moth-eaten pattern is used to classify a radiolucent lesion.

(a) *Moth-eaten pattern* is used to classify a radiolucent lesion. Target lesion is used to classify a radiopaque lesion.

(b) *Moth-eaten pattern* is used to classify a radiolucent lesion. Multifocal confluent is used to classify a radiopaque lesion.

(c) *Moth-eaten pattern* is used to classify a radiolucent lesion. Ground glass is used to classify a radiopaque lesion.

REF: p. 426

---

10. A unilocular lesion with corticated borders is usually indicative of a _____ process.
   a. benign slow-growing
   b. benign rapidly growing
   c. malignant slow-growing
   d. malignant rapidly growing

Answer: a

Correct: A unilocular lesion with corticated borders is usually indicative of a benign slow-growing process.

Incorrect:

(b) A unilocular lesion with corticated borders is usually indicative of a benign *slow-growing* process. Unilocular lesions tend to be small and nonexpansile. A unilocular lesion with noncorticated borders appears fuzzy or ill defined and may represent either a benign or a malignant process.

(c) A unilocular lesion with corticated borders is usually indicative of a *benign* slow-growing process. Unilocular lesions tend to be small and nonexpansile. A unilocular lesion with noncorticated borders appears fuzzy or ill defined and may represent either a benign or a malignant process.

(d) A unilocular lesion with corticated borders is usually indicative of a *benign slow-growing* process. Unilocular lesions tend to be small and nonexpansile. A unilocular lesion with noncorticated borders appears fuzzy or ill defined and may represent either a benign or a malignant process.

REF: p. 427

---

11. Unilocular lesions tend to be:
   a. Small and expansile
   b. Small and nonexpansile
   c. Large and expansile
   d. Large and nonexpansile

Answer: b

Correct: Unilocular lesions tend to be small and nonexpansile.

Incorrect:

(a) Unilocular lesions tend to be small and *nonexpansile*.

(c) Unilocular lesions tend to be *small and nonexpansile*.

(d) Unilocular lesions tend to be *small* and nonexpansile.

REF: p. 426

---

12. The term _____ refers to a radiolucent lesion located around the crown of an impacted tooth.
   a. periapical
   b. inter-radicular
   c. pericoronal
   d. edentulous zone

Answer: c

Correct: The term *pericoronal* refers to a radiolucent lesion located around the crown of an impacted tooth.

Incorrect:

(a) The term *pericoronal* refers to a radiolucent lesion located around the crown of an impacted tooth. Periapical refers to a lesion located around the apex of a tooth.

(b) The term *pericoronal* refers to a radiolucent lesion located around the crown of an impacted tooth. Inter-radicular refers to a lesion located between the roots of adjacent teeth.

(d) The term *pericoronal* refers to a radiolucent lesion located around the crown of an impacted tooth. Edentulous zone refers to a lesion located in an area without teeth.

REF: p. 428

---

13. Radiopaque lesions may occur in:
   a. Bone but not soft tissue
   b. Soft tissue but not bone
   c. Neither bone nor soft tissue
   d. Either bone or soft tissue

Answer: d

Correct: Radiopaque lesions may occur in either bone or soft tissue.

Incorrect:

(a) Radiopaque lesions may occur in *either bone or soft tissue*.

(b) Radiopaque lesions may occur in *either bone or soft tissue*.

(c) Radiopaque lesions may occur in *either bone or soft tissue*.

REF: p. 430

---

14. The term _____ refers to a well-defined, localized radiopaque area surrounded by a uniform radiolucent halo.
   a. focal opacity
   b. target lesion
   c. multifocal confluent
   d. ground glass

Answer: b

Correct: The term *target lesion* refers to a well-defined, localized radiopaque area surrounded by a uniform radiolucent halo. A benign cementoblastoma is an example of a radiopacity that can be described as a target lesion.

Incorrect:
  (a) The term *target lesion* refers to a well-defined, localized radiopaque area surrounded by a uniform radiolucent halo. A focal opacity is a well-defined, localized radiopaque lesion on a radiograph, but it is not surrounded by a uniform radiolucent halo.
  (c) The term *target lesion* refers to a well-defined, localized radiopaque area surrounded by a uniform radiolucent halo. A multifocal confluent radiopaque pattern can be described as multiple radiopacities that appear to overlap or flow together.
  (d) The term *target lesion* refers to a well-defined, localized radiopaque area surrounded by a uniform radiolucent halo. A ground-glass pattern can be described as a granular or pebbled radiopacity that resembles pulverized glass.

REF: p. 430

15. Condensing osteitis is an example of a lesion that can be described as:
  a. A focal opacity
  b. A target lesion
  c. Multifocal confluent
  d. Ground glass

Answer: a
Correct: Condensing osteitis is an example of a lesion that can be described as a focal opacity.
Incorrect:
  (b) Condensing osteitis is an example of a lesion that can be described as *a focal opacity*. A benign cementoblastoma is an example of a radiopacity that can be described as a target lesion.
  (c) Condensing osteitis is an example of a lesion that can be described as *a focal opacity*. Diseases such as osteitis deformans and florid osseous dysplasia exhibit a multifocal confluent radiopaque pattern.
  (d) Condensing osteitis is an example of a lesion that can be described as *a focal opacity*. Diseases such as osteitis deformans and osteopetrosis may radiographically exhibit a ground-glass appearance.

REF: p. 430

16. A ground-glass appearance of bone is associated with which of the following diseases?
  a. Condensing osteitis
  b. Osteosarcoma
  c. Fibrous dysplasia
  d. Benign cementoblastoma

Answer: c
Correct: A ground-glass appearance of bone is associated with fibrous dysplasia.
Incorrect:
  (a) A ground-glass appearance of bone is associated with *fibrous dysplasia*. Condensing osteitis is an

example of a radiopaque lesion that can be described as a focal opacity. Focal opacity refers to a well-defined, localized radiopaque lesion on a radiograph.
  (b) A ground-glass appearance of bone is associated with *fibrous dysplasia*. Osteosarcoma is an example of a radiopaque, irregular, ill-defined lesion.
  (d) A ground-glass appearance of bone is associated with *fibrous dysplasia*. Benign cemetoblastoma is an example of a radiopaque lesion that can be described as a target lesion.

REF: p. 431

17. Which of the following would be an example of a mixed lucent-opaque lesion?
  a. Compound odontoma
  b. Osteitis deformans
  c. Chondrosarcoma
  d. Florid osseous dysplasia

Answer: a
Correct: A compound odontoma would be an example of a mixed lucent-opaque lesion.
Incorrect:
  (b) A *compound odontoma* would be an example of a mixed lucent-opaque lesion. Osteitis deformans is an example of a lesion with either a multifocal confluent or a ground-glass radiopaque appearance.
  (c) A *compound odontoma* would be an example of a mixed lucent-opaque lesion. Chondrosarcoma is an example of an irregular, ill-defined radiopaque lesion.
  (d) A *compound odontoma* would be an example of a mixed lucent-opaque lesion. Florid osseous dysplasia is an example of a lesion with a multifocal confluent radiopaque pattern.

REF: p. 432

18. Which of the following is an example of a soft tissue opacity?
  a. Osteitis deformans
  b. Sialolith
  c. Chondrosarcoma
  d. Florid osseous dysplasia

Answer: b
Correct: A sialolith is an example of a soft tissue opacity.
Incorrect:
  (a) A *sialolith* is an example of a soft tissue opacity. It is a calcification within the duct of a salivary gland. Osteitis deformans is a bony opacity found in the jaw.
  (c) A *sialolith* is an example of a soft tissue opacity. It is a calcification within the duct of a salivary gland. Chondrosarcoma is a malignant tumor of cartilage.
  (d) A *sialolith* is an example of a soft tissue opacity. It is a calcification within the duct of a salivary

gland. Florid osseous dysplasia is an abnormal proliferation of bone.

REF: p. 432

CHAPTER 31   IDENTIFICATION OF RESTORATIONS, DENTAL MATERIALS, AND FOREIGN OBJECTS

MULTIPLE CHOICE

1. According to the text, if questions arise as to what is seen on a radiograph concerning dental restorations, materials, or foreign objects, _____ can be used to obtain additional information.
   a. verbal inquiry of the patient
   b. clinical examination of the patient
   c. an Internet search
   d. a textbook reference

Answer: b

Correct: According to the text, if questions arise as to what is seen on a radiograph concerning dental restorations, materials, or foreign objects, clinical examination of the patient can be used to obtain additional information.

Incorrect:
   (a) According to the text, if questions arise as to what is seen on a radiograph concerning dental restorations, materials, or foreign objects, *clinical examination of the patient* can be used to obtain additional information. Verbal inquiry of the patient can be attempted, but some patients are unreliable historians. If radiographs are interpreted without the patient present, some important clinical information is not available.
   (c) According to the text, if questions arise as to what is seen on a radiograph concerning dental restorations, materials, or foreign objects, *clinical examination of the patient* can be used to obtain additional information. An Internet search may be useful for background information, but if radiographs are interpreted without the patient present, some important clinical information is not available.
   (d) According to the text, if questions arise as to what is seen on a radiograph concerning dental restorations, materials, or foreign objects, *clinical examination of the patient* can be used to obtain additional information. A textbook reference may be useful for background information, but if radiographs are interpreted without the patient present, some important clinical information is not available.

REF: p. 438

2. Because metallic restorations absorb x-rays, the area of the film that corresponds to their location remains unexposed, and the metallic restorations appear completely _____ on a dental radiograph.
   a. radiosensitive
   b. radioresistant
   c. radiopaque
   d. radiolucent

Answer: c

Correct: Because metallic restorations absorb x-rays, the area of the film that corresponds to their location remains unexposed, and the metallic restorations appear completely radiopaque on a dental radiograph.

Incorrect:
   (a) Because metallic restorations absorb x-rays, the area of the film that corresponds to their location remains unexposed, and the metallic restorations appear completely *radiopaque* on a dental radiograph. Radiosensitivity refers to the relative sensitivity of a tissue or organ to damage from radiation and is not a property of restorations, metallic or otherwise.
   (b) Because metallic restorations absorb x-rays, the area of the film that corresponds to their location remains unexposed, and the metallic restorations appear completely *radiopaque* on a dental radiograph. Radioresistance refers to the relative resistance of a tissue or organ to damage from radiation and is not a property of restorations, metallic or otherwise.
   (d) Because metallic restorations absorb x-rays, the area of the film that corresponds to their location remains unexposed, and the metallic restorations appear completely *radiopaque* on a dental radiograph. Nonmetallic restorations may vary in radiographic appearance from radiolucent to slightly radiopaque, depending on the density of the material.

REF: p. 438

3. Of the nonmetallic restorations, _____ is the most dense and least radiolucent.
   a. unfilled acrylic
   b. filled acrylic
   c. composite
   d. porcelain

Answer: d

Correct: Of the nonmetallic restorations, porcelain is the most dense and least radiolucent.

Incorrect:
   (a) Of the nonmetallic restorations, *porcelain* is the most dense and least radiolucent. Acrylic is the least dense and most radiolucent. Manufacturers may add radiopaque materials such as barium to acrylic and composite materials to enhance visualization.
   (b) Of the nonmetallic restorations, *porcelain* is the most dense and least radiolucent. Acrylic is the least dense and most radiolucent. Manufacturers may add radiopaque materials such as barium to acrylic and composite materials to enhance visualization.
   (c) Of the nonmetallic restorations, *porcelain* is the most dense and least radiolucent. Acrylic is the least dense and most radiolucent. Manufacturers may add radiopaque materials such as barium

191

to acrylic and composite materials to enhance visualization.

REF: p. 438

4. Which of the following is the most common restorative material used in dentistry?
   a. Porcelain
   b. Cast gold
   c. Amalgam
   d. Acrylic

Answer: c

Correct: Amalgam is the most common restorative material used in dentistry.

Incorrect:
   (a) Porcelain is used as a restorative material, but amalgam is the most common restorative material used in dentistry.
   (b) Cast gold is used as a restorative material, but amalgam is the most common restorative material used in dentistry.
   (d) Acrylic is used as a restorative material, but amalgam is the most common restorative material used in dentistry.

REF: p. 438

5. Amalgam overhangs can be described as extensions of amalgam seen on dental radiographs beyond the crown portion of a tooth located in the _____ region.
   a. buccal
   b. lingual
   c. interproximal
   d. occlusal

Answer: c

Correct: Amalgam overhangs can be described as extensions of amalgam seen on dental radiographs beyond the crown portion of a tooth located in the interproximal region.

Incorrect:
   (a) Amalgam overhangs can be described as extensions of amalgam seen on dental radiographs beyond the crown portion of a tooth located in the *interproximal* region. Amalgam extensions on buccal restorations may often be observed clinically; however, they are not often seen on dental radiographs because the radiograph is a two-dimensional representation of a three-dimensional object and depth perception is lost.
   (b) Amalgam overhangs can be described as extensions of amalgam seen on dental radiographs beyond the crown portion of a tooth located in the *interproximal* region. Amalgam extensions on lingual restorations may often be observed clinically; however, they are not often seen on dental radiographs because the radiograph is a two-dimensional representation of a three-dimensional object and depth perception is lost.
   (d) Amalgam overhangs can be described as extensions of amalgam seen on dental radiographs beyond the

crown portion of a tooth located in the *interproximal* region. Amalgam extensions on occlusal restorations may occasionally be observed; however, they do not contribute to bone loss.

REF: p. 439

6. The greatest potential negative consequence of an amalgam overhang is:
   a. Unesthetic contour
   b. Destruction of interproximal bone
   c. Impingment of the interdental papilla
   d. Stretching of periodontal ligament fibers

Answer: b

Correct: The greatest potential negative consequence of an amalgam overhang is destruction of interproximal bone.

Incorrect:
   (a) Unesthetic contour is a negative consequence of an amalgam overhang, but destruction of interproximal bone is the greatest potential negative consequence because it is a permanent condition.
   (c) Impingement of the interdental papilla is a negative consequence of an amalgam overhang, but destruction of interproximal bone is the greatest potential negative consequence because it is a permanent condition.
   (d) Stretching of periodontal ligament fibers is a negative consequence of an amalgam overhang, but destruction of interproximal bone is the greatest potential negative consequence because it is a permanent condition.

REF: p. 439

7. A large, well-adapted radiopaque restoration with smooth borders is probably:
   a. Silver amalgam
   b. Gold
   c. Porcelain
   d. Stainless steel

Answer: b

Correct: A large, well-adapted radiopaque restoration with smooth borders is probably gold.

Incorrect:
   (a) A large, well-adapted radiopaque restoration with smooth borders is probably *gold*. Silver amalgam two-surface and multisurface restorations are characterized by their irregular outlines or borders.
   (c) A large, well-adapted radiopaque restoration with smooth borders is probably *gold*. Unlike metallic restorations, which appear totally radiopaque, porcelain restorations are slightly radiopaque and resemble the radiodensity of dentin.
   (d) A large, well-adapted radiopaque restoration with smooth borders is probably *gold*. Stainless steel crowns are prefabricated, and their outlines and margins appear very smooth and regular; often, however, these crowns do not appear to fit the tooth well.

REF: p. 440

8. Post and core restorations can be seen in _____ treated teeth.
   a. periodontally
   b. orthodontically
   c. endodontically
   d. nonendodontically

Answer: c
Correct: Post and core restorations can be seen in endodontically treated teeth.
Incorrect:
   (a) Post and core restorations can be seen in *endodontically* treated teeth.
   (b) Post and core restorations can be seen in *endodontically* treated teeth.
   (d) Post and core restorations can be seen in *endodontically* treated teeth.
REF: p. 441

9. Porcelain restoration are:
   a. Radiolucent
   b. Slightly radiolucent
   c. Slightly radiopaque
   d. Radiopaque

Answer: c
Correct: Porcelain restorations are slightly radiopaque.
Incorrect:
   (a) Porcelain restorations are *slightly radiopaque.*
   (b) Porcelain restorations are slightly *radiopaque.*
   (d) Porcelain restorations are *slightly* radiopaque.
REF: p. 441

10. A thin radiopaque line outlining the prepared tooth may be evident on a dental radiograph of an all-porcelain crown. This thin line represents:
    a. Die spacer
    b. Cement
    c. An air pocket
    d. A metal substructure

Answer: b
Correct: A thin radiopaque line outlining the prepared tooth may be evident on a dental radiograph of an all-porcelain crown. This thin line represents cement.
Incorrect:
   (a) A thin radiopaque line outlining the prepared tooth may be evident on a dental radiograph of an all-porcelain crown. This thin line represents *cement.* Die spacer is placed to provide space for the cement layer.
   (c) A thin radiopaque line outlining the prepared tooth may be evident on a dental radiograph of an all-porcelain crown. This thin line represents *cement.*
   (d) A thin radiopaque line outlining the prepared tooth may be evident on a dental radiograph of an all-porcelain crown. This thin line represents *cement.* A metal substructure blocks the x-rays and produces a radiopaque area on the film.
REF: p. 441

11. A porcelain-fused-to-metal crown appears:
    a. Uniformly radiopaque
    b. Uniformly radiolucent
    c. To have two radiographic components. The metal component appears completely radiopaque, and the porcelain component appears slightly radiopaque.
    d. To have two radiographic components. The metal component appears completely radiolucent, and the porcelain component appears slightly radiolucent.

Answer: c
Correct: A porcelain-fused-to-metal crown appears to have two radiographic components. The metal component appears completely radiopaque, and the porcelain component appears slightly radiopaque.
Incorrect:
   (a) A porcelain-fused-to-metal crown appears *to have two radiographic components.* The metal component appears completely radiopaque, and the porcelain component appears slightly radiopaque.
   (b) A porcelain-fused-to-metal crown appears *to have two radiographic components.* The metal component appears completely radiopaque, and the porcelain component appears slightly radiopaque.
   (d) A porcelain-fused-to-metal crown appears to have two radiographic components. The metal component appears *completely radiopaque,* and the porcelain component appears *slightly radiopaque.*
REF: p. 441

12. Some manufacturers of composite materials add radiopaque particles to their products to help the viewer differentiate a composite restoration from:
    a. An amalgam restoration
    b. Dental caries
    c. A cast gold restoration
    d. A porcelain-fused-to-metal crown

Answer: b
Correct: Some manufacturers of composite materials add radiopaque particles to their products to help the viewer differentiate a composite restoration from dental caries.
Incorrect:
   (a) Some manufacturers of composite materials add radiopaque particles to their products to help the viewer differentiate a composite restoration from *dental caries.* Historically, some composite restorative materials were radiolucent, making it difficult at times to differentiate the restoration from decay. An amalgam restoration is very radiopaque. Adding radiopaque particles to composite materials would diminish rather than increase the differentiation of a composite restoration from amalgam.

(c) Some manufacturers of composite materials add radiopaque particles to their products to help the viewer differentiate a composite restoration from *dental caries*. Historically, some composite restorative materials were radiolucent, making it difficult at times to differentiate the restoration from decay. A cast gold restoration is very radiopaque. Adding radiopaque particles to composite materials would diminish rather than increase the differentiation of a composite restoration from a cast gold restoration.

(d) Some manufacturers of composite materials add radiopaque particles to their products to help the viewer differentiate a composite restoration from *dental caries*. Historically, some composite restorative materials were radiolucent, making it difficult at times to differentiate the restoration from decay. A porcelain-fused-to-metal crown is very radiopaque. Adding radiopaque particles to composite materials would diminish rather than increase the differentiation of a composite restoration from a porcelain-fused-to-metal crown.

REF: p. 443

13. A base material appears _____. If compared with amalgam, the base material appears _____ radiodense.
   a. radiolucent; more
   b. radiolucent; less
   c. radiopaque; more
   d. radiopaque; less

Answer: d
Correct: A base material appears radiopaque. If compared with amalgam, the base material appears less radiodense.
Incorrect:
   (a) A base material appears *radiopaque*. If compared with amalgam, the base material appears *less* radiodense.
   (b) A base material appears *radiopaque*. If compared with amalgam, the base material appears less radiodense.
   (c) A base material appears radiopaque. If compared with amalgam, the base material appears *less* radiodense.
REF: p. 444

14. Diatorics are found in:
   a. Silver point endodontic fillings
   b. Gutta percha endodontic fillings
   c. Anterior porcelain denture teeth
   d. Anterior acrylic denture teeth

Answer: c
Correct: Diatorics are found in anterior porcelain denture teeth.

Incorrect:
   (a) Diatorics are found in *anterior porcelain denture teeth*. They are used to retain the denture teeth in the acrylic denture base material.
   (b) Diatorics are found in *anterior porcelain denture teeth*. They are used to retain the denture teeth in the acrylic denture base material.
   (d) Diatorics are found in *anterior porcelain denture teeth*. They are used to retain the denture teeth in the acrylic denture base material.
REF: p. 445

15. Diatorics are:
   a. Color sources
   b. Metal retention pins
   c. Identification dots
   d. Orthodontic brackets

Answer: b
Correct: Diatorics are metal retention pins.
Incorrect:
   (a) Diatorics are *metal retention pins*.
   (c) Diatorics are *metal retention pins*.
   (d) Diatorics are *metal retention pins*.
REF: p. 445

16. With intraoral films, patients should be instructed to remove:
   (1) Necklaces
   (2) Eyeglasses
   (3) Nose jewelry
   (4) Patient napkin chains
      a. 1, 2, 3, 4
      b. 1, 2, 3
      c. 2, 3, 4
      d. 2, 3

Answer: d
Correct: With intraoral films, patients should be instructed to remove eyeglasses and nose jewelry.
Incorrect:
   (a) With intraoral films, patients should be instructed to remove *eyeglasses* and *nose jewelry*. Necklaces and patient napkin chains would be outside the field for an intraoral film, but not for an extraoral film.
   (b) With intraoral films, patients should be instructed to remove *eyeglasses* and *nose jewelry*. Necklaces and patient napkin chains would be outside the field for an intraoral film, but not for an extraoral film.
   (c) With intraoral films, patients should be instructed to remove *eyeglasses* and *nose jewelry*. Necklaces and patient napkin chains would be outside the field for an intraoral film, but not for an extraoral film.
REF: p. 446

CHAPTER 32   INTERPRETATION OF DENTAL CARIES

MULTIPLE CHOICE

1. In the practice of dentistry, _____ is probably the most frequent reason for taking dental radiographs.
   a. periodontitis
   b. caries
   c. impacted teeth
   d. orthodontia

Answer: b
Correct:
Incorrect: In the practice of dentistry, caries is probably the most frequent reason for taking dental radiographs.
   (a) In the practice of dentistry, *caries* is probably the most frequent reason for taking dental radiographs.
   (c) In the practice of dentistry, *caries* is probably the most frequent reason for taking dental radiographs.
   (d) In the practice of dentistry, *caries* is probably the most frequent reason for taking dental radiographs.
REF: p. 456

2. A radiograph is most useful for detection of _____ caries.
   a. buccal
   b. lingual
   c. occlusal
   d. interproximal

Answer: d
Correct: A radiograph is most useful for detection of interproximal caries.
Incorrect:
   (a) Buccal caries are typically found using the explorer during the clinical examination.
   (b) Lingual caries are typically found using the explorer during the clinical examination.
   (c) Occlusal caries are typically found using the explorer during the clinical examination.
REF: p. 456

3. A carious lesion appears _____ on a dental radiograph.
   a. radiopaque
   b. radiolucent
   c. white
   d. clear

Answer: b
Correct: A carious lesion appears radiolucent (dark or black) on a dental radiograph.
Incorrect:
   (a) A carious lesion appears *radiolucent* (dark or black) on a dental radiograph. Demineralization and destruction of the hard tooth structures result in a loss of tooth density in the area of the lesion. Decreased density allows greater penetration of x-rays in the carious area. A radiopaque (light or white) area would be caused by due to increased rather than decreased density.
   (c) A carious lesion appears *radiolucent* (dark or black) on a dental radiograph. Demineralization and destruction of the hard tooth structures result in a loss of tooth density in the area of the lesion. Decreased density allows greater penetration of x-rays in the carious area. A radiopaque (light or white) area would be caused by due to increased rather than decreased density.
   (d) A carious lesion appears *radiolucent* (dark or black) on a dental radiograph. Demineralization and destruction of the hard tooth structures result in a loss of tooth density in the area of the lesion. Decreased density allows greater penetration of x-rays in the carious area. A radiopaque (light or white) area would be due to increased rather than decreased density.
REF: p. 457

4. The _____ radiograph is the radiograph of choice for the evaluation of caries.
   a. periapical
   b. bite-wing
   c. panoramic
   d. occlusal

Answer: b
Correct: The bite-wing radiograph is the radiograph of choice for the evaluation of caries.
Incorrect:
   (a) The *bite-wing* radiograph is the radiograph of choice for the evaluation of caries. A periapical radiograph using the paralleling technique can also be used for evaluation of dental caries;, however, day-in and day-out most practitioners rely on bite-wing films for the evaluation of caries in posterior teeth.
   (c) The *bite-wing* radiograph is the radiograph of choice for the evaluation of caries. Although panoramic films are superior to periapical or bite-wing films for visualization of the entire head and jaws, the resolution is less than that seen with intraoral films. In fact, a panoramic film is typically supplemented with bite-wing films to create a full mouth series.
   (d) The *bite-wing* radiograph is the radiograph of choice for the evaluation of caries. The steep vertical angulation of an occlusal film largely precludes utilization for the detection of caries.
REF: p. 457

5. Caries found between two teeth is termed _____ caries.
   a. occlusal
   b. buccal
   c. lingual
   d. interproximal

Answer: d

Correct: Caries found between two teeth is termed inter-proximal caries.

Incorrect:

  (a) Caries found between two teeth is termed *inter-proximal* caries. Occlusal caries involves the chewing surface of the posterior teeth.

  (b) Caries found between two teeth is termed *inter-proximal* caries. Buccal caries involves the buccal tooth surface.

  (c) Caries found between two teeth is termed *inter-proximal* caries. Lingual caries involves the lingual tooth surface.

REF: p. 457

---

6. On a dental radiograph, interproximal caries is typically seen at or just below the:
  a. Marginal ridge
  b. Contact point
  c. Cementoenamel junction
  d. Crest of the alveolar bone

Answer: b

Correct: On a dental radiograph, interproximal caries is typically seen at or just below the contact point.

Incorrect:

  (a) On a dental radiograph, interproximal caries is typically seen at or just below the *contact point*.

  (c) On a dental radiograph, interproximal caries is typically seen at or just below the *contact point*.

  (d) On a dental radiograph, interproximal caries is typically seen at or just below the *contact point*.

REF: p. 457

---

7. _____ interproximal caries extends less than halfway through the thickness of enamel.
  a. Incipient
  b. Moderate
  c. Advanced
  d. Severe

Answer: a

Correct: Incipient interproximal caries extends less than halfway through the thickness of enamel.

Incorrect:

  (b) *Incipient* interproximal caries extends less than halfway through the thickness of enamel. Moderate interproximal caries extends more than halfway through the thickness of enamel but does not involve the dentinoenamel junction (DEJ).

  (c) *Incipient* interproximal caries extends less than halfway through the thickness of enamel. Advanced interproximal caries extends to or through the DEJ and into dentin but does not extend through the dentin more than half the distance toward the pulp.

  (d) *Incipient* interproximal caries extends less than halfway through the thickness of enamel. Severe interproximal caries extends through enamel, through the dentin, and more than half the distance toward the pulp.

REF: p. 458

---

8. A Class _____ lesion is an advanced interproximal lesion.
  a. I
  b. II
  c. III
  d. IV

Answer: c

Correct: A Class III lesion is an advanced interproximal lesion.

Incorrect:

  (a) A Class *III* lesion is an advanced interproximal lesion. A Class I lesion is incipient interproximal caries. A Class I lesion is seen in enamel only.

  (b) A Class *III* lesion is an advanced interproximal lesion. A Class II lesion is moderate interproximal caries. A moderate lesion is seen in enamel only.

  (d) A Class *III* lesion is an advanced interproximal lesion. A Class IV lesion is severe interproximal caries. A severe lesion involves both enamel and dentin and may appear clinically as a cavitation in the tooth.

REF: p. 458

---

9. _____ occlusal caries cannot be seen on a dental radiograph and must be detected clinically with an explorer.
  (1) Incipient
  (2) Moderate
  (3) Severe
    a. 1, 2, 3
    b. 1, 3
    c. 2, 3
    d. 1 only

Answer: d

Correct: Incipient occlusal caries cannot be seen on a dental radiograph and must be detected clinically with an explorer.

Incorrect:

  (a) *Incipient* occlusal caries cannot be seen on a dental radiograph and must be detected clinically with an explorer.

  (b) *Incipient* occlusal caries cannot be seen on a dental radiograph and must be detected clinically with an explorer.

  (c) *Incipient* occlusal caries cannot be seen on a dental radiograph and must be detected clinically with an explorer.

REF: p. 458

---

10. Caries that involves the buccal or lingual surface appears as a small, _____ area.
  a. triangular radiolucent
  b. circular radiolucent

c. triangular radiopaque
d. circular radiopaque

Answer: b
Correct: Caries that involves the buccal or lingual surface appears as a small, circular radiolucent area.
Incorrect:
(a) Caries that involves the buccal or lingual surface appears as a small, *circular* radiolucent area.
(c) Caries that involves the buccal or lingual surface appears as a small, *circular radiolucent* area.
(d) Caries that involves the buccal or lingual surface appears as a small, circular *radiolucent* area.
REF: p. 460

11. Which of the following statements is *true* of root surface caries?
   a. Root surface caries involves the loss of enamel.
   b. Root surface caries is clinically difficult to detect on exposed root surfaces.
   c. Root surface caries appears as a cupped-out or crater-shaped radiolucency just below the cementoenamel junction (CEJ).
   d. Root surface caries appears as a cupped-out or crater-shaped radiolucency just above the CEJ.

Answer: c
Correct: Root surface caries appears as a cupped-out or crater-shaped radiolucency just below the CEJ.
Incorrect:
(a) Root surface caries appears as a cupped-out or crater-shaped radiolucency just below the CEJ. Root surface caries involves only the roots of teeth. No involvement of enamel occurs.
(b) Root surface caries appears as a cupped-out or crater-shaped radiolucency just below the CEJ. Root surface caries is easily detected on exposed root surfaces.
(d) Root surface caries appears as a cupped-out or crater-shaped radiolucency just *below* the CEJ. Enamel is found above the CEJ and no involvement of enamel occurs with root
REF: p. 462

12. Rampant caries is typically seen in children with _____ dietary habits or in adults with _____ salivary flow.
   a. poor; increased
   b. poor; a decreased
   c. good; increased
   d. good; a decreased

Answer: b
Correct: Rampant caries is typically seen in children with poor dietary habits or in adults with a decreased salivary flow.
Incorrect:
(a) Rampant caries is typically seen in children with poor dietary habits or in adults with *a decreased* salivary flow.

(c) Rampant caries is typically seen in children with *poor* dietary habits or in adults with *a decreased* salivary flow.
(d) Rampant caries is typically seen in children with *poor* dietary habits or in adults with *a* decreased salivary flow.
REF: p. 462

CHAPTER 33 INTERPRETATION OF PERIODONTAL DISEASE

MULTIPLE CHOICE
1. In health, the lamina dura around the roots of the teeth appears as a(n) _____ line.
   a. dense radiolucent
   b. dense radiopaque
   c. intermittent radiolucent
   d. intermittent radiopaque

Answer: b
Correct: In health, the lamina dura around the roots of the teeth appears as a dense radiopaque line.
Incorrect:
(a) In health, the lamina dura around the roots of the teeth appears as a dense *radiopaque* line.
(c) In health, the lamina dura around the roots of the teeth appears as a *dense radiopaque* line.
(d) In health, the lamina dura around the roots of the teeth appears as a *dense* radiopaque line.
REF: p. 467

2. The normal healthy alveolar crest is located approximately _____ mm apical to the cementoenamel junction.
   a. 0.5 to 1.0
   b. 1.0 to 1.5
   c. 1.5 to 2.0
   d. 2.0 to 2.5

Answer: c
Correct: The normal healthy alveolar crest is located approximately 1.5 to 2.0 mm apical to the cementoenamel junction.
Incorrect:
(a) The normal healthy alveolar crest is located approximately *1.5 to 2.0* mm apical to the cementoenamel junction.
(b) The normal healthy alveolar crest is located approximately *1.5 to 2.0* mm apical to the cementoenamel junction.
(d) The normal healthy alveolar crest is located approximately *1.5 to 2.0* mm apical to the cementoenamel junction.
REF: p. 467

3. The normal periodontal ligament space appears as a _____ line.
   a. thin radiopaque
   b. thin radiolucent
   c. thick radiopaque
   d. thick radiolucent

197

Answer: b
Correct: The normal periodontal ligament space appears as a thin radiolucent line.
Incorrect:
 (a) The normal periodontal ligament space appears as a thin *radiolucent* line.
 (c) The normal periodontal ligament space appears as a *thin radiolucent* line.
 (d) The normal periodontal ligament space appears as a *thin* radiolucent line.
REF: p. 467

4. The periodontal ligament space is located between the root of the tooth and the:
 a. Crest of alveolar bone
 b. Lamina dura
 c. Cementum
 d. Spongy bone

Answer: b
Correct: The periodontal ligament space is located between the root of the tooth and the lamina dura.
Incorrect:
 (a) The periodontal ligament space is located between the root of the tooth and the *lamina dura.*
 (c) The periodontal ligament space is located between the root of the tooth and the *lamina dura.*
 (d) The periodontal ligament space is located between the root of the tooth and the *lamina dura.*
REF: p. 467

5. Radiographs permit the evaluation of _____ in the detection of periodontal disease.
 a. pocket depth
 b. soft tissue
 c. inflammation
 d. bone

Answer: d
Correct: Radiographs permit the evaluation of bone in the detection of periodontal disease.
Incorrect:
 (a) Radiographs permit the evaluation of *bone* in the detection of periodontal disease. They cannot be used to determine pocket depth.
 (b) Radiographs permit the evaluation of *bone* in the detection of periodontal disease. They cannot be used to determine the condition of soft tissue; the clinical examination provides information about the soft tissue.
 (c) Radiographs permit the evaluation of *bone* in the detection of periodontal disease. They cannot be used to determine inflammation.
REF: p. 468

6. The _____ radiograph using the _____ technique is the film of choice for the evaluation of periodontal disease.
 a. bite-wing; paralleling
 b. bite-wing; bisecting
 c. periapical; paralleling
 d. periapical; bisecting

Answer: c
Correct: The periapical radiograph using the parallcling technique is the film of choice for the evaluation of periodontal disease.
Incorrect:
 (a) The *periapical* radiograph using the paralleling technique is the film of choice for the evaluation of periodontal disease. The horizontal bite-wing alone should not be used to document periodontal disease. The vertical bite-wing radiograph can be used to examine bone levels and is best used as a posttreatment or follow-up film.
 (b) The *periapical* radiograph using the *paralleling* technique is the film of choice for the evaluation of periodontal disease. The horizontal bite-wing alone should not be used to document periodontal disease. The vertical bite-wing radiograph can be used to examine bone levels and is best used as a posttreatment or follow-up film.
 (d) The periapical radiograph using the *paralleling* technique is the film of choice for the evaluation of periodontal disease. If the bisecting technique is used to expose periapical radiographs, a dimensional distortion of bone is seen because of the vertical angulation used.
REF: p. 468

7. The _____ of adjacent teeth can be used as a plane of reference in determining the pattern of bone loss present.
 a. marginal ridge height
 b. cementoenamel junctions (CEJs)
 c. pulp chambers
 d. thickness of cementum

Answer: b
Correct: The cementoenamel junctions (CEJs) of adjacent teeth can be used as a plane of reference in determining the pattern of bone loss present.
Incorrect:
 (a) The *cementoenamel junctions* (CEJs) of adjacent teeth can be used as a plane of reference in determining the pattern of bone loss present. With horizontal bone loss, the bone loss occurs in a plane parallel to the CEJs of the adjacent teeth. With vertical bone loss, the bone loss does not occur in a plane parallel to the CEJs of adjacent teeth. The marginal ridge height is not used to determine the pattern of bone loss.

(c) The *cementoenamel junctions* (CEJs) of adjacent teeth can be used as a plane of reference in determining the pattern of bone loss present. With horizontal bone loss, the bone loss occurs in a plane parallel to the CEJs of the adjacent teeth. With vertical bone loss, the bone loss does not occur in a plane parallel to the CEJs of adjacent teeth. The pulp chambers are not used to determine the pattern of bone loss.

(d) The *cementoenamel junctions* (CEJs) of adjacent teeth can be used as a plane of reference in determining the pattern of bone loss present. With horizontal bone loss, the bone loss occurs in a plane parallel to the CEJs of the adjacent teeth. With vertical bone loss, the bone loss does not occur in a plane parallel to the CEJs of adjacent teeth. The thickness of cementum is not used to determine the pattern of bone loss.

REF: p. 469

8. Generalized bone loss occurs evenly throughout the dental arches, including greater than _____ of the sites involved.
   a. 10%
   b. 20%
   c. 30%
   d. 50%

Answer: c
Correct: Generalized bone loss occurs evenly throughout the dental arches, including greater than 30% of the sites involved.
Incorrect:
   (a) Generalized bone loss occurs evenly throughout the dental arches, including greater than *30%* of the sites involved. Localized bone loss occurs in isolated areas, specifically less than 30% of the sites involved.
   (b) Generalized bone loss occurs evenly throughout the dental arches, including greater than *30%* of the sites involved. Localized bone loss occurs in isolated areas, specifically less than 30% of the sites involved.
   (d) Generalized bone loss occurs evenly throughout the dental arches, including greater than *30%* of the sites involved. Localized bone loss occurs in isolated areas, specifically less than 30% of the sites involved.

REF: p. 469

9. The severity of bone loss is measured by the:
   a. Pocket depth
   b. Recession
   c. Amount of inflammation
   d. Clinical attachment loss

Answer: d
Correct: The severity of bone loss is measured by the clinical attachment loss.

Incorrect:
   (a) The severity of bone loss is measured by the *clinical attachment loss*. This is considered to be a more significant clinical parameter than pocket depth.
   (b) The severity of bone loss is measured by the *clinical attachment loss*. Recession may involve many factors, including toothbrushing technique and bruxism, and does not necessarily involve bone loss.
   (c) The severity of bone loss is measured by the *clinical attachment loss*. The amount of inflammation does not necessarily reflect or determine bone loss.

REF: pp. 469 & 471

10. Using the measurements of clinical attachment loss (CAL), moderate bone loss is defined as a loss of _____ mm.
   a. 1 to 2
   b. 2 to 3
   c. 3 to 4
   d. more than 5 mm

Answer: c
Correct: Moderate bone loss is defined as a loss of 3 to 4 mm.
Incorrect:
   (a) Slight bone loss is defined as a loss of *1 to 2* mm.
   (b) A measurement of *2 to 3* mm falls between slight and moderate bone loss.
   (d) Severe bone loss is defined as a loss *more than 5* mm.

REF: p. 473

11. ADA Case Type II is:
   a. Gingivitis
   b. Mild or slight periodontitis
   c. Moderate periodontitis
   d. Advanced or severe periodontitis

Answer: b
Correct: ADA Case Type II is mild or slight periodontitis.
Incorrect:
   (a) ADA Case Type I is *gingivitis*.
   (c) ADA Case Type III is *moderate periodontitis*.
   (d) ADA Case Type IV is *advanced or severe periodontitis*.

REF: p. 471

12. Calculus _____ on a dental radiograph.
   a. appears radiolucent
   b. appears radiopaque
   c. does not appear
   d. appears dark or black

Answer: b
Correct: Calculus appears radiopaque on a dental radiograph.

199

Incorrect:
- (a) Calculus *appears radiopaque* on a dental radiograph.
- (c) Calculus *appears radiopaque* on a dental radiograph.
- (d) Calculus *appears radiopaque* on a dental radiograph.

REF: p. 473

CHAPTER 34 INTERPRETATION OF TRAUMA AND PULPAL AND PERIAPICAL LESIONS

MULTIPLE CHOICE

1. Root fractures occur most often in the _____ region.
- a. maxillary central incisor
- b. mandibular central incisor
- c. maxillary molar
- d. mandibular molar

Answer: a

Correct: Root fractures occur most often in the maxillary central incisor region.

Incorrect:
- (b) Root fractures occur most often in the *maxillary* central incisor region.
- (c) Root fractures occur most often in the maxillary *central incisor* region.
- (d) Root fractures occur most often in the *maxillary central incisor* region.

REF: p. 480

2. The _____ radiograph is the film of choice for the evaluation of mandibular fractures.
- a. occlusal
- b. periapical
- c. bite-wing
- d. panoramic

Answer: d

Correct: The panoramic radiograph is the film of choice for the evaluation of mandibular fractures.

Incorrect:
- (a) The *panoramic* radiograph is the film of choice for the evaluation of mandibular fractures. An occlusal film is too small and is not in the right plane for visualization of jaw fractures.
- (b) The *panoramic* radiograph is the film of choice for the evaluation of mandibular fractures. A periapical film is too small for visualization of jaw fractures.
- (c) The *panoramic* radiograph is the film of choice for the evaluation of mandibular fractures. A bite-wing film is too small for visualization of jaw fractures.

REF: p. 480

3. Luxation is:
- a. The abnormal displacement of teeth
- b. Used to describe fragments of bone following traumatic injury
- c. Hemorrhage, or bleeding
- d. Swelling or edema

Answer: a

Correct: Luxation is the abnormal displacement of teeth.

Incorrect:
- (b) Spicule is used to describe fragments of bone following traumatic injury.
- (c) Luxation can cause hemorrhage or bleeding, but is actually the abnormal displacement of teeth.
- (d) Luxation can cause swelling or edema, but is actually the abnormal displacement of teeth.

REF: p. 481

4. Teeth that have been luxated should be evaluated by a(n) _____ radiograph.
- a. bite-wing
- b. periapical
- c. occlusal
- d. panoramic

Answer: b

Correct: Teeth that have been luxated should be evaluated by a periapical radiograph.

Incorrect:
- (a) Teeth that have been luxated should be evaluated by a *periapical* radiograph and examined for root and adjacent alveolar bone fractures, damage to the periodontal ligament, and pulpal problems. The bite-wing film does not permit visualization of the apex of the tooth.
- (c) Teeth that have been luxated should be evaluated by a *periapical* radiograph and examined for root and adjacent alveolar bone fractures, damage to the periodontal ligament, and pulpal problems. The occlusal film may reveal the apex of some anterior teeth, but the roots of many teeth are severely foreshortened.
- (d) Teeth that have been luxated should be evaluated by a *periapical* radiograph and examined for root and adjacent alveolar bone fractures, damage to the periodontal ligament, and pulpal problems. The panoramic film does not have the resolution of a periapical film, making it difficult to rely on alone for evaluation of a luxated tooth.

REF: p. 481

5. _____ is the complete displacement of a tooth from alveolar bone.
- a. Luxation
- b. Intrusion
- c. Extrusion
- d. Avulsion

Answer: d

Correct: Avulsion is the complete displacement of a tooth from alveolar bone.

Incorrect:
- (a) *Avulsion* is the complete displacement of a tooth from alveolar bone. *Luxation* is the abnormal displacement of teeth.
- (b) *Avulsion* is the complete displacement of a tooth from alveolar bone. *Intrusion* refers to the abnormal displacement of teeth into bone.

(c) *Avulsion* is the complete displacement of a tooth from alveolar bone. *Extrusion* refers to the abnormal displacement of teeth out of bone.

REF: p. 482

6. _____ resorption is a process seen with the normal shedding of primary teeth.
   a. Physiologic
   b. Pathologic
   c. External
   d. Internal

Answer: a
Correct: Physiologic resorption is a process seen with the normal shedding of primary teeth.
Incorrect:
   (b) *Physiologic* resorption is a process seen with the normal shedding of primary teeth. *Pathologic* resorption is a regressive alteration of tooth structure observed when a tooth is subjected to abnormal stimuli.
   (c) *Physiologic* resorption is a process seen with the normal shedding of primary teeth. *External* resorption is seen along the periphery of the root surface and is often associated with reimplanted teeth, abnormal mechanical forces, trauma, chronic inflammation, tumors and cysts, impacted teeth, or idiopathic causes.
   (d) *Physiologic* resorption is a process seen with the normal shedding of primary teeth. *Internal* resorption occurs within the crown or root of a tooth and involves the pulp chamber, pulp canals, and surrounding dentin. Precipitating factors such as trauma, pulp capping, and pulp polyps are believed to stimulate the internal resorption process.

REF: p. 482

7. _____ is a diffuse calcification of the pulp chamber and pulp canals of teeth.
   a. Pulpal sclerosis
   b. Pulpal obliteration
   c. Pulp stones
   d. Internal resorption

Answer: a
Correct: Pulpal sclerosis is a diffuse calcification of the pulp chamber and pulp canals of teeth.
Incorrect:
   (b) *Pulpal sclerosis* is a diffuse calcification of the pulp chamber and pulp canals of teeth. A tooth with pulpal obliteration does not appear to have a pulp chamber or pulp canals.
   (c) *Pulpal sclerosis* is a diffuse calcification of the pulp chamber and pulp canals of teeth. On a dental radiograph, pulp stones appear as round, ovoid, or cylindrical radiopacities.
   (d) *Pulpal sclerosis* is a diffuse calcification of the pulp chamber and pulp canals of teeth. Internal

resorption appears as a round-to-ovoid radiolucency in the midcrown or midroot portion of a tooth.

REF: p. 483

8. Teeth that exhibit pulpal obliteration:
   a. Require extraction
   b. Require endodontic therapy
   c. Require occlusal restoration
   d. Do not require treatment

Answer: d
Correct: Teeth that exhibit pulpal obliteration do not require treatment.
Incorrect:
   (a) Teeth that exhibit pulpal obliteration *do not require treatment*
   (b) Teeth that exhibit pulpal obliteration *do not require treatment*
   (c) Teeth that exhibit pulpal obliteration *do not require treatment*

REF: p. 483

9. Pulp stones _____ cause symptoms and _____ require treatment.
   a. do; do
   b. do; do not
   c. do not; do
   d. do not; do not

Answer: d
Correct: Pulp stones do not cause symptoms and do not require treatment.
Incorrect:
   (a) Pulp stones *do not* cause symptoms and *do not* require treatment.
   (b) Pulp stones *do not* cause symptoms and do not require treatment.
   (c) Pulp stones do not cause symptoms and *do not* require treatment.

REF: p. 483

10. Which of the following is a periapical radiolucency?
    a. Hypercementosis
    b. Condensing osteitis
    c. Periapical cyst
    d. Sclerotic bone

Answer: c
Correct: A periapical cyst is a periapical radiolucency.
Incorrect:
    (a) A *periapical cyst* is a periapical radiolucency. Hypercementosis is a periapical radiopacity.
    (b) A *periapical cyst* is a periapical radiolucency. Condensing osteitis is a periapical radiopacity.
    (d) A *periapical cyst* is a periapical radiolucency. Sclerotic bone is a periapical radiopacity.

REF: p. 485

11. Periapical cysts account for _____ of all cysts in the oral region.
   a. 10% to 20%
   b. 20% to 25%
   c. 25% to 50%
   d. 50% to 70%

Answer: d
Correct: Periapical cysts account for 50% to 70% of all cysts in the oral region.
Incorrect:
   (a) Periapical cysts account for *50% to 70%* of all cysts in the oral region.
   (b) Periapical cysts account for *50% to 70%* of all cysts in the oral region.
   (c) Periapical cysts account for *50% to 70%* of all cysts in the oral region.
REF: p. 485

12. A chronic periapical abscess is:
   a. Painful
   b. Usually asymptomatic
   c. Sensitive to percussion
   d. Sensitive to heat

Answer: b
Correct: A chronic periapical abscess is usually asymptomatic.
Incorrect:
   (a) A chronic periapical abscess is *usually asymptomatic.*
   (c) A chronic periapical abscess is *usually asymptomatic.*
   (d) A chronic periapical abscess is *usually asymptomatic.*
REF: p. 486

13. The periapical abscess:
   a. Refers to a tooth with an infection in the pulp
   b. Is a purulent inflammation within the periodontal tissues
   c. Is treated with deep scaling and debridement
   d. Both b and c

Answer: a
Correct: The periapical abscess refers to a tooth with an infection in the pulp.
Incorrect:
   (b) The periapical abscess *refers to a tooth with an infection in the pulp.* The periodontal abscess is a purulent inflammation within the periodontal tissues.
   (c) The periapical abscess *refers to a tooth with an infection in the pulp.* Treatment of the periapical abscess includes drainage and endodontic therapy or extraction. The periodontal abscess is treated with deep scaling and debridement.
   (d) The periapical abscess *refers to a tooth with an infection in the pulp.* The periodontal abscess is a

purulent inflammation within the periodontal tissues. Treatment of the periapical abscess includes drainage and endodontic therapy or extraction. The periodontal abscess is treated with deep scaling and debridement.
REF: p. 486

14. _____ is a well-defined radiopacity that is seen below the apex of a nonvital tooth with a history of a long-standing pulpitis.
   a. Condensing osteitis
   b. Periodontal abscess
   c. Sclerotic bone
   d. Periapical abscess

Answer: a
Correct: Condensing osteitis is a well-defined radiopacity that is seen below the apex of a nonvital tooth with a history of a long-standing pulpitis.
Incorrect:
   (b) *Condensing osteitis* is a well-defined radiopacity that is seen below the apex of a nonvital tooth with a history of a long-standing pulpitis. A periodontal abscess is a purulent inflammation within the periodontal tissues.
   (c) *Condensing osteitis* is a well-defined radiopacity that is seen below the apex of a nonvital tooth with a history of a long-standing pulpitis. Sclerotic bone is a well-defined radiopacity that is seen below the apices of vital, noncarious teeth.
   (d) *Condensing osteitis* is a well-defined radiopacity that is seen below the apex of a nonvital tooth with a history of a long-standing pulpitis. With an acute periapical abscess, no radiographic change may be evident. A chronic periapical abscess appears as a round or ovoid, apical radiolucency with poorly defined margins.
REF: p. 487

15. Condensing osteitis is seen _____ the apex of a _____ tooth.
   a. below; vital
   b. below; nonvital
   c. above; vital
   d. above; nonvital

Answer: b
Correct: Condensing osteitis is seen below the apex of a nonvital tooth.
Incorrect:
   (a) Condensing osteitis is seen below the apex of a *nonvital* tooth.
   (c) Condensing osteitis is seen *below* the apex of a *nonvital* tooth.
   (d) Condensing osteitis is seen *below* the apex of a nonvital tooth.
REF: p. 487

16. Condensing osteitis _____ vary in size and shape and _____ appear to be attached to the tooth root.
   a. may; does
   b. may; does not
   c. may not; does
   d. may not; does not

Answer: b
Correct: Condensing osteitis may vary in size and shape and does not appear to be attached to the tooth root.
Incorrect:
   (a) Condensing osteitis may vary in size and shape and *does not* appear to be attached to the tooth root.
   (c) Condensing osteitis *may* vary in size and shape and *does not* appear to be attached to the tooth root.
   (d) Condensing osteitis *may* vary in size and shape and does not appear to be attached to the tooth root.
REF: p. 487

17. The treatment for condensing osteitis is:
   a. Extraction
   b. Root canal therapy
   c. Osseous recontouring
   d. No treatment is necessary

Answer: d
Correct: No treatment is necessary for condensing osteitis.
Incorrect:
   (a) Extraction is not the treatment for condensing osteitis. There is no treatment.
   (b) Root canal therapy is not the treatment for condensing osteitis. There is no treatment.
   (c) Osseous recontouring is not the treatment for condensing osteitis. There is no treatment.
REF: p. 487

18. _____ is the most common periapical radiopacity observed in adults.
   a. Hypercementosis
   b. Sclerotic bone
   c. Condensing osteitis
   d. Pulpal sclerosis

Answer: c
Correct: Condensing osteitis is the most common periapical radiopacity observed in adults.

Incorrect:
   (a) *Condensing osteitis* is the most common periapical radiopacity observed in adults.
   (b) *Condensing osteitis* is the most common periapical radiopacity observed in adults.
   (d) *Condensing osteitis* is the most common periapical radiopacity observed in adults.
REF: p. 487

19. Condensing osteitis most frequently involves the _____ tooth.
   a. mandibular premolar
   b. mandibular molar
   c. maxillary premolar
   d. maxillary molar

Answer: b
Correct: Condensing osteitis most frequently involves the mandibular molar tooth.
Incorrect:
   (a) Condensing osteitis most frequently involves the mandibular *molar* tooth.
   (c) Condensing osteitis most frequently involves the *mandibular molar* tooth.
   (d) Condensing osteitis most frequently involves the *mandibular* molar tooth.
REF: p. 487

20. Sclerotic bone is seen below the apices of _____ teeth.
   a. vital, carious
   b. vital, noncarious
   c. nonvital, carious
   d. nonvital, noncarious

Answer: b
Correct: Sclerotic bone is seen below the apices of vital, noncarious teeth.
Incorrect:
   (a) Sclerotic bone is seen below the apices of vital, *noncarious* teeth.
   (c) Sclerotic bone is seen below the apices of *vital, noncarious* teeth.
   (d) Sclerotic bone is seen below the apices of *vital,* noncarious teeth.
REF: p. 487